Lower Limb and Leg Ulcer Assessment and Management

Lower Limb and Leg Ulcer Assessment and Management

Edited by

ABY MITCHELL
GEORGINA RITCHIE
ALISON HOPKINS

WILEY Blackwell

Registered Offices
John Wiley & Sons, Inc., 111 River Street, Hoboken, NJ 07030, USA
John Wiley & Sons Ltd, The Atrium, Southern Gate, Chichester, West Sussex,
PO19 8SQ, UK

For details of our global editorial offices, customer services, and more information
about Wiley products visit us at www.wiley.com.

Library of Congress Cataloging-in-Publication Data Applied for:

Paperback ISBN: 9781119908210
ePDF: 9781119908227
ePUB: 9781119908234
oBook: 9781119908241

Cover Design: Wiley
Cover Image: © medejaja/Adobe Stock Photos

Set in 10/12pt STIXTwoText by Straive, Pondicherry, India
Printing and Binding: CPI Group (UK) Ltd, Croydon, CR0 4YY

C9781119908210_160524

In remembrance of Hugo

Professor Hugo Partsch, 1938–2023
Doctor, researcher, scientist
A humble and generous mentor
Founder of the International Compression Club
Who ignited for many a lifelong fascination with compression therapy
Thank you

Contents

CHAPTER 8
Clinical Management of the Lower Limb 353
Georgina Ritchie

CHAPTER 9
Lifelong Management 405
Jane Harry

List of Contributors

Sarah Bradbury RN, BSc(Hons), MSc
Clinical Research Director
Welsh Wounds Innovation Centre
Pontyclun, UK

Rona Frances Campbell Podiatrist, BSc(Hons), MSc
Clinical Lead Podiatry &
Biomechanics
Accelerate CIC
London, UK

Deborah Chester-Bessell Nurse BSc(Hons)
Learning and Teaching Fellow
University of Salford
Salford, UK

Rhodri Harris RN, BSc, LTA Cert (Lip)
Advanced Lymphoedema
Specialist Nurse
Accelerate CIC
London, UK

Jane Harry RN, Dip Nurs, BSc, MSc
Tissue Viability Specialist
Service Team Leader
Berkshire Healthcare Foundation
Trust
Wokingham, UK

Juliet Herbert RN, DipHE
Advanced Lymphoedema
Specialist Nurse
Accelerate CIC
London, UK

Alison Hopkins MBE RN FQNI MSc
Chief Executive
Accelerate CIC
London, UK

Gabriela Korn RGN, MSc
Advanced Specialist Wound
Care Nurse
Accelerate CIC
London, UK

Kirsten Mahoney RGN, BSc, MSc, IP
Senior Tissue Viability
Nurse and
Clinical Operational Programme
Improvement Lead
Welsh Wounds Innovation Centre
Pontyclun, UK

Aby Mitchell RGN, MSc, PG Cert, BA, FHEA
Senior Lecturer in Nursing
Education
King's College London
London, UK

Joseph Montgomery
Customer Services Lead
Accelerate CIC
London, UK

Caitriona O'Neill RGN
Director of Clinical Services and
Lymphoedema
Accelerate CIC
London, UK

**Georgina Ritchie RN, DN,
QN, MEd, FHEA**
Director of Education
Accelerate CIC
London, UK

**Charlotte Smith RN,
SCPHN, MEd**
Senior Lecturer and Healthy
University Advisor
Faculty of Health and Wellbeing
University of Central
Lancashire
Preston, UK

Heidi Sandoz RN, BSc
Tissue Viability Clinical Nurse
Specialist Lead Nurse
Hertfordshire Community
NHS Trust
Welwyn Garden City, UK

Karen Staines RN, QN, BSc
Director of Research and
Wound Care
Accelerate CIC
London, UK

**Hayley Turner-Dobbin
RN, QN, MSc**
Clinical Delivery Lead
Accelerate CIC
London, UK

**Fran Worboys RGN, BSc, Dip
Nurs, Dip HE**
Consultant Clinical Nurse
Specialist in Tissue Viability
Accelerate CIC
London, UK

Foreword

Wound care is predominantly a nursing issue. It is a vital and highly skilled field of nursing practice that is routinely delivered in the community, every day of the year, to hundreds of thousands of individuals in homes and clinics, where it is unseen and rarely celebrated.

This book lifts the veil on the management of leg ulcers, with evidence-informed approaches to providing excellent care. It is written by a team of experts for nurses, principally for the district nursing service, but it will also be highly beneficial to all nurses working in general practice, in care homes and in domiciliary care where they are also responsible for leg ulcer care.

Nurses ensure that care is personalised to the individual they are caring for and this book provides a framework for practice that recognises the holistic, person-centred nature of nursing assessments and nursing work. It brings together a guide to practice along with the supporting evidence, to enable learning and critical thinking on assessment techniques, diagnosis, selection of the most appropriate intervention, evaluation, potential referral and review.

Nurses providing care for people in a home environment know that it is not only expert skills that are needed to provide the most appropriate care for the leg ulcer, but also seeing the person in the context of the environment in which they live. In addition to undertaking a physical assessment of the wound and surrounding skin condition to ensure that the most appropriate therapeutic intervention is prescribed, nurses observe mobility, continence, hydration, nutritional status, levels of self-care and the warmth and living conditions of the home, including the potential for personal care and elevation of legs as required.

With highly developed skills in communication and personalised care, nurses provide the most appropriate therapeutic intervention as part of a shared decision-making process, considering the person's lifestyle, employment status and psychological and social situation. This is complex work – and nurses make it look easy, all the while utilising skills of critical thinking and holistic assessment to determine the best approach for leg ulcer care to propose to the individual. They also know when to refer to the multidisciplinary team for additional assessment, with an understanding of the benefits of working in a wider team of clinical professionals.

This perfectly formed reference, provided as a very practical pocketbook to accompany the nurse in practice, challenges the reader to think differently about leg ulcer care. The text changes the narrative about leg ulcer healing and prevention, with references to causing harm to the very people being cared for through inappropriate interventions or sub-therapeutic 'doses' of compression therapy. It places the person being cared for at the centre and provides an accessible and supportive reference for all nurses in clinical practice delivering leg ulcer care for the communities they serve.

The development of this book by United Kingdom experts in the field of leg ulcer management is timely, with the National Wound Care Strategy Programme (NWCSP) in England having been published in 2018 and the learning from this continuing to be rolled out. The book brings into sharp focus a world in which leg ulcer management can be rapidly and radically improved through education and the application of best practice.

My congratulations to every member of the Accelerate CIC team, the Welsh Wounds Innovation Centre, King's College London and the nurses working in the National Health Service who have contributed their expertise to this book. I very much look forward to seeing the tangible impact flowing through the nurses working in the community setting, and most importantly to the individuals they care for.

Dr Crystal Oldman CBE RN RHV EdD MSc MA FRCN
Chief Executive of The Queens Nursing Institute

Preface

Often people peruse a book with the question 'Is this for me?' So what is your purpose in picking up this book? What are you hoping to gain or change? You certainly must have an interest in leg ulcers, otherwise you would not have sought out or reached for this book.

Simply because of that interest, the authors are interested in you, in your ambition and in what changes you want to be part of. This book has been written with you in mind. You are likely a community nurse or therapist who wants to manage people with lower limb conditions more effectively, and perhaps you would like to place a greater emphasis on partnership working with your patients and colleagues. With our collaborative experience and clinical expertise, gained in the classroom and in the mentoring of specialists, our aim is to help you increase your knowledge and skill set so that you can improve the lives of your patients and bring about the change the healthcare system and our citizens deserve.

Lower limb management is not just for nurses; it needs to involve multidisciplinary teams. There is certainly a groundswell of change being advocated in the world of leg ulcer management and the authors are keen to support this. Improving understanding and developing specialist skills require teamwork, so Accelerate CIC has partnered with key allies in the NHS, King's College London and the Welsh Wounds Innovation Centre to write this book. This has been an exciting collaboration to be part of.

As I write this preface, I am reminded that this is my 35th year of a focus on improving the lives of people with leg ulcers. It is exciting to see recent developments and the establishment of the National Wound Care Strategy. There is a growing body of evidence about the costs of wound care for both people and the health economy; there is a recognition of the drain that unhealed leg ulcers are on our resources and lives. I do believe we are making national progress. Yet the story underpinning leg ulcer management can sometimes feel as if nothing has changed since I started my journey in 1989. The health system continues to perpetuate avoidable patient harm through system paralysis and a lack of understanding of the extent of the damage to patients and clinicians.

And this harm is avoidable. The system must focus on developing skilled practitioners, optimising compression therapy, safeguarding escalation to specialist practitioners and ensuring that access for biomechanical assessment is addressed. If not, then our patients may well continue to suffer life-changing events, potentially leading to sepsis and even death. This is completely unnecessary, and we do not need more research to tell us what to do to prevent this or how to improve the lives of our citizens. The resources used to prop up a poor system are costly to all.

Unfortunately we have a narrative that reinforces a negative view of people with leg ulcers. I have witnessed 35 years of a damaging story, a powerful and influential narrative that has led to an acceptance of chronicity and to delays in treatment, allowing non-healing wounds to hit crisis point with inadequate resources to manage them. This false narrative says that leg ulcers are inevitably 'chronic', that it is the non-compliance of patients that hinders healing and that nurses should be afraid of doing harm by using compression. Products have been adapted to reflect this false narrative; there has been a growth in sub-optimal compression devices alongside hundreds of unnecessary wound dressings designed to promote the healing that has so far eluded us.

Meanwhile the prevalence of non-healing persists and grows, using up 50% of community nursing workload. This all-pervasive story hinders the healing of lower limb wounds and is the reason behind the writing of this book. The book aims to bring together the multidisciplinary knowledge and insight required to effectively manage lower limb conditions, and it aims to support you, the practitioner, in developing the courage you need to counter this pervasive narrative. Together we can indeed improve lower limb management by simply using our skills and knowledge.

This level of understanding is necessary to create confidence in your growing expertise. It will enable you to have good conversations with your patients and to consider the next steps in partnership with them. The language this book promotes should give you clarity, confidence and courage alongside professional humility – recognising that we have much to learn from our patients. This book will hopefully assist in growing your resolution to deliver the expert compassionate care required alongside confidence to challenge the system. Your expanding knowledge will enable you to act as an advocate for your patients and your colleagues, and to champion an improved health system.

I want to give my heartfelt thanks to all the contributors for their time freely given. I feel privileged and blessed to have been part of this book. A very special thanks need to be offered to my fellow editors, Georgina Ritchie and Aby Mitchell; the book simply would not have been published without their tireless support, energy and enthusiasm.

Alison Hopkins MBE RN FQNI MSc

Acknowledgements

Thank you to Accelerate CIC members and patients.

A heartfelt thanks to members of Accelerate CIC who provided unwavering support throughout the writing of this book.

A special thank you to the Accelerate CIC patients who were brave and kind enough to allow us to photograph and share pictures of their wounds and lower limbs. Without their contribution, learning and understanding lower limb management would not be possible.

The editors of this book wish to thank the contributors for their input into the writing of this book.

Juliet Herbert
Hayley Turner-Dobbin
Gabriela Korn
Heidi Sandoz
Deborah Chester-Bessell

Introduction

ALISON HOPKINS AND JOSEPH MONTGOMERY

In order to understand the placement of and need for this textbook, it is critical that practitioners understand the resources being used in the management of the lower limb. In order to improve outcomes for patients, we need to critically appraise the resources being used, the waste in the health system and where to focus our attention. Resource management is also part of excellent system management. Unfortunately the collection and analysis of system and patient data concerning those with wounds are not routinely accessible and providers often have to rely on the data of others or studies to make conclusions about their local provision. This has created much paralysis in our commissioning landscape. However, there is some local data that can be accessed and this introduction sets the scene and clarifies the role the insights can play in improving care delivery. Dressing spend will reduce when best practice is utilised and wound chronicity avoided. Thus clinical improvements as a result of increasing readers' knowledge and skills in leg ulcer management will create a profound and positive impact on the health economy.

THE WOUND CARE BURDEN

During 2017 and 2018 it was estimated that more than one million people in the United Kingdom had an active ulcer on the lower limb (Guest et al. 2020). This equates to 2% of the population and is a 37% increase from the prevalence data recorded in 2012 (Guest et al. 2020). More than 50% of these patients were recorded as having venous leg ulceration and approximately 36% of all lower limb wounds did not

Lower Limb and Leg Ulcer Assessment and Management, First Edition.
Edited by Aby Mitchell, Georgina Ritchie, and Alison Hopkins.
© 2024 John Wiley & Sons Ltd. Published 2024 by John Wiley & Sons Ltd.

have a documented diagnosis. This lack of accurate diagnosis indicates that a significant proportion of the population is likely to experience delayed wound healing associated with the absence of effective treatment. The cost of lower limb ulceration cannot be underestimated, as experiencing a leg ulcer is known to be associated with a negative effect on the biopsychological, spiritual and socioeconomic aspects of patients' health, well-being and quality of life.

Treatment and management of leg ulcers are expensive, and the financial costs of wounds overall are well documented. Approximately £8.3 billion per year are spent on wound management, of which £2.7 billion is associated with managing healed wounds and £5.6 billion is associated with managing unhealed wounds (Guest et al. 2020). In terms of practitioner time, this equates to 54.4 million district or community nurse visits per year, 28.1 million practice nurse appointments and 53.6 million healthcare support worker visits (Guest et al. 2020). It is estimated that 50% of community nursing caseloads is attributed to lower limb wounds (Hopkins and Samuriwo 2022). Missing from the picture is health economics data about the amount of money and time spent by patients, their families and support networks in managing their wounds.

For practitioners this so-called 'big data' can feel disconnected from day-to-day practice, but effective resource management is an area that practitioners can influence, through learning about local needs and patterns, choosing the right management plan, analysing and understanding available data and working effectively to be aware of sustainability. Front-line healthcare practitioners are well positioned to make a difference in resource management and environmental sustainability (Ritchie 2019) for the benefit of the local health economy.

Effective management of resources, whether that is clinical consumables, human time or a commitment to environmental sustainability, has the potential to underpin effective leg ulcer management. When managing resources for the population of citizens who have wounds, it is necessary to be cognisant of the resources being used, those that are obvious and measurable, as well as where we are data poor. This is an important area for practitioners to appreciate and lead on, whatever level of change they are attempting to create, from developing a basic business case to those who wish to promote system-level change. Table I.1 highlights areas of data that could support a strategy to improve resource management.

TABLE I.1 Data for insight into the use of healthcare resources.

Understanding the burden on the local workforce such as frequency of
dressing and nursing activity per week.

The dressing spend per resident for the borough and comparing to others.

Identifying unwarranted variation such as use of compression therapy or
antimicrobials across teams.

Identifying the types of wounds on the caseload and proportion of bilateral
leg ulcers.

Obtaining data on urgent admissions for cellulitis and the impact of
unmanaged oedema.

THE COST OF SUB-OPTIMAL WOUND CARE

Dressing prescription costs are a known resource within community
services alongside the awareness that waste is prevalent and there is
a chronic lack of adherence to formularies. This brings an opportunity for cost control and reduction often led by medicines management teams. Less known or understood is the extent of time spent on
delivering wound care; this has been reviewed in some studies (Guest
et al. 2020; Hopkins and Samuriwo 2022) but it is rare for an area to
know accurately how many hours of practitioner time are spent on
care delivery. This prevents the development of a comprehensive
workforce strategy that will utilise an effective skill mix for the
successful management of patient need.

The successful management of lower leg wounds and lymphoedema is very dependent on the skillful use of dressings, compression
bandages and compression garments. When evidence based care is
utilised for people with leg ulcers, this has a positive effect on spend
and patient outcomes, as well as practitioner time. Hopkins and
Samuwiro (2022) found that more nursing time was spent on lower
limb management when compression was not used; non-use of compression increased nursing activity by 37%. Analysis of the usage and
costs of dressings, compression bandages and compression garments
bring insights to direct care delivery at the front line, as well as
improving the system-wide population health management. Yet the
insightful management of dressings and bandages as a critical
resource remains a rarity in resource management.

TABLE I.2 Tips on how practitioners can develop good resource management practices.

Identify a person with sub-optimal management of leg ulcers; explore the resources used in time and dressings, the number and costs of infections and admission. Describe an alternative journey for this person and identify the impact on cost reduction.

Use the insights developed through dressing analysis with terminology that targets the commissioners' understanding and focuses on population health, such as 'unwarranted variation', 'inequity', 'sub-optimal care', 'unplanned admission'.

Highlight the need for budget holders to invest in robust, high-quality education, rejecting a 'see one, do one' approach to lower limb management that perpetuates the cycle of sub-optimal care and ineffective resource management.

Look at your caseload of all those with lower leg wounds of all types. Establish how many are using compression therapy and whether this is optimal.

Collecting local data on practitioner time, dressing and bandage usage and unplanned admissions remains a difficult task but can provide profound insights into the evidence of sub-optimal care and unwarranted variation. Persuading commissioners of the worth of investment remains problematic and hence the need for the National Wound Care Strategy to provide a framework for evidence production and business cases. While data may be lacking, enthusiastic local leaders can help commissioners or nursing leaders make system-changing decisions. Table I.2 offers some tips for how practitioners can develop good resource management practices.

CLASSIFICATION OF DRESSING PRODUCTS

Dressings are classified according to their primary purpose, with the exception of some antimicrobial products. Categorising products, as in Table I.3, is beneficial when reviewing the use of dressings and

TABLE I.3 Product classification.

Classification	Generic examples
Absorbent	Hydrofibre, supra-absorbents
Antimicrobial	Products with Ag (silver) layer or specific antimicrobial properties
Bandage	Crepe or retention bandage
Compression bandage systems	Individual bandages, multicomponent kits, hosiery kits
Debridement	Skin or wound cleansing wipes or pads, often with microfibres
Dressing packs	Including gloves and aprons to aid good infection control practices
Film	Film only
Foam	Adhesive or non-adhesive hydrophilic polyurethane foams
Gauze	Packs of simple gauze
Hydrocolloid	Hydrocolloid of various thicknesses
Hydrogel	Debriding gel
Irrigation	Saline and other wound cleansers
Non-adherent	Wound contact layers
Negative pressure wound therapy	Various manufacturers
Other (consumables)	Forceps, scissors, probes
Paste bandage	Impregnated bandages or tubular bandages
Pressure-offloading devices	Footwear
Simple dressings	Non-adherent pads with adhesive tape or film
Tubular bandage	Used under bandages
Wadding	Sub-bandage wadding
Hosiery/wraps	Hosiery, split into garments and wraps and by compression class

spending attributed to them. This method provides a quick overview of the most-used or highest-spending products and brings insight at a glance, while highlighting where further analysis is needed.

Displaying spend and usage in this manner to those using the scheme can stimulate conversation and debate about what this means for them and how their clinical decisions are shaping their dressing and bandage spend.

DRESSING PRODUCT ANALYSIS

Top 10 Dressing Products

An example of a typical annual spend in dressings across the classifications can be seen in Figure I.1.

Foam, absorbent and antimicrobial dressings will normally feature within the first five highest-spending classifications.

In areas where a dressings optimisation scheme is actively managed, the insights from the analysis should create a change in usage. A strategy for optimising dressings is linked to delivering evidence based care; effective management of oedema will see an increase in compression products and a reduction in use of bandages (crepe and retention). Monitoring product use across teams will also establish other areas of unwarranted variation.

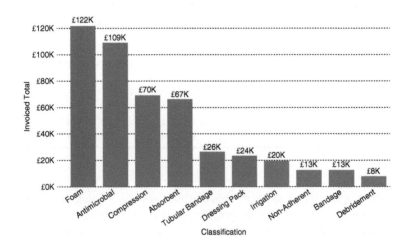

FIGURE I.1   Typical annual spend across wound management classifications.

Foam dressings combined with an online dressing optimisation system are often considered the first choice for even simple wounds as they are easy to use and comfortable. While they are essential for pressure ulcers, they are not always required for simple surgical or traumatic wounds. Encouraging a suitable switch to simple dressings such as non-adherent pads with film or tape adhesive is cost effective.

Antimicrobial spending is excessive in the example in Figure I.1 and needs to be understood and reduced through a coordinated action plan that combines effective management of wounds with a local anti-microbial strategy.

The use of absorbent dressing often benefits from greater exploration; excessive use, and certainly of the large sizes can point to inadequate lower limb management. Large absorbent dressings or pads are primarily used for lymphorrhoea or large bilateral leg ulcers; excessive use can suggest that oedema is not being addressed properly, especially if the analysis also demonstrates a high use of crepe in proportion to compression.

ONLINE NON PRESCRIPTION SERVICES

Prescribing is an essential component of effective clinical management in many areas of healthcare and non-medical prescribing in particular has been demonstrated to have many positive outcomes for practitioners and patients (Nuttall and Rutt-Howard 2019). The last 15 years have seen a number of online non prescription services developed by dressing manufacturers. Accelerate CIC has developed an independent online system that supports effective dressing optimisation through analysis and insight development; as an agnostic system there are no industry requirements for particular dressings to be present on the formulary allowing greater choice and control. Within leg ulcer management a dressing optimisation scheme (DOS) can be an effective way to deliver the insights required in order to manage resources successfully ensuring good prescribing practices that are not adversely affected by patient or colleague expectations, the organisational culture, as well as external influences such as pharmaceutical companies and the media (Ritchie 2019). While a dressing optimisation scheme does not eliminate the influences entirely, it can support their minimisation or regulation.

An online dressing optimisation system reduces waste. As the dressing or product is procured off prescription it is no longer the property of the patient but of the healthcare organisation. Therefore, a box could be opened and distributed across multiple patients or places of treatment. Additionally, as these items are owned by the local health organisation and fall under one budget for all services, if a dressing is no longer required or is likely to expire without being used, it can be utilised within the same organisation, infection control issues permitting. Orders made under the dressing optimisation scheme can also be returned to the supplier if they have not been opened and the account is credited. The system prevents people from continuing to collect or receive dressings direct to their homes without oversight. Regular reviews by a practitioner are completed to ensure that the patient's needs have not changed and that what they are using is still appropriate thereby preventing a wasteful build up of products in the home.

Access to dressings is managed through the agreed wound formulary, which is easily visible and accessible in the online system. Due to the ease of access it is critical that product sizes are restricted and products kept to a minimum; unusual products or sizes are restricted to a clinical lead or specialist nurse for authorisation and monitoring.

A benefit of an online non prescription service is that people with wounds do not pay for their dressings or compression garments via this system. This is significant for working adults and to those suffering due to the cost of living crisis. If the person is in supported self-management, products are given to them as required.

Traditional prescriptions can create waste and delays in getting the right product to the right patient on time; delays in this system are common but rarely captured or monitored. An online system has far greater transparency allowing for monitoring and improvement processes. For practice nurses, leg ulcer clinics and nursing homes, delivery direct to the team is simple and easy to manage, although a storage area is required. For community nurses visiting people with wounds in their own homes, it is more difficult (Kilborn and Hopkins 2017); community nurses are required to provide dressings from the store or nursing base. The advantage is that nurses have what they need when they need it but they are required to be the provider of the dressings. Bringing clarity about the benefits and challenges at the outset of changing to an online system is critical so that expectations are clear. The savings through waste reduction and the insights into use should both contribute to a quality improvement programme and reduction in variation. The savings realised should be invested back into the system, through either additional nursing roles or specific equipment to improve service delivery.

The analysis that can be obtained from the dressing spend within a service or trust is often not understood or examined. The provision of insightful data can improve resource management and inform practice; linking this to population health management, reduction in variation and education of practitioners will deliver significant opportunities for the health of the system and for improvement in the lives of both people with wounds and practitioners. Significant savings can be made when the spend across the system is brought together and analysed.

CONCLUSION

This book will guide you through the physiology of the venous, arterial and lymphatic systems; the pathophysiology of lymphoedema, chronic oedema and lipoedema; lower limb and leg ulcer assessment; pain and clinical management; personalised care; and prevention of recurrence. The aim is to support clinicians in leg ulcer clinical decision-making, inform practice and underpin the case for systemic change. Improved outcomes for patients can be evidenced within the data on dressings, compression and hosiery use.

REFERENCES

Guest, J., Fuller, G., and Vowden, P. (2020). Cohort study evaluating the burden of wounds to the UK's National Health Service in 2017/2018: update from 2012/2013. *BMJ Open* 10: e045253. https://doi.org/10.1136/bmjopen-2020-045253.

Hopkins, A. and Samuriwo, R. (2022). Comparison of compression therapy use, lower limb wound prevalence and nursing activity in England: a multisite audit. *Journal of Wound Care* 31 (12): 1016–1028.

Kilborn, C. and Hopkins, A. (2017). Dressing optimisation strategy: meeting the needs of the patient and population. *Nurse Prescribing* 14 (4): 188–191.

Nuttall, D. and Rutt-Howard, J. (2019). *The Textbook of Non-Medical Prescribing*, 3e. Chichester: Wiley-Blackwell.

Ritchie, G. (2019). What nurses can do to combat the dangers of air pollution. *Journal of Community Nursing* 33 (2): 10.

CHAPTER 1

Aetiology

ABY MITCHELL

NORMAL VENOUS FUNCTION

The venous system is an important part of the circulatory system. The heart may be the principal organ that pumps blood around the body, but it is the vascular system that transports the blood throughout the system. Blood flows through arteries and arterioles transporting oxygen, nutrients and other substances essential for cellular metabolism and homeostatic regulation. Veins and venules are responsible for carrying deoxygenated (oxygen-depleted) blood towards the heart. The exceptions to this are the pulmonary arteries (which carry deoxygenated blood) and the pulmonary veins (which carry oxygenated blood) (Blanchflower and Peate 2021). Capillaries are tiny blood vessels that form a delicate network near most parts of the body tissues and connect arteries and veins; they are unable to withstand high pressure. Their thin walls allow oxygen, nutrients, carbon dioxide and waste products to pass to and from tissue cells. Figure 1.1 illustrates blood flow, which is from the capillaries to the venules (Figure 1.2). Venules are porous and composed mainly of endothelium and fibroblast cells. Substances such as water, solutes and white blood cells are able to move in and out of the vessel in the extracellular fluid.

Lower Limb and Leg Ulcer Assessment and Management, First Edition.
Edited by Aby Mitchell, Georgina Ritchie, and Alison Hopkins.
© 2024 John Wiley & Sons Ltd. Published 2024 by John Wiley & Sons Ltd.

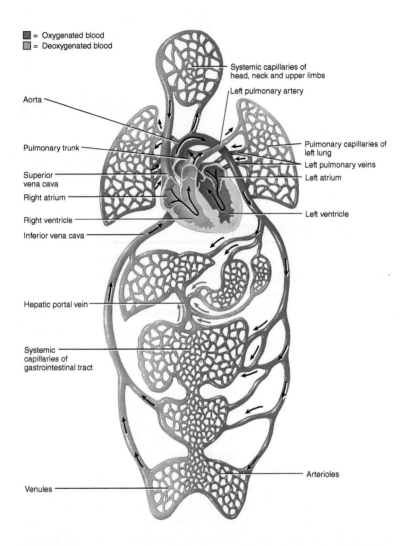

FIGURE 1.1 Transportation of blood around the body. Peate (2021) / John wiley & Sons.

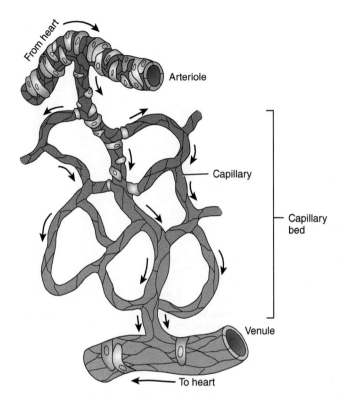

FIGURE 1.2 Blood flow from capillaries to venules. Peate (2021) / John wiley & Sons.

Venules unite to form veins. They contain three layers from the inside out:

- Tunica interna
- Tunica media
- Tunica externa

The walls of veins are thinner compared to arteries and contain less elastic, collagenous tissue and smooth muscle. Veins have a

As the muscles move and contract, the blood is pushed towards the heart

Skeletal striated muscles

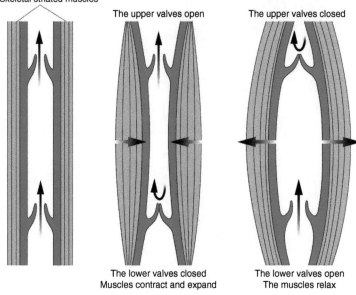

The upper valves open   The upper valves closed

The lower valves closed   The lower valves open
Muscles contract and expand   The muscles relax

FIGURE 1.3   One-way bicuspid valves.

larger lumen compared to arteries. Some veins, most commonly in the lower extremities, contain one-way paired semilunar bicuspid valves. Their function is to prevent any backward reflux of blood towards the capillaries – allowing blood only to flow back towards the heart (Figure 1.3).

The superficial venous system includes the great and lesser saphenous veins as well as the anterior, posterior and superficial accessory saphenous veins. Superficial leg veins run between the dermis and muscle fascia. The deep venous systems are located below the muscle facia and contain the femoral vein, the common femoral vein, the deep femoral vein and the popliteal vein, as well as the anterior and posterior tibial veins and the fibular veins. The two systems are linked by perforating veins that pass through the muscle fascia.

Veins in the leg are classified into three main categories:

- The deep vein (can withstand high pressures during muscle contraction).
- The superficial veins (not designed to withstand prolonged high pressures).
- The perforator veins.

Lying deep in the muscles of each leg is a deep vein that runs the length of the leg. In the calf this is also known as the anterior tibial vein, in the knee the popliteal vein and in the thigh the femoral vein. These are all sections of the deep vein. In the groin, the deep vein joins the common iliac vein, which leads to the vena cava and eventually the heart (Figure 1.4).

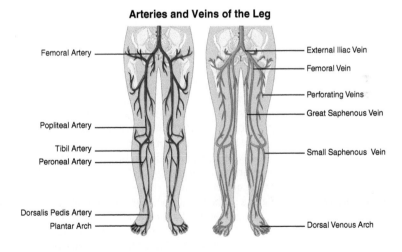

FIGURE 1.4   The venous system of the leg.

There are numerous superficial veins that lie outside the muscle just below the skin. They comprise:

- Long saphenous veins – originate from the medial malleolus (inner ankle) and empty into the femoral vein.
- Short saphenous veins – run from the lateral malleolus (outer ankle) and empty into the popliteal vein.

There are also tributaries of these veins.

The perforator veins pass through the muscles, transporting blood from the superficial system into the deep vein. These are located at regular intervals along the leg and are particularly abundant in the ankle.

VEINS IN ACTION

The veins have an important job forcing blood upwards towards the heart against gravity. Table 1.1 depicts all the mechanisms of action that facilitate this.

TABLE 1.1 Mechanisms of action.

Heart	The heart exerts a mild 'pull' on the veins due to the pressure gradient between the right atrium (pressure is around 0 mmHg) and the venous system. This is sufficient to produce some blood flow back to the heart when the person is horizontal, but insufficient in aiding venous return when upright
Veins	Dilate and contract
Respirator pump	Plays a limited role in venous return. During inspiration the diaphragm pushes against the abdomen, causing a rise in pressure in the intra-abdominal veins. At the same time, the pressure in the thorax falls (pressure also falls in the intra-thoracic veins and right atrium) and blood is drawn from the abdominal cavity into the thorax. The deeper the inspiration, the greater the venous return

TABLE 1.1 (Continued)

Calf muscle and foot pumps	These are the most important mechanisms for aiding venous return. The foot pump (contraction of the plantar muscles during movement) squeezes and empties veins in the foot. During exercise, the calf muscle contracts, compressing the deep vein and forcing the displacement of blood. The one-way valves prevent blood from refluxing, forcing the flow upwards against gravity. When the muscles relax the deep vein expands, which causes pressure to drop below that of the superficial veins. The resulting pressure gradient draws blood via the perforator veins from the superficial veins into the deep vein. As exercise continues, muscle contraction squeezes the refilled vein, forcing blood towards the heart. This is a continuous cycle

Source: Adapted from Moffatt et al. (2007).

It is important to note that the effectiveness of the calf muscle and foot pumps depends on healthy one-way valves and good ankle function/movement. Valve incompetence and limited ankle movement are major contributors to the development of venous disease and non-healing leg ulceration (see Chapter 4).

BLOOD PRESSURE IN VEINS AND CAPILLARIES

- Blood pressure in the capillary network is around 5–15 mmHg.
- Blood pressure in veins fluctuates according to position and level of activity for each individual.
- When a person is standing, venous pressure is equal to the weight of the volume of blood from the foot to the right side of the heart, which is about 80–100 mmHg. This falls to 10–20 mmHg when the calf muscle and foot pumps empty the veins during exercise.
- The values in the perforating veins that connect the superficial veins to the deep veins prevent reflux. Pressure in the superficial veins remains low (Grey and Patel 2022).
- Venous blood pressure is reduced when the person lies horizontally.

VENOUS DISEASE

Venous disorders are thought to be a major cause of morbidity and decreased health-related quality of life (White and Ryjewski 2005). Venous leg ulcers (VLUs) are typically long-lasting, and there is a high risk of recurrence that can have a negative impact on a patient's quality of life (Green et al. 2014). VLUs arise from chronic venous insufficiency (CVI) in the lower limb. The prevalence of VLUs in adults over 18 years rose to 1 per 100 individuals in 2017/2018 (Guest et al. 2020). In the United Kingdom, complex wounds such as VLUs are mostly treated by community nursing teams (Urwin et al. 2022). The estimated national cost of treating a VLU in the United Kingdom is £102 million, with a per-person annual cost of £4787.70 (Urwin et al. 2022). The average cost per person of treating a VLU is estimated at £166.39 (Urwin et al. 2022). The cost of managing an unhealed VLU is thought to be 4.5 times more than managing a healed VLU (£3000 per healed VLU and £135 000 per unhealed VLU) (Guest et al. 2018). Subsequent studies have identified a decrease in healing rates for VLUs in 2020 and 2021 by 16% and 42%, respectively, following the COVID-19 pandemic (Guest and Fuller 2023). The pandemic appears to have had a deleterious impact on the health of patients with VLU (Guest and Fuller 2023).

Venous disease occurs when the calf muscle pump and foot muscle pumps are unable to effectively empty veins. This results in venous hypertension (increased pressure in the veins). This is often due to valve incompetence allowing blood to flow backwards ('reflux') towards capillaries as well as forwards towards the heart. Valve incompetence in the deep vein causes increased pressure on the valve below and the corresponding perforator vein valve. As a result, these valves also become incompetent, causing the superficial veins to varicose and leading to disease progression (Figure 1.5). The same effect happens whether the primary incompetence occurs in the perforator or superficial veins.

Chronic venous hypertension causes an above-normal rise in pressure within the capillaries (which are not capable of withstanding high pressure). Although capillaries are very porous, their pores are normally too small to allow for larger molecules and blood cells to pass into the surrounding tissue. If there is a rise in pressure the

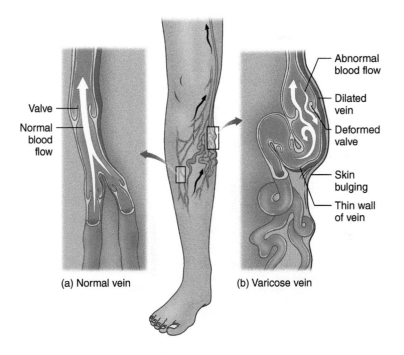

Valve

Normal blood flow

Abnormal blood flow

Dilated vein

Deformed valve

Skin bulging

Thin wall of vein

(a) Normal vein

(b) Varicose vein

FIGURE 1.5   (a, b) Varicose veins.

capillaries swell, stretching their delicate walls, which increases the size of the pores and allows blood products to leak into the surrounding tissue.

PATHOPHYSIOLOGY OF CHRONIC VENOUS DISEASE

Evidence suggests that chronic venous disease (CVD) is primarily a blood pressure–driven inflammatory disease. The sequence of events is not fully understood and may be different for each patient depending on the risk factors involved (Figures 1.6 and 1.7) (Mansilha and Sousa 2018).

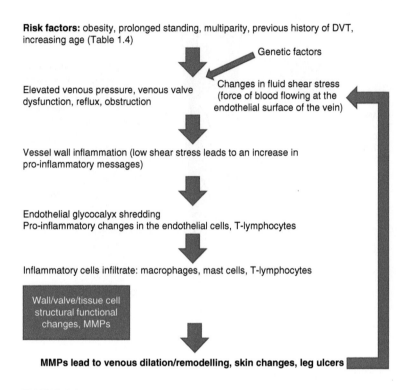

Risk factors: obesity, prolonged standing, multiparity, previous history of DVT, increasing age (Table 1.4)

Genetic factors

Elevated venous pressure, venous valve dysfunction, reflux, obstruction

Changes in fluid shear stress (force of blood flowing at the endothelial surface of the vein)

Vessel wall inflammation (low shear stress leads to an increase in pro-inflammatory messages)

Endothelial glycocalyx shredding
Pro-inflammatory changes in the endothelial cells, T-lymphocytes

Inflammatory cells infiltrate: macrophages, mast cells, T-lymphocytes

Wall/valve/tissue cell structural functional changes, MMPs

MMPs lead to venous dilation/remodelling, skin changes, leg ulcers

FIGURE 1.6   DVT, deep vein thrombosis; MMP, matrix metalloproteinase.

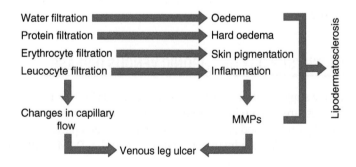

Water filtration → Oedema
Protein filtration → Hard oedema
Erythrocyte filtration → Skin pigmentation
Leucocyte filtration → Inflammation

Lipodermatosclerosis

Changes in capillary flow

MMPs

Venous leg ulcer

FIGURE 1.7   Consequences of glycocalyx and endothelium changes in venules and capillaries. MMP, matrix metalloproteinase.

THEORIES OF TISSUE DAMAGE

The progression from venous hypertension to leg ulceration is not fully understood. Several theories exist as to how this happens:

- Fibrin cuff theory (Browse and Burnard 1982; Herrick et al. 1992).
- White cell trapping theory (Coleridge-Smith et al. 1988).
- Mechanical theory (Chant 1988).
- 'Trap' growth factor theory (Higley et al. 1995).

Fibrin Cuff Theory

Venous hypertension causes capillary distension that results in endothelial pore dilation, allowing fibrinogen to leak through. Layers of fibrin are laid down as cuffs along the capillary wall. This causes a diffusion barrier inhibiting oxygen and nutrient transfer, leading to atrophic skin, tissue hypoxia, induration, liperdermatosclerosis and ulceration (Figure 1.8). In addition, chronic inflammation occurs due to extracellular proteins and leucocytes.

White Blood Cell Theory

White cells adhere to (are trapped by) the endothelium of the capillaries as a result of venous hypertension. The accumulation and activation of trapped white blood cells in patients with venous hypertension release toxic metabolites, tumour necrosis factor (TNF, a pro-inflammatory cytokine) and proteolytic enzymes that cause vascular destruction and lead to increased vascular permeability. Leucocytes become trapped in the capillaries in static blood and obstruct the flow. Monocytes become active, causing skin damage by the release of cytokines. Increased permeability leads to fibrin cuff formation, as in the fibrin cuff theory.

Mechanical Theory

High pressure in the capillary bed leads to oedema, which increases tissue pressure and stretches the skin. It is thought that ulceration arises from tissue ischaemia. Tissue ischaemia is a restriction on the blood supply of tissues. This causes a shortage of oxygen and glucose required for cellular metabolism.

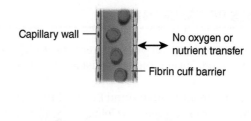

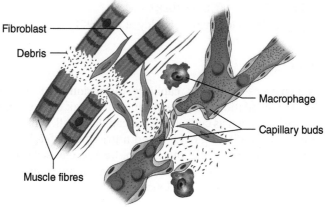

FIGURE 1.8   Fibrin cuff theory.

'Trap' Growth Factor Theory

An extension of the fibrin cuff theory suggests that growth factors and inflammatory cells are trapped in the fibrin cuff, preventing their normal function in epidermal tissue repair.

None of these theories has been proven conclusively, yet there is evidence to support them all and a combination of causes is therefore suspected. Other theories suggest that lymphatic angiopathy and capillary network abnormalities may be causes of leg ulceration.

A VLU is defined as a break in the skin below the knee, which has not healed within two weeks (National Institute for Health and Care Excellence 2023). The main cause of VLU is an increase in pressure over time, impaired blood flow and damage to the valves in the veins, resulting in physiological changes leading to skin breakdown

TABLE 1.2   Disease pathology.

Venous disease	A condition of the lower limb that can be caused by structural or functional damage as a result of venous insufficiency
Venous insufficiency	A condition that affects venous return from the lower limb to the heart. This is commonly caused by valve incompetence. Venous insufficiency can affect the superficial or deep venous system
Superficial venous incompetence	The same as venous insufficiency but relating only to the superficial venous system (e.g. valve incompetence in the long or short saphenous vein)
Venous hypertension	A condition that causes an abnormal increase in pressure within the veins due to sustained venous incompetence
Venous leg ulcer	An individual with venous incompetence that is evidenced and supported by venous duplex ultrasound

Source: Adapted from Wounds UK (2022).

and poor healing. Understanding disease pathology is essential for assessment and treatment (Table 1.2).

CHRONIC VENOUS INSUFFICIENCY

CVI in the lower limbs is one of the most common conditions in adults in the Western world, with a prevalence of 25–40% and 10–20% in women and men, respectively (Shammeri et al. 2014). However, it is recognised that the way CVI is defined can affect statistics (Shammeri et al. 2014). CVI accounts for 60–80% of leg ulcer cases (National Institute for Health and Care Excellence 2023). CVI refers to functional changes that occur in the lower limbs due to persistent elevated venous pressures. Commonly the result is venous reflux due to faulty valve function. Classification of venous insufficiency is difficult due to the broad spectrum of venous complaints, which range from minor blemishes to chronic venous ulcers. The CEAP (Clinical-Etiology-Anatomy-Pathophysiology) system is an internationally

TABLE 1.3   Features of venous ulcers.

History	Patients have a history of varicose veins, deep vein thrombosis, venous insufficiency, or venous/valve incompetence
Common site	Medial gaiter/lower leg
Edges	Sloping/irregular
Wound bed	Sloughy
Exudate	High level
Pain	Often associated with excessive oedema or infection
Oedema	Usually associated with limb oedema
Chronic venous insufficiency– associated features	Varicose eczema, lipodermatosclerosis, atrophie blanche
Treatment	Compression therapy

Source: Adapted from Grey and Patel (2022).

accepted standard for describing patients with venous disease (see Chapter 5).

According to Grey and Patel (2022), 95% of venous ulcers are located in the gaiter region around the malleoli. Ulcers can be small or circumferential. The ulcer bed is a mixture of fibrin and granulation surrounded by an irregular, sloping edge. Features of venous ulcers are described in Table 1.3.

RISK FACTORS FOR VENOUS INSUFFICIENCY

Venous insufficiency is thought to be caused by several risk factors that need to be assessed as part of a holistic assessment (see Table 1.4)

ARTERIAL DISEASE

Prevalence studies consistently suggest that 20% of patients with leg ulcers have arterial disease (Nelson and Adderley 2016). The notable factor about the prevalence of arterial disease is that despite the low percentage rates compared to venous disease, the number of people increases significantly with advancing age. It is therefore likely

TABLE 1.4 Risk factors for venous insufficiency.

Family history	Some evidence suggests that venous disease is hereditary. This could include any relatives who had/have a history of venous disease or oedema
Previous trauma	Leg injury inclusive of fractures, broken bones, soft tissue injuries, drug use, phlebitis and any other injury that can damage veins, impair mobility or cause DVT
Previous surgery	Previous surgery to the leg including fractures or flap surgery that cause damage to veins, lymphatics, ankle mobility or gait
Deep vein thrombosis (DVT)	History of major surgery that may have caused DVT, including abdominal surgery or orthopaedic surgery, prolonged immobility. Any clotting disorders, previous long-distance travel, pregnancy and the oral contraceptive pill. The effects of DVT can manifest over decades after the event
Varicose veins	Swollen and enlarged veins caused by malfunctioning valves
Mobility	The calf muscle relies on good ankle function to pump blood back to the heart through the veins. Patients with calf muscle wastage due to poor mobility, long-term bandaging, arthritis and ulcer pain are less likely to reduce venous hypertension through exercise
Obesity	Patients who are overweight are more at risk of venous disease. This increases pressure on valves by the increase in hydrostatic pressure (pressure exerted by a fluid at rest due to the force of gravity) in veins of the lower extremities and abdomen
Pregnancy	Pregnancy causes increased abdominal pressure and hormonal changes can affect the muscle layer within veins, making them more vulnerable to becoming varicosed
Age	Increasing age affects patients' mobility. Patients find it hard to mobilise, particularly if they suffer from other conditions such as arthritis
Occupation	Jobs that require prolonged sitting and standing appear to increase the risk of venous disease. This is presumed to be due to prolonged pressure in the veins
Chronic constipation	Chronic constipation increases the amount of pressure on the veins that can lead to valve damage

TABLE 1.5   Basic clinical descriptors of arterial leg ulcers.

Site	Lower leg, foot, malleoli, toes, area of pressure
Shape	Can be round, well demarcated with a punched-out appearance
Depth	Can be deep with exposed underlying structures, e.g. bone, tendon
Edges	Raised or cliff-like
Tissue type	Devitalised tissue (sloughy/necrotic) granulation is pale if present
Surrounding skin	Cool, colour changes depending on skin tone: paler than normal skin tone, or bluish skin that appears shiny

considering the ageing population that prevalence rates will increase further (Nelson and Adderley 2016). Arterial leg ulcers have several basic clinical descriptors (Table 1.5) and it is important for healthcare practitioners to understand these to aid in diagnosis.

Patients who present with arterial disease must be screened for the presence of peripheral arterial occlusive disease (POAD) and healthcare professionals should be able to recognise the risk factors for POAD. In order to assess for the presence of POAD it is important to understand normal arterial function.

In the human body there are several different kinds of blood vessels. Arteries and arterioles are the vessels that transport oxygen-rich (oxygenated) blood around the body away from the heart to all cells and organs. Arteries play a crucial role in distributing not only oxygen but also nutrients, hormones and other substances throughout the body that are essential for cellular metabolic and homeostatic regulation (Blanchflower and Peate 2021). Capillaries are tiny blood vessels that link the arterial and venous systems by forming a delicate network of vessels close to body tissues. Blood vessels dilate, constrict and pulsate to deliver blood, which begins and ends at the heart.

Arteries

The arterial system has two interrelated haemodynamic functions:

- It acts as a network to deliver an adequate supply of oxygenated blood from the left ventricle of the heart to peripheral tissues.

This is dictated by metabolic activity and termed the 'conduit function'.

- It acts as a filter to dampen blood flow and pressure oscillations to sustain adequate blood pressure and flow during diastole to ensure that peripheral organ perfusion is at a steady flow and pressure. This is termed the 'cushioning and dampening function' (London and Pannier 2010).

Other functions include cardiovascular haemostasis. When the sensors in the body detect an increase in core temperature, the vessels dilate to allow increased blood to pass through them, releasing excess heat and cooling the body. This works in reverse when the vessels constrict to conserve heat.

All blood vessels except for capillaries have three distinct layers (Figure 1.9):

- Tunica externa (outer layer) – composed largely of collagen fibres that protect and support vessels and secure them to surrounding tissues. The tunica externa is involved in healing after injury,

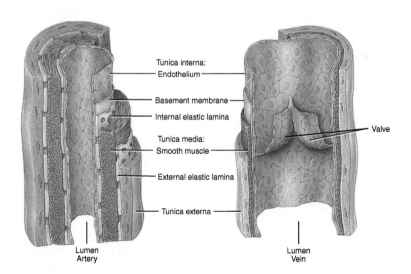

FIGURE 1.9 Layers of the arteries and veins.

immunity and maintenance of vascular tone (Blanchflower and Peate 2021). A variety of special types of cells are located in the tunica externa that are involved in immune function: macrophages (effector cells in the innate immune response), lymphocytes (B-lymphocytes make antibodies and T-lymphocytes help to kill tumour cells) and dendritic cells (boost immune responses by showing antigens to other cells in the immune system). Stem cells and fibroblasts are also found in the tunic externa and are involved in healing after injury. Cells that originate in the tunica externa have been found to migrate to the tunica media (middle layer) and tunica intima (inner layer) during repair after vessel damage (McCance et al. 2018).

- Tunica media (middle layer) – contains smooth muscle and elastic tissue and is innervated by the sympathetic nervous system (SNS). Activation of the SNS constricts arteries and arterioles (resistance vessels), which increases vascular resistance and decreases distal blood flow. When this occurs, vascular resistance causes arterial pressure to increase throughout the body (Tucker et al. 2022). As blood vessels constrict or dilate, the blood pressure increases or decreases respectively.
- Tunica interna (inner layer) – lined with endothelium, making the inner surface smooth and minimising friction as blood travels through the vessels.

Arteries can be divided into three main groups:

- Elastic arteries – thick walls found near the heart, e.g. the aorta.
- Muscular arteries – smooth muscle capable of greater vasoconstriction and vasodilation. Distribute blood to specific organs and parts of the body.
- Arterioles – determine the amount of blood flowing into organs and tissues.

The endothelium lines all the vessels and makes up the main part of the capillary wall. The role of the endothelium is significant in maintaining arterial pressure. It manages this by producing and releasing factors (i.e. nitric oxide) that have a relaxing effect on the smooth muscle of the artery, resulting in vasodilation and endothelins that have a constrictive effect (Blanchflower and

TABLE 1.6   Functions of arteries in the leg.

Femoral artery	Main blood supply to the lower body. Starts in the upper thigh near the groin and continues down the back of the knee. The femoral artery branches to supply the lower limbs with blood
Deep femoral artery	Branches from the femoral artery and supplies blood to the femur, hip, buttocks and tissues deep in the thigh
Popliteal artery	Located behind the knee in the popliteal fossa and is a direct extension of the superficial femoral artery. Supplies blood to the soleus, gastrocnemius, plantaris and distal portions of the hamstring muscles
Posterior tibial artery	Supplies blood to the posterior crural compartment
Anterior tibial artery	Responsible for blood supply of the anterior crural compartment. It is important to note that at the anterior aspect of the ankle joint, the anterior tibial artery becomes the dorsalis pedis artery

Peate 2021). In a healthy arterial network, the highly elastic walls and normal endothelial function ensure the sufficient flow of blood around the body.

The main arteries in the leg are depicted in Figure 1.9. These include the femoral artery, deep femoral artery, popliteal artery, posterior tibial artery and anterior tibial artery. These arteries are responsible for providing a rich supply of oxygenated blood and nutrients to the lower limb. Their functions are described in Table 1.6.

Peripheral Arterial Disease

PAOD is the failure of arteries to deliver sufficient blood to a particular part of the body, which results in oxygen starvation (tissue ischaemia) and cellular death. Over a prolonged period, this will lead to poorly nourished skin that is vulnerable to infection, skin that has a reduced ability to repair and the development of arterial leg ulcers. In most cases of PAOD atherosclerotic plaques narrow the artery lumen, reducing blood flow to the distal extremity (Zematitis et al. 2022). Reduced blood flow can result in thigh or calf pain when walking due to temporary ischaemia of the leg muscles during exertion. Walking pain as a result of PAOD is referred to as intermittent claudication (Zematitis et al. 2022). However, many patients have either no symptoms or atypical complaints that do not conform to the definition of claudication. Conditions can develop into a threatening compromise of blood flow requiring emergency intervention.

Making an accurate diagnosis of PAOD even in asymptomatic patients can still have a significant clinical impact, acting as a marker for systemic atherosclerosis. The management of PAOD depends largely on the severity of the disease and its symptoms (Zematitis et al. 2022). Treatment options include lifestyle changes, pharmacotherapy, endovascular intervention, cardiovascular risk factor reduction and surgery (Aysert Yıldız et al. 2018; Yuksel et al. 2018; Tan et al. 2018). Lifestyle changes will include smoking cessation and an exercise programme to reduce claudication (Bevan and White Solaru 2020).

Atherosclerosis

Atherosclerosis is a common cause of arterial disease that involves the formation of fatty plaques in the interior wall of the arteries. This causes the narrowing of the lumen (stenosis), hardening of the artery and endothelial dysfunction due to lipid accumulation. This occurs mainly in the larger and medium-sized vessels, for example the aorta, its branches and the coronary arteries (Blanchflower and Peate 2021). The commonest sites in the lower limb are the lower superficial femoral artery and the aortic segments. These complications reduce pressure and the volume of blood reaching the arteries.

Atherosclerosis can also lead to heart disease and stroke. Symptoms are experienced when the lumen is occluded by 75% and depend on the presence or absence of effective collateral circulation (the body's way of working around blood blockages). Occlusion may occur in major or more distal arteries. At rest, individuals may be able to tolerate up to 70% occlusion of an artery in the lower limb. Walking or mobilising demands a higher level of oxygen in the muscles, which cannot be met if the artery is occluded (Lusis 2010).

The cause of atherosclerosis is unknown, but certain risk factors have been identified:

- Hypertension, which accelerates the progression of atherosclerosis. It is not acknowledged to be a significant risk factor on its own, but is more significant in the presence of other risk factors.
- Smoking, which damages the vascular endothelium and increases the progression rate of atherosclerosis. Exposure to smoking activates several mechanisms predisposing to atherosclerosis, including thrombosis, insulin resistance and dyslipidaemia (imbalance of lipids, such as low-density lipoprotein [LDL] levels or triglycerides being too high or high-density lipoprotein [HDL] levels too low) (Lee and Cooke 2011).
- Family history of cardiovascular, cerebrovascular or peripheral arterial disease and leg ulceration, which can be a predisposing factor for PAOD.
- Obesity, which causes chronic inflammation that contributes to inflammation and atherosclerosis, including activation of adipokines/cytokines (cell signalling molecules) and increase in aldosterone (corticosteroid hormone that stimulates the absorption of sodium by the kidneys and regulates water and salt balance) in the circulation (Henning 2021). Too much aldosterone can cause high blood pressure and the build-up of fluids in the body.
- High lipid levels in the blood, which combine with other substances to form plaque (fatty deposits) (Linton et al. 2014).
- Diabetes mellitus, in which the high serum glucose levels cause vascular damage (Blanchflower and Peate 2021).
- Lifestyle – regular exercise involving at least 150 minutes of moderate activity per week is thought to increase HDL levels ('good' cholesterol) and protect against atherosclerosis (National Institute of Health and Care Excellence 2016).
- Alcohol – constant heavy drinking can age arteries prematurely, interfering with the blood flow and affecting the elasticity of the arterial walls.
- Gender – the incidence of atherosclerosis appears to be higher in men under 70 but similar for both sexes over 70. Oestrogen has a protective effect in reducing LDL cholesterol (McCance et al. 2018).

- Stress – biological and immune responses associated with stress may predispose patients to atherosclerosis.
- Age – increased age increases the risk of atherosclerosis.

Acute Arterial Thrombus or Embolism

A thrombus is an unstable atheromatous plaque that can originate from an area of diseased artery and can result in thrombus formation, for example atrial fibrillation. When the thrombus becomes mobilised it gets lodged in a smaller artery, causing occlusion (Mutirangura et al. 2009). Fat and air can also embolise. Assessments of patients suspected of a thrombus should include the six Ps (Smith and Lilie 2023):

- Pain
- Pallor
- Paraesthesia (burning or prickling sensation)
- Paralysis
- Pulseless
- Poikilothermia (inability to maintain a constant core temperature independent of the ambient temperature)

Inflammatory Vascular Disease

This is a rare, progressive, degenerative disease that affects small and medium-sized arteries and veins. The artery wall becomes inflamed due to an occlusion that is surrounded by non-specific immune cells, which deprive healthy cells local to the occlusion of oxygen and nutrients (Blanchflower and Peate 2021). This results in tissue ischaemia and symptoms such as intermittent claudication – fatigue, cramping, numbness, pain, tingling and weakness in a muscle group. It is aggravated by exercise and relieved by rest. Chronic ischaemia results in persistent ischaemic rest pain.

The majority of patients with leg ulcers have some degree of venous disease. The presence of venous disease suggests that the ulcer is likely to be of venous origin. Peripheral arterial disease is the second most common cause of ulceration, and all patients should be screened for signs and symptoms of arterial disease. There are many factors that contribute to the risk of venous or arterial disease

TABLE 1.7   Risk factors for venous and arterial disease.

	Venous	Arterial
Smoker		X
High cholesterol		X
Hypertension		X
Previous DVT	X	
Pregnancy	X	
Varicose veins	X	
Oedema localised		X
Oedema to lower limb	X	
Capillary refill <3 seconds	X	
Hyperaemia on limb elevation (pole test)		X
Intermittent claudication		X
Rest pain on limb elevation		X
Cool toes (consider Reynaud's phenomenon)		X
IV drug abuse	X	
Obesity	X	
Men		X
Women	X	
Ulcer below ankle		X
Punched out ulcer (cliff edges)		X
Shiny hairless limb (not from hair removal)		X
Hairy lower limb/toes	X	
Family history of arterial disease		X
Family history of venous disease	X	
Cardiac/stroke or TIA		X
Staining of limb –haemosiderin. Will not disappear but may fade, so could then be arterial	X	

DVT, deep vein thrombosis; IV, intravenous; TIA, transient ischaemic attack.

(Table 1.7). It is essential that healthcare practitioners are aware of these to inform assessment diagnosis and treatment.

THE SKIN

The skin is the largest organ in the body, accounting for 15% of all body weight. It is integral to both physical and psychosocial health and can have an impact on quality of life (Wounds UK 2018). In a

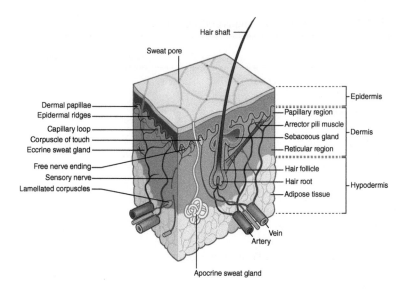

FIGURE 1.10   The layers of the skin.

healthy individual, the skin is strong, resilient and repairs easily. It consists of three layers (Figure 1.10). The epidermis (outer layer) provides a waterproof barrier. The dermis lies beneath the epidermis, has a rich blood supply and contains tough connective tissue, hair follicles, sweat glands and sensory nerve endings. The hypodermis (deep subcutaneous tissue) is made of fat and connective tissue.

The functions of the skin include the following (Mitchell 2022):

- Protection: intact skin acts as a protective barrier and prevents internal tissues from trauma, ultraviolet light, toxins, pathogens and allergens, and changes in environmental temperature.
- Barrier to infection: part of this is the physical barrier, but also the presence of sebum, a natural antibiotic chemical in the epidermis, and a surface acidic environment.
- Sensory perception: nerve endings in the skin respond to painful stimuli, temperature, vibrations, touch and itch.

- Temperature regulation: the rich blood supply in the skin can act as a 'heat dump' to enable body cooling. The subcutaneous fat acts as a heat source and heat insulation.
- Production of vitamin D and melanin: vitamin D is important for bone development; melanin is responsible for colouring the skin and protecting from sunlight and radiation damage.
- Communication: the skin is a sensory organ that enables communication through touch and physical appearance.

The skin is constantly exposed to injury and any wounding to the skin compromises function and integrity.

WOUND HEALING

Wounds can be divided into two sub-categories, 'acute' and 'chronic'. All leg ulceration will begin as a new or acute wound when the break in the integrity of the skin first occurs, yet often people with new ulceration do not present to clinical services until much later when the wound has been there for some time. There has been a drive nationally to challenge the use of the word 'chronic' in leg ulceration; this is mirrored in the long-term condition management world where terms such as 'chronic disease management' have been rejected in favour of 'long-term conditions management'. This adaption of the description is rationalised by the argument that the use of the term 'chronic' is negative and relates to the normalisation of delayed wound healing (Hopkins and Ritchie 2021). As discussed later in this book, the underlying cause of leg ulceration is indeed a long-term condition, requiring lifelong management, but with the correct treatment the episode of leg ulceration need not be a long-standing condition in itself.

Leg ulcers are often complex due to factors such as wound location. Simply put, this is due to the effects of gravity: a wound on the arm has less gravity to overcome than a wound on the leg. On first presentation to a healthcare professional many person-centred complexities (for example co-morbidities, medications, health beliefs) and system-level complexities (workforce, finances and staffing issues) will have led to an already established wound that will require proactive clinical treatment with the correct dose of compression therapy to promote healing (EWMA 2008).

PHASES OF WOUND HEALING

Wound healing is commonly described in four stages (Table 1.8). In every wound type, the healing process runs through a cascade of phases that partly overlap in time, and so while described here as a linear process, it is important to acknowledge the overlap of phases and also the possibility that in wounds that have become hard to heal, there is potential for a wound to have become 'stuck' in one of the phases of wound healing. Most commonly in hard-to-heal wounds the wound has become trapped in the inflammatory phase.

Haemostasis

The first phase is known as the vascular phase. Following initial wounding the degree of blood loss is controlled by a series of events. The blood and lymphatic vessels undergo vasoconstriction of the capillaries to slow and reduce the flow of blood to the wounded area and the production of a fibrinous blood clot. Haemostasis can continue from the development of a wound for up to five days (Ozgok Kangal and Regan 2023). Damaged blood vessels release blood and platelets that gather, forming a blood clot in the wound. This process minimises injury and initiates the inflammatory phase (Mitchell 2020).

TABLE 1.8   Phases of wound healing.

Phase	Normal timing
Vascular (clotting)	0–5 days
Inflammatory phase (clearing-up phase)	1–7 days
Proliferative phase (rebuilding)	3–24 days
Maturation	Can take up to 2 years depending on the severity of the wound and the person's general health and well-being

Source: Adapted from Ozgok Kangal and Regan (2023).

Inflammatory Phase

The second phase is the Inflammatory response, which begins once haemostasis has been achieved. Vasodilation follows vasoconstriction, which causes hyperaemia; this presents as a red, warm, swollen area with increased pain. This usually starts within the first 24 hours of injury and can last for up to two weeks in normal wounds. For hard-to-heal wounds, this can be considerably longer. The blood vessels dilate to allow essential cells into the wound bed. Growth cells are released, which attracts the migration of phagocytic cells – neutrophils, monocytes and macrophages. The primary function of these cells is to host an immune response autolysing any bacteria, necrotic or sloughy tissue within the tissue spaces (Nguyen et al. 2009). This is known as phagocytosis. The neutrophils, monocytes and macrophages release soluble mediators such as pro-inflammatory cytokines and growth factors, which are involved in the recruitment and activation of fibroblasts and epithelial cells. These prepare the wound bed for the next phase of healing. Capillary hydrostatic pressure is increased as a result of greater blood flow and presents externally as redness and heat (Mitchell 2020), which are normal in the sequence of wound healing and should not be mistaken for wound infection at this stage (Ozgok Kangal and Regan 2023; Reinke and Sorg 2012). The effectiveness of normal blood osmotic pressure increases capillary permeability, which leads to protein-rich fluid leaking into the interstitial tissue. The viscosity of the blood increases as the fluid moves out of the capillaries, slowing down the flow. This results in the blood cells clumping together, forcing white cells to move towards the endothelium of the vessels and causing swelling and pain. During this process, there is an increased demand for nutrients and oxygen to the wounded area, which increases the individual's core body temperature and metabolic rate.

Proliferation Phase

The third phase is the proliferative phase (also known as rebuilding), which occurs at between 3 and 24 days and can be sub-divided into the granulation stage and the re-epithelisation stage. It is a complex process where fibroblasts and growth factors are released from the surrounding tissues and rapidly multiply.

- Granulation: angiogenesis is the formation of new blood cells. This process ensures that the nutrients, gas and metabolic exchange are provided for granulation tissue formation, which is essential for wound healing. The fibroblasts from surrounding tissues activate growth factors released in the inflammatory phase. These produce a collagen-rich matrix through replication, which builds strength and elasticity in the wound (Mitchell 2020). The red, velvety appearance of granulation tissue on the wound bed gives an indication of healthy tissue. Dark, discoloured granulation that bleeds easily may be an indication of infection and poor vascular supply to the tissue (Peate and Stephens 2019).
- Contraction: a push/pull effect to contract the wound edges is created by the myofibroblasts.
- Epithelisation: once healthy granulation tissue is laid down, the re-epithelisation stage can begin (Gantwerker and Hom 2012). The epithelial cells change shape to migrate across the wound bed, forming islands of epithelisation that in time multiply to cover the wound. Once migration has completed and the wound has closed, the epithelial cells reattach themselves to the basement membrane.

Maturation Phase

Also known as remodelling, this is the final stage of wound healing. The granulation tissue matures into a scar and tissue tensile strength is increased. This phase can take up to two years to complete. It involves the reorganisation and maturation of the collagen fibres to maximise tensile strength. This strength will most likely only remain at 80% of the strength of unwounded skin (Ozgok Kangal and Regan 2023). The collagen fibres reorganise themselves and cross-link to strengthen and remodel the scar tissue to complete the wound-healing process. Once the wound has progressed through all four phases it is healed. However, it is important to remember that scar tissue is always vulnerable, and for a leg ulcer the underlying pathophysiology that has caused the ulceration remains and requires lifelong management to prevent reoccurrence (see Chapter 9).

An understanding of wound healing is essential for the overall assessment of a wound to identify the stage of healing, or indeed if the ulcer has become 'trapped', perhaps in the inflammatory stage. It is also important to be able to recognise abnormal wound healing, which may be indicative of more unusual ulceration, discussed in Chapter 3.

CONCLUSION

A good understanding of the vascular system and associated disorders is important for healthcare professionals so they can gather all the information needed to aid diagnosis, complete lower limb assessments, plan treatment and care, and educate patients.

REFERENCES

Aysert Yıldız, P., Özdil, T., Dizbay, M. et al. (2018). Peripheral arterial disease increases the risk of multidrug-resistant bacteria and amputation in diabetic foot infections. *Turkish Journal of Medical Sciences* 48 (4): 845–850.

Bevan, G. and White Solaru, K. (2020). Evidence based medical management of peripheral arterial disease. *Arteriosclerosis, Thrombosis, and Vascular Biology* 40 (3): 541–553.

Blanchflower, J. and Peate, I. (2021). *Fundamentals of Applied Pathophysiology: An Essential Guide*. Chichester: Wiley-Blackwell.

Browse, N.L. and Burnard, K.G. (1982). The cause of venous ulceration. *Lancet* ii: 243–245.

Chant, A.D.P. (1988). Tissue pressure, posture and venous ulceration. *Lancet* 336: 1050–1051.

Coleridge-Smith, P.D., Thomas, P., Scurr, J.M., and Dormandy, J.A. (1988). Causes of venous leg ulceration: a new hypothesis. *British Medical Journal* 296: 1726–1727.

European Wound Management Association (2008). *Hard-to-Heal Wounds: A Holistic Approach. EWMA Position Document*. London: MEP.

Gantwerker, E. and Hom, D. (2012). Skin: histology and physiology of wound healing. *Clinical Plastic Surgery* 39 (1): 85–97. https://doi.org/10.1016/j.cps.2011.09.005.

Green, J., Jester, R., McKinley, R. et al. (2014). The impact of chronic venous leg ulcers: a systematic review. *Journal of Wound Care* 23: 601–612. https://doi.org/10.12968/jowc.2014.23.12.601.

Grey, E. and Patel, K. (2022). Venous and arterial leg ulcers. In: *ABC of Wound Healing*, 2e (ed. A. Price), 34–40. Chichester: Wiley.

Guest, J.F. and Fuller, G.W. (2023). Cohort study assessing the impact of COVID-19 on venous leg ulcer management and associated clinical outcomes in clinical practice in the UK. *BMJ Open* 13 (2): e068845.

Guest, J.F., Fuller, G.W., and Vowden, P. (2018). Venous leg ulcer management in clinical practice in the UK: costs and outcomes. *International Wound Journal* 15: 29–37. https://doi.org/10.1111/iwj.12814.

Guest, J., Fuller, G., and Vowden, P. (2020). Cohort study evaluating the burden of wounds to the UK's National Health Service in 2017/2018: update from 2012/2013. *BMJ Open* 10: e045253. https://doi.org/10.1136/bmjopen-2020-045253.

Henning, R. (2021). Obesity and obesity-induced inflammatory disease contribute to atherosclerosis: a review of the pathophysiology and treatment of obesity. *American Journal of Cardiovascular Disease* 11 (4): 504–529.

Herrick, S.E., Sloan, P., McGurk, M. et al. (1992). Sequential changes in histological pattern and extracelluar matrix deposition during the healing of chronic venous ulcers. *American Journal of Pathology* 14 (5): 1085–1095.

Higley, H.R., Ksander, G.A., Gerhardt, C.O., and Falanga, V. (1995). Extravasion of macromolecules and possible trapping of transferring growth factor in ulceration. *British Journal of Dermatology* 132: 79–85.

Hopkins, A. and Ritchie, G. (2021). The legs matter campaign: the need to change culture not dressings. *Wounds UK* 17 (2): 23–24.

Lee, J. and Cooke, P. (2011). The role of nicotine in the pathogenesis of atherosclerosis. *Atherosclerosis* 215 (2): 281–283. https://doi.org/10.1016/j.atherosclerosis.2011.01.003.

Linton, M., Yancey, P., Davies, S. et al. (2014). *The Role of Lipids and Lipoproteins in Atherosclerosis*. Bethesda, MD: National Library of Medicine.

London, G. and Pannier, B. (2010). Arterial functions: how to interpret the complex physiology. *Nephrology Dialysis Transplantation* 25 (12): 3815–3823.

Lusis, A. (2010). Atherosclerosis. *Nature* 407 (6801): 233–241.

Mansilha, A. and Sousa, J. (2018). Pathophysiological mechanisms of chronic venous disease and implications for venoactive drug therapy. *International Journal of Molecular Sciences* 19 (6): 1669.

McCance, K.L., Huether, S.E., Brashers, V.L., and Rote, N.S. (2018). *Pathophysiology: The Biologic Basis for Disease in Adults and Children*, 8e. St Louis, MO: Mosby.

Mitchell, A. (2020). Assessment of wounds in adults. *British Journal of Nursing* 29 (20): S18–S24.

Mitchell, A. (2022). Skin assessment in adults. *British Journal of Nursing* 31 (5): 274–278.

Mutirangura, P., Ruangsetakit, C., Wongwanit, C. et al. (2009). Clinical differentiation between acute arterial embolism and acute arterial thrombosis of the lower extremities. *Journal of the Medical Association of Thailand* 92 (7): 891–897.

National Institute for Health and Care Excellence (2016). Physical activity: brief advice for adults in primary care. Public health guideline [PH44]. https://www.nice.org.uk/guidance/ph44

National Institute for Health and Care Excellence (2023). Leg ulcer – venous. https://cks.nice.org.uk/topics/leg-ulcer-venous

Nelson, E. and Adderley, U. (2016). Venous leg ulcers. *British Medical Journal Clinical Evidence* 2016: 1902.

Nguyen, D.T., Orgill, D.P., and Murphy, G.F. (2009). The pathophysiologic basis for wound healing and cutaneous regeneration. In: *Biomaterials for Treating Skin Loss* (ed. D.P. Orgill and G.F. Murphy), 25–57. Cambridge: Woodhead Publishing.

Ozgok Kangal, M. and Regan, J. (2023). Wound healing. In: *StatPearls*. Treasure Island, FL: StatPearls Publishing https://www.ncbi.nlm.nih.gov/books/NBK535406.

Peate, I. and Stephens, M. (2019). *Wound Care at a Glance*, 2e. Chichester: Wiley-Blackwell.

Reinke, J.M. and Sorg, H. (2012). Wound repair and regeneration. *European Surgical Research* 49: 35–43. https://doi.org/10.1159/000339613.

Shammeri, O., AlHamdan, N., Al-hothaly, B. et al. (2014). Chronic venous insufficiency: prevalence and effect of compression stockings. *International Journal of Health Sciences* 8 (3): 231–236.

Smith, D. and Lilie, C. (2023). Acute arterial occlusion. In: *StatPearls*. Treasure Island, FL: StatPearls Publishing https://www.ncbi.nlm.nih.gov/books/NBK441851.

Tan, M.N.A., Lo, Z.J., Lee, S.H. et al. (2018). Review of transmetatarsal amputations in the management of peripheral arterial disease in an Asian population. *Annals of Vascular Diseases* 11 (2): 210–216.

Tucker, W., Arora, Y., and Mahajan, K. (2022). *Anatomy, Blood Vessels*. Bethesda, MD: National Library of Medicine.

Urwin, S., Dumville, J.C., Sutton, M. et al. (2022). Health service costs of treating venous leg ulcers in the UK: evidence from a cross-sectional survey based in the northwest of England. *BMJ Open* 12: e056790. https://doi.org/10.1136/bmjopen-2021-056790.

White, J. and Ryjewski, C. (2005). Chronic venous insufficiency. *Perspectives in Vascular Surgery and Endovascular Therapy* 17 (4): 319–327. https://doi.org/10.1177/153100350501700406.

Wounds UK (2018). Best practice statement: Maintaining skin integrity. https://wounds-uk.com/best-practice-statements/maintaining-skin-integrity

Wounds UK (2022). Best practice statement: Holistic management of venous leg ulceration (second edition). https://wounds-uk.com/best-practice-statements/holistic-management-venous-leg-ulceration-second-edition

Yuksel, A., Velioglu, Y., Cayir, M.C. et al. (2018). Current status of arterial revascularization for the treatment of critical limb ischemia in infrainguinal atherosclerotic disease. *International Journal of Angiology* 27 (3): 132–137.

Zematitis, M., Boll, J., and Dreyer, M. (2022). Peripheral arterial disease. In: *StatPearls*. Treasure Island, FL: StatPearls Publishing https://www.ncbi.nlm.nih.gov/books/NBK430745.

CHAPTER 2

Lymphoedema and Chronic Swelling

CAITRIONA O'NEILL AND RHODRI HARRIS

FUNCTION OF THE LYMPHATIC SYSTEM

The lymphatic system is considered a complement of both the circulatory and immune systems. It keeps fluid levels balanced and protects the body against infections. Often referred to in lay terms as the drainage pipe of the circulatory system, unlike the circulatory system (which is closed) the lymphatic system is a blind-ended system that is responsible for the uptake of lymphatic fluid from the interstitial space arising from the blood vascular system. Lymphatic fluid that fills the lymph vessels is pushed around the body by a combination of contractions of the smooth muscular walls of the blood vessels and flexing and relaxing of the striated muscle in the body during movement (Urner et al. 2018).

Like the arteries that send the blood flow out to the body and the veins that return it, the lymphatic system is a system-wide transport network. It has three main functions:

- Facilitating tissue fluid balance and recycling of fluid and proteins (Negrini and Moriondo 2011; Bazigou and Makinen 2013).
- Filtering and production of lymphocytes (Margaris and Black 2012).

Lower Limb and Leg Ulcer Assessment and Management, First Edition.
Edited by Aby Mitchell, Georgina Ritchie, and Alison Hopkins.
© 2024 John Wiley & Sons Ltd. Published 2024 by John Wiley & Sons Ltd.

■ Providing a mechanism for lipid absorption from the gut into the circulatory system (Goswami et al. 2020).

The initial lymphatics or lymphatic capillaries are microscopic vessels that form web-like networks in the interstitial spaces (spaces between body organs and tissues). These capillaries branch out within the tissues and interweave around the capillary beds to take in excess fluid and particles that leak from blood capillaries into the tissue and return it to the circulatory system. Lymphatic capillaries have a single lining called an endothelium, making them permeable to absorb fluid. They are made up of overlapping sections that prevent fluid from leaking back out again (Goswami et al. 2020). Lymphatic capillaries are attached to surrounding tissues by anchoring filaments, causing a pull on the initial lymphatics as well as the tissues, allowing fluid into them (Negrini and Moriondo 2011). The initial lymphatics are activated to varying degrees by the mechanical forces of surrounding anatomy such as organs, muscles and vessels, which are further enhanced by external stimulation (Gordon and Morgan 2007). For an overview of the key components of the anatomy of the lymphatic system, see Table 2.1 and Figures 2.1 and 2.2.

Lymphoedema is chronic swelling owing to failure or incompetence of the lymphatic system, which results in an imbalance between

TABLE 2.1 Anatomy of the lymphatic system.

Precollectors	Connect the initial lymphatics to the collecting lymphatics and are partially contractile and partially permeable like the lymphatic capillaries (Margaris and Black 2012)
Collecting lymphatics	Made up of valve-segregated, smooth muscle cell–lined lymphangions that syphon fluid from one section to the next
Lymph nodes	Small bean-shaped structures that filter substances that travel through the lymphatic fluid. They contain lymphocytes (white blood cells) that help fight infection and disease (Goswami et al. 2020)
Lymphatic trunks	Where the smaller lymphatic 'branches' converge into larger lymphatic vessels that drain larger regions. Lymphatic trunks merge until the lymph enters the two lymphatic ducts

TABLE 2.1 (Continued)

Lymphatic ducts	The right duct drains lymph from the upper right quadrant of the body and the remainder of the body drains to the cisterna chyli, which then transports lymph back into the venous system via the thoracic duct. These ducts act as highways to the major venous junctions between both the left and right internal jugular and subclavian veins (Goswami et al. 2020)
Lymphocytes	White blood cells play a major role in immunity, fighting pathogens. These are made in the primary lymphatic organs – the thymus and bone marrow – and develop further in the secondary lymphatic organs, including the spleen, Peyer's patches, appendix, tonsils and lymph nodes (Margaris and Black 2012)
Lymphatic fluid	Known as 'lymph', this is produced from the filtration of the blood in the arteries and leaks from the capillaries to soak the cells of interstitial tissue. As excess fluid drains from cells and tissues throughout the body, lymphatic fluid collects waste products, toxins and abnormal cells (Urner et al. 2018). These include lipids and vitamins from the digestive tract and molecules such as large protein molecules and cellular debris. The lymphatic system is responsible for transporting 100% of the lymphatic fluid from the interstitial space back into the bloodstream. The fluid is then transported alongside the waste products to the lymph nodes, the 'filtering stations' in which lymphocytes destroy bacteria and viruses (Levick and Michel 2010)
	Only 10% of the lymph fluid was understood to be returned through the lymphatic system and most was reabsorbed by the venous system. This was based on the Starling principle. Recent evidence and revision of the Starling principle have provided a greater understanding of lymph fluid transport and a change in understanding that 100% of the lymphatic fluid is reabsorbed at the peripheral end from the interstitial tissue. This change in the theory is based mainly on the endothelial glycocalyx, which lines the capillary wall. These structures are similar to fine hair on the inner capillary wall, which creates an exclusion whereby fluid cannot go back to the venous side of the system as the glycocalyx is opposing the reabsorption (Michel et al. 2020; Woodcock and Woodcock 2012)

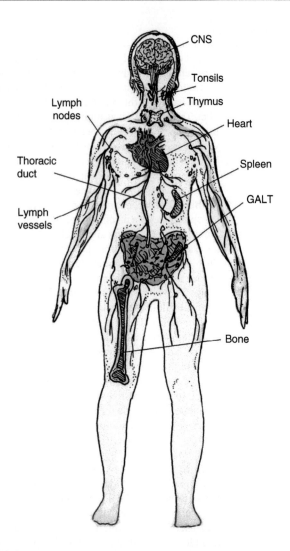

FIGURE 2.1 Lymphatics in humans. The system consists of serially connected networks of vessels and lymph nodes, and lymphoid organs, such as the thymus, bone marrow, spleen, gut-associated lymphoid tissue (GALT), lymph nodes and tonsils. Lymphatics play essential roles in maintaining tissue fluid homoeostasis and immune surveillance and responses. CNS (central nervous system).

Source: Al-Kohafi et al. (2017). Reproduced with permission.

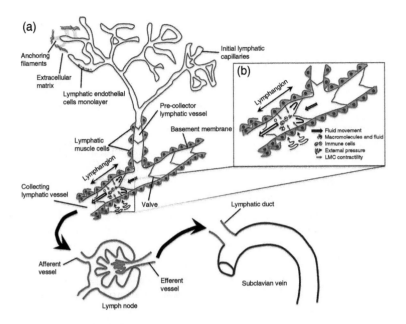

FIGURE 2.2 Lymphatic vessels. (a) Initial lymphatic capillaries are blind-ended vessels comprising a single layer of lymphatic endothelial cells, surrounded by a minimal basement membrane without muscular investment. The basal aspect of initial lymphatics are linked to the surrounding extracellular matrix by a series of anchoring filaments. Pre-collecting lymphatics transfer lymph collected in initial lymphatic capillaries into collecting lymphatics. The collecting lymphatics act as connections between initial lymphatics as well as the lymph nodes, and between lymph nodes and the blood vascular circulation. The walls of collecting lymphatics are infused with layers of smooth muscle cells and unidirectional lymphatic valves in the lumen of collecting lymphatics. (b) Lymphangions are segmented chambers located between two valves that are functional propulsive units within lymphatic collecting vessels that often show an ability to contract phasically (as well as tonically). *Source:* Al-Kohafi et al. (2017). Reproduced with permission.

capillary filtration and lymphatic drainage from the interstitial space. It is essentially a problem of 'low output' by the lymphovascular system due to a failure in lymphatic transport (International Society of Lymphology 2013, p. 52). The result is an accumulation of lymphatic fluid that cannot drain and leads to chronic swelling. It is most common in the lower or upper limbs, although other areas including the head, neck, breast and genitalia can also be affected. It can occur in persons of any age.

PREVALENCE AND KEY FACTS

Lymphoedema has a significant impact on the population, society, and on the wider health and social care system. England currently spends more than £178 million on admissions due to lymphoedema (National Lymphoedema Partnership 2019). It is a common problem that can cause a serious impact on quality of life with a risk of hospitalisation. It is important to understand the size of the problem and varying profiles within a population to appreciate how the lives of people living with lower limb swelling will be restricted, including activities of daily living and psychosocial impacts. It is also necessary to understand the challenges for health services and health professionals responsible for caring for people with lymphoedema.

Lymphoedema is an underestimated health problem and remains widely unrecognised (NLP 2019, p. 6). Moffatt et al. (2017) estimated the prevalence in the United Kingdom to be close to 3.93 per 1000 population, while Thomas and Morgan (2017) found the prevalence in Wales to be as high as 6.4 per 1000 population. The incidence is higher in women (Moffatt et al. 2019, p. 151) and increases with age (NLP 2019, p. 8). People with certain underlying conditions or medical or surgical histories have a higher risk of lymphoedema. Inadequate management of people with lymphoedema of the leg greatly increases the risk of lower limb cellulitis, a serious sequela often requiring hospital admission, which adds greatly to the cost of health service provision. In 2011–2012, there were an estimated 55 000 hospital admissions for lower limb cellulitis in England, with an average length of stay of 10 days (Atkin 2016). In a study of patients admitted to acute services for cellulitis, lymphoedema was a significant factor, with an average length of stay of 6.06 bed days (for cellulitis of limbs only) (Moffatt et al. 2017).

Many people are living in the community with undiagnosed lymphoedema or with unrecognised early signs of lymphoedema. Primary care and community nurses are often in a position to identify signs, particularly early signs. While a diagnosis requires the involvement of specialists, primary care can play an important part in recognition, referral and management after diagnosis (National Lymphoedema Partnership 2019). The prevalence of lymphoedema can be characterised as follows:

- 6 per 1000 across a population will have chronic swelling.
- 20% of patients following breast cancer will develop lymphoedema.
- 30% of all patients will have had an episode of cellulitis prior to diagnosis.
- 20–50% of those with deep vein thrombosis (DVT) will require compression due to post-thrombotic symptoms.
- Older age significantly increases the prevalence (Appelen et al. 2017; National Lymphoedema Partnership 2019; Moffatt et al. 2017).

When describing lymphoedema it is defined within two categories (see Table 2.2):

- Primary lymphoedema
- Secondary lymphoedema

The majority of lymphoedema presentations that are seen within a community setting will sit within the secondary component and may have both elements of damage to the system and overload to the system. This creates a mixed picture:

- Scenario 1: Significant venous insufficiency and immobility (overload), but also DVT in one leg (damage).
- Scenario 2: Surgery to the lower limb, e.g. coronary artery bypass graft (damage) and renal impairment, decreasing mobility (overload).
- Scenario 3: Surgery related to cancer requiring groin node dissection (damage), also leading to very poor mobility and not getting to bed overnight or maintaining a full night's rest in bed (overload).

While lymphoedema is defined as primary and secondary lymphoedema for simplicity, it can also be sub-divided into obstructive and non-obstructive lymphoedema (Table 2.3).

TABLE 2.2   Types of lymphoedema.

Type of lymphoedema	What has happened to the system?	When does it appear?	What occurs?
Primary lymphoedema	An intrinsic defect of the system whereby the anatomy is affected by the vessels being too small, too large or absent. There may be a genetic link for some	At birth, but commonly in adolescence or in the early years of adulthood	Failure of the lymphatic system to function due to a defect whereby the vessels are too small, too large or absent and the system becomes overwhelmed
Secondary lymphoedema/ chronic oedema	Damage or overload to the lymphatic system due to an external cause such as cancer treatment, trauma, venous disease, wounds or other causes	At any age where there has been damage or overload	Failure of the lymphatic system to function due to damage or overload

TABLE 2.3   Obstructive and non-obstructive causes of lymphoedema.

Obstructive cause	Damage	The consequence of damage or intrinsic defect to lymphatic vessels or lymph nodes, or lymph node removal
Non-obstructive causes	Overload	Causes include those that are the result of immobility, venous incompetence, lymphovenous stasis or hypoproteinaemia

Source: Adapted from Lymphoedema Framework, 2019: 31.

'Chronic oedema' is often used interchangeably with the term 'lymphoedema'. Oedema results from an imbalance between capillary filtration and lymphatic drainage from the interstitial space. Although the term 'lymphoedema' suggests that the oedema is caused by a lymphatic abnormality, in every case of chronic oedema there will be some impairment of lymphatic drainage, either through an underlying abnormality (primary or secondary) or through lymphatic failure as a result of the capacity of the lymphatics being overloaded or damaged. The degree to which the lymphatics are or become affected may influence the clinical presentation of oedema, the subcutaneous tissues and skin. Where there is an impairment of lymphatic drainage, over time the fluid component of oedema may become replaced by fibrosis and/or adipose tissue (National Lymphoedema Partnership 2015).

Fibrosis is the thickening, hardening or scarring of tissues in the body and is part of the body's natural healing process. It is the formation of a thickened collagen bundle and sclerosis of skin lymphatic vessels (Kataru et al. 2019) and may be a result of surgery or other medical treatments such as radiation therapy, or have other causes such as injury, infection or inflammation. Unlike superficial wounds, surgical wound scars tend to run deeper and can extend from the skin to bones and organs. These scars can become hard and inflexible, obstructing lymphatic circulation, which contributes to a form of fibrosis that is related to lymphoedema: lymphostatic fibrosis. Fibrosis occurs in both primary and secondary lymphoedema in most areas of the body and is more frequently seen in long-standing lymphoedema. Fibrotic tissues feel very dense to the touch, are nonpliable and increase the thickness of the skin.

Treating surgical fibrosis can affect the process of scar hardening, which lessens lymphatic obstruction. Treating lymphoedema lessens lymph stasis, which lowers the development of fibrosclerotic fibrosis (Azhar et al. 2020). In the case of prolonged swelling, an inflammatory process is occurring that is representative of the lymphatic fluid being chronically congested, and after a while this attracts fat cells that bind to the surrounding tissues. Over time the tissues become firmer as the lymphostatic fibrosis process begins, leading to firm tissue.

CAUSES OF AND RISK FACTORS

- Lower limb lymphoedema – associated with several forms of cancer, including gynaecological malignancies such as cervical, endometrial, ovarian and vulvar cancers in women (Dessources et al. 2020), prostate and penile cancers in men and melanoma of the lower limbs (Paskett et al. 2012; National Cancer Control Programme (Ireland) 2015).

- Lymphoedema of the arm – associated with breast cancers that require surgical removal of the underarm (axillary) lymph nodes, and generally involves chemotherapy and radiotherapy (Bromham et al. 2017, pp. 2–3). More than 20% of women who survive breast cancer are estimated to develop arm lymphoedema, with a higher risk in women who need extensive surgery and are overweight or obese (DiSipio et al. 2013).

- Wounds – the presence of a wound is the greatest independent risk factor for lymphoedema, while obesity and heart failure are also important independent risk factors (Moffatt et al. 2019).

- Cellulitis – lymphoedema is associated with a history of cellulitis, and the presence of lymphoedema substantially increases the risk of cellulitis (Mortimer and Rockson 2014, p. 919). One study of lymphoedema patients in southwest London found that 29% of patients experienced at least one episode of cellulitis over the period of one year, with 17% requiring hospitalisation (Moffatt et al. 2003). A more recent Canadian study reported that 72.06% of patients attending a wound management clinic had suffered from cellulitis (Keast et al. 2019). A cost burden of £178 million is aligned to acute hospital admissions for lymphoedema-related cellulitis (National Lymphoedema Partnership 2019).

- Risk factors that increase prevalence – cancer, increased age, obesity, heart failure and neurological defects, particularly those impacting mobility (Quéré et al. 2019) (Table 2.4).

- Other risk factors – trauma such as burns, orthopaedic trauma or surgery, abdominal surgery and long-standing skin disorders; damage to the venous system such as varicose veins, DVT, varicose vein stripping and chronic venous insufficiency, which may reduce lymphatic motility; and immobility, which reduces muscular function of the venous and lymphatic systems (NLP 2019, p. 9).

TABLE 2.4   Risk factors for lymphoedema.

Risk factor	Impact on system	Cause
Obesity overload of the system	Increased abdominal girth causes pressure on the lymphatic vessels in the groin, reducing lymphatic and venous return	Overload
Decreased mobility including paralysis	Mobility is required for venous and lymphatic return	Overload
Age	Can occur at any time, however the risk increases with age and is linked to an increase of co-morbidities and decreased mobility	Overload
Cancer	Cancer treatment, i.e. radiotherapy or surgery, or obstruction from tumour	Damage
Wounds	Disruption of skin integrity	Damage
Recurrent cellulitis	Inflammatory response to the skin and subcutaneous tissue	Damage and/ or overload
Venous thromboembolism/ thrombosis	Obstruction in the venous system	Damage and/ or overload
Chronic venous insufficiency/ venous ulceration/ venous surgeries	Reduced transit through the venous and lymphatic system; skin integrity may be affecting the mechanics	Overload and/or damage
Dermatitis/eczema	Disruption of skin integrity	Damage
Scarring	Disruption of skin integrity and subcutaneous tissue	Damage
Trauma	May affect the mechanics of the lymphatic system, including, but not exclusive to, burns, orthopaedic trauma or surgery, abdominal surgery	Damage
Hereditary	Malformation of the lymphatics	Intrinsic defect

The main causes of swelling will often be a combination of several factors (Tables 2.5 and 2.6). Reviewing the groups that sit within the higher-risk categories for swelling highlights that these high-risk groups would be prevalent within a community nursing or primary care environment.

TABLE 2.5 Underlying causes of swelling.

Overload (non-obstructive)	Damage (obstructive)
Dependency	Malformation of the lymphatic system
Venous disease	Tumour obstructing lymph vessels/nodes
Paralysis	Surgery
Cardiac failure	Radiotherapy
Renal failure	Metastatic disease
Obesity	Deep vein thrombosis
	Filariasis

TABLE 2.6 Common factors that will influence and contribute to the oedema.

Factors to consider	Why?
Low serum albumin	Without enough albumin, the body cannot keep fluid from leaking out of the blood vessels
Anaemia	The low concentration of haemoglobin causes a reduced inhibition of basal endothelium-derived relaxing factor activity and leads to generalised vasodilation. The consequent low blood pressure may be the stimulus for neurohormonal activation and salt and water retention
Hypothyroidism	Hypothyroidism induces a decreased basal metabolism and thermogenesis, an accumulation of hyaluronic acid and a decreased renal flow, all factors leading to water retention
Rheumatoid arthritis	Lymphatic obstruction occurs by fibrin degradation of inflammatory products that block the lymphatic channels. There is also a link to drug-induced and decreased mobility for some people

TABLE 2.6　(Continued)

Factors to consider	Why?
Drug-induced	Many pharmacological agents modify the activity of ion channels and other protein structures in lymph muscle cells to disrupt the cyclic contraction and relaxation of lymph vessels, thereby compromising lymph flow and predisposing to the development of lymphoedema (Largeau et al. 2021)
Lipoedema	Lipoedema as a condition on its own does not always present with swelling. Consideration links additional risk factors with decreased mobility, concurrent obesity and venous insufficiency. In addition, there is a theory that the increased subcutaneous fat may delay the initial lymphatic drainage routes

ASSESSMENT, DIAGNOSIS AND STAGING

Many patients in the community experience early or more advanced signs of lymphoedema that can be overlooked (Moffatt et al. 2017, 2019; Quéré et al. 2019; Nørregaard et al. 2019; Gordon et al. 2019). It is therefore important to be vigilant for signs of lymphoedema when assessing or treating patients in primary care, especially those at high risk, for example patients with any wound. Lymphoedema is prevalent in lower limb wounds and also has a higher prevalence in those with post-surgical, cancer-related, arterial or vascular conditions, obesity, impaired mobility and with diabetes. Specialist lymphoedema services should always be involved in the diagnosis of primary lymphoedema (British Lymphology Society 2016). However, it is essential that all healthcare professionals follow the principles of early recognition and prompt assessment.

While patients with lymphoedema may require a diagnosis from a specialist for appropriate treatment and management, this does not negate early-stage recognition and first-line assessment and management within the more generic community and primary care setting. Diagnosis is also important to slow the progression of the disease and prevent the development of co-morbidities, to minimise negative impacts on the person's quality of life and to ameliorate the physical and psychosocial problems associated with lymphoedema. Diagnosis and intervention at an early stage of the disease are more effective than once the disease has progressed to a more severe form (British Lymphology Society 2020, p. 2). A late diagnosis can increase the need for healthcare services and increase the risk of a convoluted patient journey.

Symptoms of Lymphoedema

- Swelling present for three months or longer.
- Swelling that does not reduce overnight or on elevation.
- Skin changes – thickened, dry, dilated lymph vessels.
- Tissue changes in consistency, becoming firm/hard, may be non-pitting.
- Recurrent infections.

Simple diagnosis summary questions:

- When did it start?
- Was it sudden or gradual?
- Is it bilateral or unilateral?
- Where is the oedema? At the distal end of the limb or near the trunk?
- Have systemic causes been ruled out? (For example, sudden acute swelling, underlying heart failure or renal impairment, unilateral onset, underlying malignancy, DVT or infection.)
- What does the skin look and feel like?
- How significant is the swelling? And how far does it extend?
- Is there shape distortion?
- Are any triggers noted? (For example, a new medication and sudden swelling, a new diagnosis, decreased mobility or a recent traumatic wound.)
- Is there a history of cellulitis or lymphorrhoea (lymph fluid leaking on the skin)?

Diagnosis

A full assessment combining the past medical history and lymphoedema history, including family history and cellulitis history, should be complemented by a physical examination. It should include staging consideration to exclude any systemically driven causes that have been investigated or may require further investigation to rule them out. The assessment aims to support a differential diagnosis by pulling all the key components together.

Step 1: Medical History

A full medical history of the patient is required, including the personal history of lymphoedema, a history of travel to areas where filariasis is endemic, past inguinal or axillary lymphadenectomy or radiation, a history of severe obesity (body mass index [BMI] > 50 kg/m²) or cellulitis. Other important indications of lymphoedema are the site of swelling onset and presentation of the swelling, considering whether the swelling is distal or proximal to the trunk (Greene and Goss 2018, p. 12) (Table 2.7).

TABLE 2.7 Medical history to support diagnosis of lymphoedema.

Past medical history	Identify if there is any direct link or trigger to the presentation of the swelling, for example cancer diagnosis, venous disease, previous surgery or a history of deep vein thrombosis (DVT)
History of onset/site of swelling	When did it start? Was it gradual or sudden? Was it linked to a medical cause or was there an external trigger, such as trauma, an insect bite or a period of immobility? N.B. Check if there was intermittent swelling in the past even if it was not bothersome. What body area is affected and is this distal or proximal, whole limb, trunk?
Age of onset	Consider age of onset – prevalence increases with age linked to immobility and concurrent co-morbidities. In cases first line is to exclude any cause for concern such as cancer, DVT and infection. Once excluded, consider if this could be a primary lymphoedema

(Continued)

TABLE 2.7 (Continued)

Allergies	Note all allergies and sensitives as this may affect the ability to manage and require consideration with compression and skin care products
Diet and nutritional status	Obesity is a direct risk factor. Being underweight and unexpected weight loss may link to general poor health or to a direct systemic concern. Both may link to general poor nutritional status and ill health
Sleep pattern	Not sleeping in bed or having a poor night's rest will link to dependency-related swelling
Mobility	Any decrease or alteration in mobility may impact and contribute to swelling
Lifestyle (drugs/alcohol)	Consider if there is intravenous drug use, which can cause damage. Alcohol consumption is linked to liver damage and associated low albumin. Both link to poor nutritional status in some cases
Medication	There are many drugs that can trigger swelling or have a negative impact on existing swelling. Some of these are discussed in more detail in Chapter 8. The most commonly used drugs that can cause oedema are calcium channel blockers, e.g. amlodipine; non-steroidal anti-inflammatory drugs (NSAIDs), e.g. ibuprofen; corticosteroids, e.g. prednisolone; and hormones and related compounds, e.g. tamoxifen (Pal et al. 2022)
Family history	Family history may link to a predisposition and primary lymphoedema or to other existing medical risk factors, e.g. venous insufficiency (Brouillard et al. 2021; Ho et al. 2018)
Cellulitis history and lymphorrhoea	Identifying cellulitis episodes and repeated episodes can be linked directly as there is a higher lifetime prevalence of cellulitis in those with swelling. It also correlates to delays in therapeutic management. Cellulitis can be as high as 37% lifetime prevalence for those with lymphoedema (Vignes et al. 2022; Burian et al. 2021). If there has been any episode of lymphorrhoea (leaking) this will represent a high risk of cellulitis, as the skin integrity is breached and represents unmanaged lymphoedema

Lymphoedema History

History taking of the lymphoedema onset and its presentation are required as part of a holistic assessment. Where it is noted that there has been a sudden onset of swelling, this may relate to an underlying systemic cause and thus require a systemic medical assessment in the first instance. Longer-standing gradual swelling with an identified linked reason for venous insufficiency and decreasing mobility, with no systemic concerns or identified medical history and gradual presentation, will lend itself to an easier diagnosis as the identification is clear. Any swelling noted that is proximal to the trunk and unilateral would be a cause for concern and necessitate a medical assessment to out rule any red flags, such as an underlying malignancy not yet diagnosed or a reoccurrence, DVT or cellulitis. In addition, a family history of lymphoedema where there has been a diagnosis of primary lymphoedema may provide a link to a primary lymphoedema, as in some cases this can be inherited. If the presentation of swelling is of sudden onset, there is significant deterioration of the oedema that was otherwise stable or swelling close to the trunk with no clear identifying factors, all systemic causes should be ruled out from a medical perspective as part of exclusion (for example cardiac failure, renal impairment, undiagnosed malignancy or DVT) and a subsequent specialist assessment would be required (Gasparis et al. 2020).

Cellulitis and Lymphorrhoea History

Capturing a detailed history of cellulitis episodes alongside any hospital admissions linked to the onset of the condition will aid in consideration of the diagnosis and management plan; new or repeated episodes demonstrate delayed identification or sub-therapeutic management. Lymphorrhoea represents the most critical component of unmanaged lymphoedema. Patients who are leaking will have a higher risk of cellulitis infection (skin integrity is breached and the oedema is not controlled). Similar to cellulitis, unmanaged lymphorrhoea also directly correlates with late intervention or assessment or with sub-therapeutic management. Approximately 10% of palliative patients will be symptomatic with lymphorrhoea due to the overwhelming fluid retention as part of the end-of-life process (Real et al. 2016). Repeated infection due to poorly managed oedema is resource intensive in nursing time, General Practitioner (GP) time, dressings and admissions; these healthcare costs can be avoided with effective treatment.

Step 2: Consider Other Causes and Exclusions

In addition to the screening investigations (Table 2.5), consideration should be given to the presentation of the lower limb swelling.

When swelling is first identified, it is essential that simple preliminary investigations are considered by the medical practitioner. This is in part to out rule any significant systemic root cause for the swelling; see Table 2.8. It is important to be alert for possible signs of the development of systemic problems that require urgent investigation. The critical concerns would be to out rule venous thrombosis, cancer diagnosis or reoccurrence.

Red flags to observe are:

- Pain – persistent or newly presented pain.
- Persistent neuropathic pain.
- Unusual presentations, sudden swelling or swelling proximal to the trunk with sudden onset and unresponsive.

TABLE 2.8   Unilateral or bilateral lower limb swelling.

Unilateral (single limb) swelling
- Acute deep vein thrombosis
- Post-thrombotic syndrome
- Arthritis
- Baker's cyst
- Trauma
- Presence/recurrence of carcinoma[a]

Symmetrical (bilateral) swelling
- Heart failure
- Chronic venous insufficiency
- Dependency or stasis oedema
- Renal impairment
- Hepatic impairment
- Hypoproteinaemia
- Hypothyroidism/myxoedema
- Drug-induced (e.g. calcium channel blockers, steroids, non-steroidal anti-inflammatories)
- Lipoedema

[a]Presence or recurrence of carcinoma requires direct referral to the appropriate oncology service.

- Extensive congestion swelling, which is congested, firm and unresponsive to compression.
- New venous swelling that is congested with associated venous congestion and visible telangiectasia (thread veins) or discoloration.

Step 3: Clinical Examination

Observe and record a description of the presentation of the limb and the site of the swelling. Inspect subcutaneous tissue by sight and palpation. Record a history of skin changes such as skin folds, dry skin, hyperkeratosis, papillomatosis or peau d'orange. With permission, take photographic images for the patient record. Gather context from the patient on the skin changes, the impact of these and the symptoms reported. Clinicians should look for asymmetries in the condition of the skin and signs of congestion, for example changes in skin colour or 'staining', giving particular attention to skin changes such as peau d'orange, papilloma or fibrosis (see later Table 2.10). Localised proximal swelling to the trunk or discoloration such as a red-bluish colour of the skin with the appearance of venous congestion should be considered a red flag for the presence of cancer or DVT.

A wide variety of investigations may be considered as part of exclusion considering systemic causes and to support diagnoses (Table 2.9).

TABLE 2.9 Screening and investigations.

- Full blood count (FBC)
- Urea and electrolytes (U&Es)
- Thyroid function tests (TFTs)
- Liver function tests (LFTs)
- Plasma total protein and albumin
- Fasting glucose
- Erythrocyte sedimentation rate (ESR)/C-reactive protein (CRP)
- B-natriuretic peptide
- Ultrasound, commonly abdominal ultrasound
- Venous doppler
- Venous and arterial duplex
- Chest X-ray

Source: Adapted from Lymphoedema Framework, 2006: 31

The Stemmer Sign

A positive Stemmer sign (swelling, inflammation and adipose deposition thickening the skin, making it more difficult to lift and pinch the skin on the dorsum of the hand or foot; Figure 2.3) makes lymphoedema likely, although a negative sign does not rule out early-stage lymphoedema (Greene and Goss 2018, p. 14).

The Stemmer sign is used as part of a physical examination to support the diagnosis of established lymphoedema. If the examiner cannot pinch the skin of the dorsum of the foot or hand, then this positive finding is associated with lymphoedema. Checking for a positive or negative sign as part of the physical examination allows the clinician to correlate what is presented and seen and felt alongside taking the patient's history of the onset. It is a simple check to identify that the swelling is firm and established.

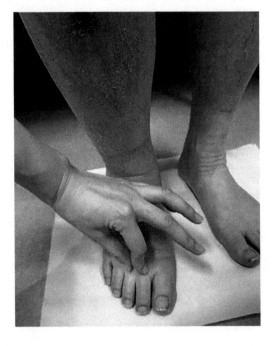

FIGURE 2.3   Stemmer sign.
Source: Reproduced by permission from Kamijo et al. 2021.

TABLE 2.10 Physical examination of the skin and tissues.

Examination of tissues and skin	Signs of lymphoedema
Texture	Tissue is soft and pitting
	Feels less elastic and firm
	Changes in consistency of the tissue or compare to a unilateral limb for comparison
	Thickened coarse skin with positive Stemmer sign
Skin changes	Skin folds, from creases in the skin predominantly noted in the toes and around or above the ankle area
	Hyperkeratosis, thickening of the outer layer of the skin, which contains a tough, protective protein called keratin
	Lymphangiectasia, a pathological dilation of lymph vessels
	Papillomatosis, characterised by the appearance of numerous papules
	Peau d'orange (French for 'orange peel skin' or, more literally, 'skin of an orange'), describing hair follicles getting buried in the oedema resembling orange peel
Temperature	Whether the limb is warmer or cooler than normal
Sensation	Consider lack of sensation or reduced sensation
Colour	Darkened skin tone or staining located to one area or bilateral can be venous congestion and will vary dependent on skin tone

The physical examination of the texture of the skin and subcutaneous tissues should note skin changes within the assessment (Table 2.10).

Simple Steps in Physical Examination

- Look – for asymmetries, skin conditions, congestion. Pay particular attention to skin changes (peau d'orange, papilloma, fibrosis).
- Touch and feel – palpation, pitting, check Stemmer sign, firmness.
- Ask questions – subjective assessment can provide essential information to form the diagnosis and future treatment plan.

TABLE 2.11   Stages of lymphoedema.

Stage 0	Clinically normal limb with abnormal lymphatic transport that is apparent only with lymphoscintigraphy
Stage 1	Early oedema responsive to limb elevation
Stage 2	Firmer tissue with fewer signs of pitting oedema unresponsive to elevation
Stage 3	Fibroadipose deposition and skin changes

Source: Adapted from International Society of Lymphology (2013) and Greene and Goss (2018), p. 12.

Step 4: Staging and Severity

The pathophysiology and staging of lymphoedema are the same whether the problem is primary or secondary (Greene and Goss 2018, p. 12) (Table 2.11).

In the initial stages of swelling, mild or fluctuating pitting oedema may be noted. Pitting oedema occurs when excess fluid in the body causes swelling that indents when pressure is applied, for example with a finger pressing down, or marks that can be noted as indents from socks. This early swelling usually resolves with elevation. As symptoms progress from Stage 1 to Stage 2, the subsidence of swelling of the affected limb becomes more and more resistant to elevation or overnight rest. This indicates that the lymphatic system is increasingly unable to maintain fluid balance by collecting and transporting fluid from the interstitial spaces to the circulation and has become congested (British Lymphology Society 2020). If symptoms progress further or are left untreated, unevenly distributed fibrosis and adipose tissue replace the interstitial fluid. Pitting oedema then becomes difficult or impossible to treat and, as a result, subcutaneous tissues become thickened and firm, with the development of deep folds and the emergence of skin changes (British Lymphology Society 2020).

According to the International Society of Lymphology (2013), the severity of oedema is classified as:

- Mild (<20% increase in limb volume)
- Moderate (20–40%)
- Severe (>40%)

Step 5: Measurements

Limb volume measurement is a method of measuring that provides a volume by percentage difference, which is mostly useful in unilateral swelling; it can be conducted with a tape measure, perometer or water displacement. For the most part and within community settings, limb volume measurement may not be attainable, thus simple measurements at key circumference points are recommended. It is noted that tape measures can be unreliable for accurate monitoring (particularly in children) because of the difficulty of measuring the same position over time and holding the tape with the same tightness (Houwen et al. 2022; Greene and Goss 2018, p. 12).

Step 6: Psychosocial Impact

The assessment must consider the negative psychosocial impact on those affected. People with lymphoedema have statistically significantly poorer social well-being, including self-perceptions of body image and appearance, and diminished sexual and social functioning. They may experience negative self-identity, emotional disturbance and psychological distress, and may feel socially isolated or marginalised, as if they are a financial burden and unsupported at work (Fu et al. 2013) (Table 2.12). Key factors that impair the quality of life in people with lymphoedema include the frequency of acute inflammatory episodes, the presence of pain, skin quality and reduced limb mobility, alongside financial concerns (Bowman et al. 2020; Morgan et al. 2005).

TABLE 2.12   Psychosocial impacts of lymphoedema.

Impact	Contributing factors
Body image disturbance	Feeling that affected limbs are ugly, unattractive, disgusting
Grief	Loss of the person's pre-lymphoedema being
Frustration, anxiety	Lack of financial support
	Burden of daily lymphoedema management
	Lack of importance accorded to lymphoedema by health services
Fear	Afraid that lymphoedema will get worse
Guilt	Feeling that the person did something themselves to cause the lymphoedema
Sadness	Having to wear unfashionable or unsexy clothes to fit the swollen limb
Depression	Need for daily management of symptoms Impairment of physical function

Source: Adapted from Fu et al. (2013).

People with lymphoedema therefore require health professionals to initiate a conversation to identify how the disease is affecting them psychosocially, and to discuss ways to manage the impact, setting realistic expectations for what can be done and the kind of support that might be available. The quality-of-life measure for limb lymphoedema (LYMQOL) (Keeley et al. 2010) is a practical tool for assessing the impact of symptoms on the patient, to help inform clinical decisions and to measure the results of progress in treatment.

MANAGEMENT CHALLENGES

Effective and appropriate management of lymphoedema requires a system-wide approach to minimise variations in outcomes and quality of care and to reduce costs. Untreated and poorly managed lymphoedema not only severely impairs patients' quality of life and increases their long-term health risks; it also has a high cost for health services and in some cases can triple the cost of treatment (Healthy London Partnership 2020). Late diagnosis can be reflective of inefficient systems and processes, which in turn can result in a convoluted patient journey leading to a negative impact from social and economic perspectives. Sub-therapeutic management for leaking legs alongside unnecessary recurrent cellulitis infections should be challenged and considered as patient harm (Atkin et al. 2021). Providing sub-therapeutic management, largely related to the sub-optimal dosage of compression, is not an efficient method for optimising nursing time (Table 2.13).

Good management includes accurate and timely diagnosis. Early recognition and prompt and effective treatment enable symptoms to be controlled and prevent escalation (Health Service Executive (Ireland) 2019, p. 33). Monitoring for signs of lymphoedema is particularly important in patients with cancer, vascular conditions or current wounds, those who use a wheelchair and the elderly (Health Service Executive (Ireland) 2019, p. 33).

Delayed or absent diagnosis can lead to inappropriate treatment, late referral to appropriate health services, the development of complications and co-morbidities, and exacerbations of the impact on the person's quality of life. It may also cause additional physical symptoms such as difficulty in moving the affected area, general discomfort and heaviness from unmanaged swelling, recurrent skin infections

TABLE 2.13 How can the complexities be addressed for a better system – what can I do as a clinician?

Risks to patient and system	Risk reduction focus	Considerations and interdependencies
Sub-therapeutic management of 'leaking legs'	Prompt assessment and therapeutic management to reduce the risk of avoidable harm and infection	Lack of therapeutic management could be considered an avoidable harm
Recurrent cellulitis	Recognition of cellulitis as an early warning sign that swelling is evident	Provision of patient education to optimise self-management
	Prompt assessment and advice on skincare and optimising oedema management to reduce the potential recurrence of cellulitis and sepsis risk and reduce harm-reducing risk factors through self-management	Raising public awareness of lower limb conditions so patients recognise when to seek help.
	Ensuring effective therapeutic compression garments to reduce recurrent infections	Improve healthcare professionals' knowledge and skills in recognition and signposting to appropriate services.
Convoluted patient journey	Ensuring a smooth pathway that reflects earlier recognition, identification, intervention and management across the pathway	Local pathways that are collaborative and seamless across primary care, community, specialist and acute services
Negative social and economic impact	Identifying where there is a multifactorial biopsychosocial negative impact on patients and the wider healthcare system and workforce	Reviewing local systems to identify gaps in provision and the negative impact on the population and workforce

(Continued)

TABLE 2.13 (Continued)

| Optimising systems, processes and resources | Identifying system pathways to ensure long-term support is available for patients to enable life-long self-management, e.g. hosiery, reassessment and review if changes in condition

Identifying pathways to support self-management, e.g. access to therapeutic compression garments in a timely manner, and patient-initiated follow-up | Multidisciplinary collaboration ensures improvements are made where harm is occurring.

Consideration for data collection, e.g. audits to identify areas of good practice or concerns

Leadership to influence and shape future systems to address health inequalities and continuous improvement |

and a change in the texture of the skin. Watery lymphorrhoea (lymph fluid) leaking from the skin and unmanaged swelling can cause a breach of skin integrity and increase the risk of infection. These complications can lead to patients experiencing psychosocial problems such as forced absence from work, isolation, absence from social activities, anxiety and depression, increasing the need for health service intervention and demand on NHS resources and economic costs.

LYMPHOVENOUS DISEASE

It is important to be alert for a number of changes in the appearance of the skin, veins and underlying tissue that indicate the presence of lymphovenous disease, a progression of lymphoedema with venous involvement. The presence of DVT and red legs indicates unmanaged or poorly managed lymphovenous disease. The most common presentation of DVT in patients with advanced cancer is asymmetrical bilateral leg oedema, but it is not limited to this group; DVT is a risk factor for those with venous disease. Progression of venous disease makes the patient's condition and treatment more complex. It is therefore important to understand the factors involved and the role of cellulitis, lymphorrhoea, inflamed or red legs and DVT so that they can be recognised, diagnosed and managed appropriately.

Cellulitis is frequently misdiagnosed (Patel et al. 2019). The signs of cellulitis are similar to those of inflamed or red legs and congestion (see later Table 2.15). However, vigilance for cellulitis is important, as it will also complicate and exacerbate lymphoedema and make treatment more difficult (see Chapter 5 for the signs of venous disease).

Lymphorrhoea

Lymphorrhoea indicates unmanaged, uncontrolled lymphoedema, and carries severe risks to the patient's health and quality of life (British Lymphology Society 2023) and utilises significant healthcare resources. Lymphorrhoea occurs because the pressure inside the tissues has become too great to contain the oedema. As a result, the lymphatic fluid leaks from the skin. This causes skin maceration and increases the risk of cellulitis. The most common place for lymphorrhoea to occur is the legs, but it can affect any area of the body.

Common triggers for lymphorrhoea are:

- Immobility and dependency.
- Non-adherence to therapeutic management.
- Health changes, such as the development of breathing difficulties or cellulitis.
- Low albumin protein level.
- Oedema at the end of life (i.e. 'leaky legs').
- Lack of recognition and ineffective management by healthcare practitioners.

Lymphorrhoea may also be a secondary symptom of cellulitis, triggered by the inflammatory response to cellulitis. Prompt management is essential to avoid the cascade of harms that may result from uncontrolled 'leaky legs'. There is a need first to establish the underlying cause of the lymphorrhoea, to inform the optimal management approach. Lymphorrhoea usually responds well and rapidly to an appropriate therapeutic intervention including skin care and compression. Once controlled, the risk of cellulitis is reduced and the patient can regain a better quality of life (Patel et al. 2019; British Lymphology Society 2023). There are signs that can increase the risk of lymphorrhoea for the more vulnerable groups (Table 2.14).

TABLE 2.14 Signs that the patient might be at increased risk of lymphorrhoea.

Recent exacerbation of poor health
Recent and sudden reduction in mobility
Taut, shiny skin
Inflammatory skin conditions
Previous lymphorrhoea
Sub-optimal management
Lymph blisters on the skin
Palliative
General systemic overload

Source: Adapted from British Lymphology Society (2023).

Red or Inflamed Legs

'Red legs' is the predominant term used to describe congestion and inflammation in the lower legs; it is a condition commonly seen in patients with chronic venous disease and chronic oedema, or lower limb dermatological conditions (Elwell 2020) and has been an important tool to differentiate between cellulitis and the inflammatory processes present. An episode of acute lipodermatoschlerosis is often misdiagnosed as cellulitis. Studies have shown that around 28–33% of patients treated for cellulitis are misdiagnosed, which subsequently leads to avoidable and costly hospitalisation and potentially hazardous use of intravenous antibiotics that may compound the evolution of antibiotic-resistant bacteria (Edwards et al. 2020). Legs need to be assessed with care, as conditions related to them may have several causes that require different treatments. The British Lymphology Society's Red Legs Pathway is a useful guide to assessment and management (Elwell 2020) and is a tool to differentiate between cellulitis and the inflammatory causes of 'red legs'.

It is important to note that the term 'red legs' is not always a useful term for darker skin tones; the expectation of redness can cause the condition to be missed. At the time of writing there is no national consensus on a new descriptor. It is recognized that there is a need to establish skills in assessing signs and symptoms in people with darker skin tones within the health care sector more broadly and lower limb management specifically (Wounds UK, 2021).

When examining the limb the aim is to recognise inflammation. In lighter skin tones the inflammation can be perceived as red or a livid dark brown due to the higher contrast. In darker skin tones, the colour change can be more subtle but also with a red or even purple hue or simply a darkening of their skin tone. Thus comparison to the other limb or another body part is critical as is asking the patient for their impression of the skin changes. Feeling for warmth or changes in texture is important.

Red legs may present either bilaterally or unilaterally. There are many possible differential diagnoses for each. Bilateral redness with wet and leaky legs indicates lymphorrhoea. If redness is unilateral, and the patient is also unwell with fever, raised temperature, pain and related symptoms, cellulitis should be considered. Cellulitis is rarely a cause of problems when redness is bilateral (British Lymphology Society and Lymphoedema Support Network 2016). For differential diagnosis see Table 2.15. For treatment of red legs see Table 2.16.

Treatment for red legs begins with daily washing with a soap substitute in warm water, followed by careful but thorough drying of the skin (patting dry) and the application of an emollient. A focus on appropriate compression therapy to address the unmanaged swelling is essential. In the event of mild swelling with no associated risk

TABLE 2.15 Differential diagnosis of red legs.

Bilateral red legs – in a well patient	Unilateral red legs – what to consider
Lipodermatosclerosis	Assess deep vein thrombosis (DVT) risk and rule out if suspected via local policy
Varicose eczema	
Gravitational dermatitis	
Contact dermatitis	Consider venous hypertension – varicosities
Fungal infection/Intertrigo in skin folds	Acute lipodermatosclerosis
Drug-induced	Phlebitis
Heat-induced redness, e.g. sunburn and radiators/open fires/hot water bottles	**Staining red flags:** In unilateral leg consider extrinsic venous compression due to undiagnosed tumour/recurrent disease – exclude with appropriate pelvic investigation/blood tests
Underlying medical condition – consider diagnosis of heart failure	DVT – exclude with venous duplex and D-dimer

Source: Adapted from Elwell (2020).

TABLE 2.16 Treatment for red legs.

Initiate skin care (wash daily with a soap substitute, dry thoroughly, moisturise with a bland emollient)

Topical steroids

Encourage exercise, e.g. chair based

Consider undersock, e.g. DermaSilk, Skinnies

Compression – class 1 British standard compression hosiery can be applied without completing an ankle brachial pressure index (ABPI) excluding those with risk factors for arterial disease and any red flags (neuropathy, swelling and misshapen legs)

If there is significant oedema or redness or the patient does not respond to class 1 British standard compression hosiery, assess vascular status using Doppler or employ the guidelines in the British Lymphology Society Position Document: Assessing Vascular Status in the Presence of Chronic Oedema and proceed to stronger compression as indicated (this may be in the form of inelastic compression bandaging, compression hosiery or wraps)

If there is failure to improve or respond or diagnostic uncertainty:
- If there is suspected peripheral arterial disease, symptomatic varicose veins or non-healing leg ulcer, refer to vascular services
- If there are concerns about skin malignancy or other skin conditions, consider referral to dermatology

---

Source: Adapted from Elwell (2020).

factors, simple class 1 British standard compression can be considered. If the swelling is more advanced, a full holistic assessment including a vascular assessment is required to ensure that the optimal dose of compression can be applied at the correct dose and correct firmness within RAL standard garment grades. In cases where the redness and congestion are persistent, this will indicate that the therapeutic dose of compression is not sufficient.

Topical Steroids

In the presence of concurrent varicose eczema, topical steroid use can be key to addressing the underlying inflammation alongside compression. The general principle is to use an ointment-based steroid at 0.1% potency, usually for one to two weeks with the emollient daily at garment changes. This should be followed by a step-down approach to alternate days, then biweekly before stopping altogether. It is not advisable to stop treatment immediately as varicose eczema can reoccur. The dose applied should be dependent on severity and presentation (Singh and Zahra 2023).

Cellulitis

Cellulitis is an acute spreading inflammation of the skin and subcutaneous tissues characterised by pain, warmth, swelling and erythema (British Lymphology Society and Lymphoedema Support Network 2016) or skin tone changes and may include blistering. In more severe cases, fever, sweats, headache and vomiting occur.

For the most part cellulitis is caused by Group A *Streptococci* (Mortimer 2000; Cox 2009). However, microbiologists consider *Staphylococcus aureus* to be the cause in some patients (Chira and Miller 2010). In lymphoedema, this may present differently than classic cellulitis and may not always be overtly symptomatic initially. Inflammatory markers (C-reactive protein [CRP], erythrocyte sedimentation rate [ESR]) may be raised. It is difficult to predict response to treatment (British Lymphology Society and Lymphoedema Support Network 2016).

If severe, cellulitis may require urgent hospital admission. Hospitalisation is necessary if there are signs of septicaemia: hypotension, tachycardia, severe pyrexia, confusion, tachypnoea or vomiting. Other possible reasons for hospitalisation are:

- Continuing or deteriorating systemic signs, with or without deteriorating local signs, after 48 hours of antibiotic treatment.
- Unresolving or deteriorating local signs, with or without systemic signs, despite trials of first- and second-line antibiotics (British Lymphology Society 2022c).

It is often difficult to differentiate cellulitis from other kinds of inflammation in the legs. Other causes of inflammation include lipodermatosclerosis, a chronic condition characterised by subcutaneous fibrosis and hardening of the skin on the lower legs (see Table 2.15); it is also known as sclerosing panniculitis and hypodermitis sclerodermaformis (Osti 2018). Cellulitis usually affects one leg only, whereas lipodermatosclerosis generally affects both legs.

TREATMENT

The treatment of lymphoedema has several aims:

- Patient education on the condition and the rationale for treatment – promoting self-care and independence and providing long-term control of the oedema.
- Improving the shape of the limb.
- Restoring functional activity and improving quality of life.
- Reducing the risk of infection and exacerbation.
- Reducing the need for hospitalisation, e.g. by preventing cellulitis through prompt assessment and management (Health Service Executive (Ireland) 2019, p. 16).

These aims should be applied alongside general health promotion interventions to attain the best long-term outcome for treatment in line with supportive self-management. Promoting movement and exercise ideally with compression is critical to ensuring venous and lymphatic drainage (Webb et al. 2019). A focus on weight maintenance and where required weight reduction strategies is important.

The treatment of both venous disease and swelling requires education of the person with lymphoedema so that they know how to take control of management themselves, with support from all professionals involved.

Skincare

Patients with lymphoedema require careful washing of the skin to ensure hygiene without compromising skin integrity. Treatment should focus on careful washing of the skin and application of emollients as well as careful management of skin folds. Emollients should be applied after washing to maintain the protective barrier. Skincare is equally important in achieving positive therapeutic outcomes. It is the first line of treatment, promoting the skin's barriers to reduce the risk of infection. Education of the patient is also important to ensure that they can take immediate action when changes in the condition or other problems arise. Changes in the skin over time due to age can impinge on the treatment of lymphoedema. With age, skin becomes less elastic and drier. Other problems such as malnutrition and chronic illnesses such as eczema affect the condition of the skin at the onset of lymphoedema. In those who are malnourished or suffering from chronic illness, their skin may also be less elastic, dryer and fragile. In the event of a concurrent dermatological condition that may affect skin integrity, this also needs to be treated; the risk of infection is greater and thus the focus on protecting the skin is essential.

Skin washing and moisturising are important opportunities to inspect the skin for signs of trauma or damage alongside monitoring for opportunistic infections such as tinea. Education for patients and carers is necessary to increase knowledge and self-care on how to wash, dry and moisturise the skin to protect it from further damage. The skin can be washed with warm, not hot, water. A non-perfumed soap substitute is recommended to minimise the risk of triggering skin sensitivities (Fife et al. 2017). The skin can be patted dry carefully after washing, without rubbing to avoid damaging fragile skin. Wash skin daily with mild soaps or skin cleansers that are moisturising, hypo-allergenic and have a neutral to slightly acid pH balance (around pH 5).

Special care is needed to wash deep folds of skin on the lymphoedematous limb. It is important to ensure that the folds are cleaned of matter that may provoke an infection. After washing, it is important to dry in between the skin folds to ensure no moisture remains that might cause maceration or moisture-associated skin damage (Mitchell and Hill 2020). It is equally important to take care not to damage fragile skin in the folds with undue abrasive rubbing with a towel.

The areas of focus are as follows:

- Fungal infections and web-space maceration – it is essential to ensure that skin creases are kept clean and dry (British Lymphology Society 2021).
- Cracks, callouses, hard skin and fissures on the feet – an appropriate moisturiser is essential to keep the skin in good condition but not leave moisture that will cause further maceration or fungal infections. A risk minimisation approach is best, with emollient creams preferred to ointments (British Lymphology Society 2021).
- Hyperkeratosis– an ointment is needed to soften and remove the hyperkeratosis, along with hydrocolloid dressings and debridement (British Lymphology Society 2021).

Emollients should be applied after bathing in the direction of hair growth to avoid folliculitis. Emollient creams are preferred for patients wearing compression hosiery, as ointments can degrade the stockings. It is important to leave the emollient to dry for some minutes before putting on the hosiery, as once the emollient is applied it can be sticky and make applying hosiery more of a challenge.

Skincare is generally recommended to be administered at night to allow for the emollient to be absorbed. However, it is important to fit in with what is suitable for the individual patient. Many people prefer to shower in the morning or might have days in the week when a morning shower is necessary. Whichever regimen is adopted, it needs to be both practical and suitable for the patient's tasks and habits of daily living, work, study and social life, as well as providing optimal care for the lymphoedema.

Patient Education

Patients require education in order to detect early signs of lymphoedema so that they can seek health professional support and treatment (Health Service Executive (Ireland) 2019). Education of the person diagnosed with lymphoedema is also necessary so that they can respond and seek help for changes in their condition, identifying early signs of infection or cellulitis and other red flags for immediate action. Barriers to lymphoedema patient education are found to be linked to the ability to self-manage (Ostby et al. 2018; Ridner et al. 2011; Alcorso and Sherman 2016). Patient education can be separated into lymphoedema-specific advice alongside general health promotion as part of the assessment and follow-up programme (Table 2.17).

COMPRESSION THERAPY AND ASSESSMENT CONSIDERATIONS

The provision of therapeutic compression is essential within the management of lymphoedema. See Chapter 8 for more information on the role and suitability of distinct types of compression therapy in venous disease and leg ulceration.

When considering the provision of compression therapy in complex lower limb lymphoedema, specialist assistance is required and is

TABLE 2.17 Lymphoedema patient education overview.

Lymphoedema-specific patient education	General health promotion
Understanding the diagnosis related to the individual	Nutritional advice
Understanding the condition and related management (skincare compression, other)	Weight management
Exercise and movement and the importance of movement for the lymphatic and venous system	Exercise
Cellulitis recognition and risk reduction	Footwear advice if lower limb
Signposting to external patient support for further information	

beyond the scope of this book. However, it is important to recognise that short-stretch non-elastic bandages are favoured in lymphoedema management, forming a firm encasement of the limb to compress the lymphatics between the muscle and the bandage to reduce the backflow of evacuated lymph and the production of interstitial fluid. This mechanically softens fibrosis and improves the efficiency of muscle and joint pumps (International Lymphoedema Framework and Canadian International Lymphoedema Framework 2010, p. 13).

Compression is applied with bandages, a wrap or hosiery. Bandaging is often used initially to swiftly reduce oedema volume, restore the limb shape, soften fibrotic tissue, reduce skin changes and eliminate lymphorrhoea. In general, a course of intensive treatment of two to four weeks is necessary to bring the lymphoedema under control and stabilise the condition of the limb. Once that is achieved, hosiery is used to prevent recurrence or deterioration of the lymphoedema for a longer term. Wraps may be used in both the intensive and maintenance stages of care. See Chapter 9 on the role of flat-knit hosiery for lymphoedema management.

If there is little improvement in the lymphoedema after four weeks of intensive compression therapy, the patient should be reassessed (Wound Care People 2019, p. 23). The compression therapy chosen should apply the same amount of pressure in the mainte-nance phase as in the intensive phase. Therefore, if a wrap has been used successfully for intensive treatment and the patient is comfort-able using it, the wrap can continue to be used for maintenance (Wound Care People 2019, p. 23).

It is necessary to determine whether the patient is suitable for compression. There are many factors to consider (Table 2.18). Com-pression is an essential part of intensive treatment, but caution is needed in some situations, such as the presence of acute cellulitis,

TABLE 2.18 Compression assessment considerations for lymphoedema.

Factors	Questions
Ability to manage and tolerate hosiery	How committed is the patient to managing and monitoring their condition?
	Does the patient need education in compression management? This is necessary in all assessments
	Does the patient's build, mobility or obesity make it difficult to self-manage compression?
	Does the patient have a supportive carer who can help appropriately?
	Does the patient consent to compression?
	Will the bandage limit bathing?
	Will the bandage prevent the patient wearing footwear or clothing?
	Is the weather too hot for the bandage to be comfortable?
	Will the patient lose faith in treatment and the therapist if the bandage or compression garment is not right the first time it is applied?
	Will the patient's ability to move be too restricted by the bandage/garment?
Skin condition	Is the skin too fragile to avoid trauma?
	Does the presence of varicose eczema or lymphorrhoea require cotton liners under the bandage?
	Does the severity of cellulitis in the acute phase require a deferral of compression for a short period?
	Is the pain or inflammation too severe for compression?
	Is the skin showing sensitivity to latex, elastane or dyes in the compression bandage?
	Does the bandage fit correctly?

TABLE 2.18 (Continued)

Factors	Questions
Lymphoedema stage and severity, shape, size and function of the limb	Does the patient need intensive therapy to restore limb shape before hosiery will be suitable? Would the distorted limb benefit from custom-made flat-knit hosiery?
Concomitant medical conditions	Will the patient's heart failure be exacerbated by compression? (Acute heart failure is a contraindication) Does neuropathy (e.g. stroke, spinal injury, spina bifida) compromise the patient's ability to feel pain?
Lower limb arterial status	Is the arterial status safe to apply compression and at what dose?

Source: Adapted from Doherty et al. (2006).

pain, reduced ability to report, psychological complications, diabetes mellitus, mild congestive heart failure, paralysis or reduced sensation. Long-term maintenance with compression garments is critical and is discussed in Chapter 9.

ADJUNCT TREATMENT MODALITIES

Manual Lymphatic Drainage

Manual lymphatic drainage (MLD) is a gentle massage technique that increases the activity of normal lymphatics and bypasses ineffective lymph vessels. As a result, MLD encourages the movement of fluid away from a fibrotic congested area of subcutaneous tissue. MLD should always be an adjunct to compression therapy and should only be performed by an appropriately trained specialist. Inappropriate massage of a lymphoedematous limb may damage tissues and exacerbate oedema by increasing capillary filtration (Lymphoedema Framework 2006, p. 29). More research is required to prove the benefits of MLD.

Self-Lymphatic Drainage

Self-lymphatic drainage (SLD) is a simplified version of MLD that is used by a patient for self-treatment and/or by their carer. The British Lymphology Society (2022a) encourages the use of SLD to maintain the benefits of MLD and encourage the continued flow of fluid through lymphatic pathways that the MLD therapist has identified as most beneficial. The benefits of SLD are unproven (Doherty and Williams 2004; Lymphoedema Framework 2006) and studies report poorer outcomes from SLD than from MLD. However, the British Lymphology Society (2022a) recommends SLD for patients in the absence of any other options to offer some relief of the psychological and physical symptoms of lymphoedema.

Contraindications to MLD and SLD include acute cellulitis, infection or erysipelas, acute or suspected (untreated) DVT and pulmonary embolism, and unstable hypertension (British Lymphology Society 2022a). The patient and/or carer must be instructed in SLD technique by an appropriately trained specialist (Table 2.19).

Other Treatment Modalities

Kinesio Tape

Kinesio taping is used to increase lymph flow, helping to stimulate the drainage of lymph away from the affected area. It can be used during the intensive or maintenance phases of care. It has been

TABLE 2.19   Requirements for self-lymphatic drainage (SLD).

Motivated patient/carer
Patient/carer sufficiently dextrous to perform SLD
Time allocated for initial teaching
Teaching is progressive and enables the patient or carer to become skilled
Written instruction is given and technique is observed
Competence in the procedure and the patient's ability to cope with
    treatment are checked regularly
Patient advised on concerns and when not to administer simple
    lymphatic drainage

Source: Adapted from Lymphoedema Framework, 2006: 31.

found to relieve tissue fluid congestion, thus improving blood and lymph circulation as well as subcutaneous lymphatic drainage. It is similar to lymphatic drainage but allows patients to receive therapeutic benefits 24 hours a day (Malicka et al. 2014). It may be contraindicated in palliative care patients if the skin is very fragile (International Lymphoedema Framework and Canadian Lymphoedema Framework 2010, p. 16).

Kinesio taping is a useful and safe option for early management of upper extremity lymphoedema in women following breast cancer treatment (Malicka et al. 2014, Pajero Otero et al. 2019).

Intermittent Pneumatic Compression

Intermittent pneumatic compression (IPC) is used widely. Aside from use in lymphoedema, it is used to prevent deep venous thrombosis in hospitalised patients and can be used in intensive, maintenance or palliative care. An inflatable plastic garment is wrapped around the limb and inflated with air from an electrical pump. Cycles of inflation and deflation for periods of 30 minutes to 2 hours give the limb a peristaltic massaging effect (Lymphoedema Framework 2006, p. 31; Zaleska et al. 2014). It is believed that IPC reduces oedema by decreasing capillary filtration, and therefore lymph formation, rather than by accelerating lymph return (Lymphoedema Framework 2006, p. 31). IPC may have benefits in addition to the reduction of oedema, including improved venous haemodynamics, reduced production of inflammatory mediators, improved microcirculation, improved arterial flow to the limb and improved wound healing (Dunn et al. 2022).

There are several contraindications that must be considered before application (Table 2.20) and IPC should only be performed by practitioners with appropriate specialist training (Lymphoedema Framework 2006, p. 31). IPC also may be useful in patients who are not gaining benefit from compression therapy (Young et al. 2021, p. 3).

Laser Therapy

Low-level laser therapy may be particularly helpful in lymphoedema of the upper limb, to reduce limb volume and tissue fibrosis (Baxter

TABLE 2.20 Contraindications to intermittent pneumatic compression.

Untreated non-pitting chronic lymphoedema
Known or suspected deep vein thrombosis
Pulmonary embolism
Thrombophlebitis
Acute skin inflammation such as cellulitis or erysipelas
Uncontrolled or severe cardiac failure
Pulmonary oedema
Ischaemic vascular disease
Active metastatic disease affecting the lymphoedematous area
Oedema at the root of the affected limb or in the adjacent trunk
Severe peripheral neuropathy

Source: Adapted from Lymphoedema Framework (2006), p. 31.

et al. 2017). However, more research is needed to confirm how laser treatment works and its benefits in lymphoedema (Lymphoedema Framework 2006, p. 51).

SURGERY

A variety of surgical options are available for lymphoedema, although access to surgery via the NHS is limited (British Lymphology Society 2022b). The options available are reconstructive microsurgery and debulking surgery. Risks associated with surgery include infection, bleeding, abnormal scarring and lymphorrhoea. Surgery should only be performed by surgeons who have experience of lymphoedema and are specialists in the lymphatic system.

Reconstructive Microsurgery

The aim of reconstructive microsurgery is to improve the functioning of the remaining lymphatic system, improve drainage, reduce swelling and reduce the patient's need for ongoing use of non-surgical treatments (British Lymphology Society 2022b). One type, lymphaticovenular anastomosis (LVA), is suitable for patients with good remaining lymphatic function. It is minimally invasive. The surgery introduces fine channels connected to veins that enable lymphatic fluid to bypass scarred or damaged tissues and return to circulation within the affected limb (Koshima et al. 2003; Campisi et al. 2007).

Lymph node transfer is more invasive and requires hospitalisation for three to five days (British Lymphology Society 2022b). It involves transplanting healthy lymph nodes from the neck or abdomen, for example, to the affected area, where over time the healthy lymph nodes regenerate lymphatics by absorbing excess fluid (British Lymphology Society 2022b).

Debulking Surgery

If the lymphoedema is advanced, the accumulating lymphatic fluid in the leg changes into fatty tissue and fibrous scar tissue through the action of proteins and growth factors in the fluid. At this stage, reconstructive surgery is not an option because it is no longer possible to redirect the fluid (Hague et al. 2020).

Lymphatic liposuction removes fatty and scar tissue that has formed in the affected limb. It requires hospitalisation for two to three days due to the high risk of serious complications. It reduces limb volume and improves limb shape. Compression hosiery needs to be worn day and night indefinitely after the operation to maintain good lymphatic function (Schaverien et al. 2018).

PALLIATIVE CARE

Lymphoedema at the end of life may be associated with long-standing lymphoedema or with other diseases such as cancer, chronic heart failure, advanced renal or liver disease, advanced neurological disease or end-stage respiratory disease. The causes are often complex. Advanced disease may impair capillary filtration as a result of venous hypertension or hypo-albuminaemia, or impaired lymphatic drainage as a result of surgery, radiotherapy, metastatic lymphadenopathy, long-standing lymphoedema or immobility (International Lymphoedema Framework and Canadian International Lymphoedema Framework 2010, p. 4) (Table 2.21). Immobility at the end of life is also a problem that may exacerbate oedema.

TABLE 2.21   End-of-life diseases associated with lymphoedema.

Disease	Symptoms and complications
Advanced pelvic cancer	Soft and pitting oedema may affect the legs, genitalia and lower abdomen Neuropathic pain, bladder spasms, fistulae, haemorrhage and malodorous exudate may be part of 'pelvic syndrome' Lymphorrhoea is also common
Chronic heart failure	Peripheral oedema More widespread oedema and ascites can occur Immobility exacerbates the symptoms
End-stage renal disease	Hypoalbuminaemia Fluid load may become intractable with dialysis
End-stage liver disease	Ascites, jaundice, hepatic encephalopathy, bleeding from oesophageal or gastric varices
Advanced neurological disease	Soft, pitting oedema Immobility promotes oedema In Parkinson disease, the weaker side usually has more oedema
End-stage respiratory disease	Extensive soft, pitting lymphoedema as a result of immobility or cor pulmonale

Source: Adapted from International Lymphoedema Framework and Canadian International Lymphoedema Framework (2010), pp. 6–7.

The prevalence of oedema at the end of life is estimated at 5–10% (International Lymphoedema Framework and Canadian International Lymphoedema Framework 2010, p. 3). The patient may experience oedema for an extended period before death, in some cases with limited access to specialist care (Real et al. 2016). Lymphoedema of the lower limbs is a common problem in palliative care patients. In an evaluation of 63 cases aged 45–97 years from a specialist palliative care oedema service, almost 9 in 10 patients had lower limb lymphoedema (Real et al. 2016). It is essential for the palliative care team to focus efforts on providing the best possible combination of effective treatments to suit the individual patient and relieve pain and discomfort as much as possible.

The aim of palliative care is to avoid further harm and to promote comfort. Early intervention is important. Many patients experience additional, preventable harm and suffering because intervention is not provided (Cobbe 2021; International Lymphoedema Framework and Canadian International Lymphoedema Framework 2010). It is therefore important to identify patients who require a palliative care approach at an early stage so that the necessary treatment regime and professional and institutional support can be put in place.

Assessment

Early assessment and intervention are essential to provide the patient with the best chance of managing symptoms well and achieving the greatest possible comfort (Lymphoedema Framework 2006). Too often patients do not present to health professionals until the lymphoedema is advanced and much more difficult to treat (Shah et al. 2016).

Assessment needs to consider the patient's priorities and goals. The cause of the lymphoedema should be diagnosed and the most appropriate treatment pathway determined that can improve symptoms. The stage of the underlying condition and the rate of progression should also be considered (International Lymphoedema Framework and Canadian International Lymphoedema Framework 2010, p. 8). It is most important to consider the symptoms' impact on the patient in several ways:

- How the symptoms affect their physical health and mobility.
- Impact on the patient's capacity to carry out daily tasks and activities.
- Impact on the patient's family situation and the availability of support and carers.
- Presence and degree of pain.

Tools such as the Palliative Care Outcome Scale (PCOS) (Sherry and McAuley 2004) or the Memorial Symptom Assessment Scale can be helpful to assess the impact of symptoms in palliative care patients (Tranmer et al. 2003). LYMQOL (Keeley et al. 2010) is also available to measure the specific impact of lymphoedema on the palliative patient's quality of life.

Management

It is likely that the palliative patient with lymphoedema will have a complex regimen combining several therapies designed to control oedema, including compression, MLD, exercises and skincare. This is sometimes referred to as complete decongestive therapy. All of these therapies need to be focused on the comfort of the palliative patient and the treatment regimen may need to be adapted (International Lymphoedema Framework and Canadian International Lymphoedema Framework 2010, p. 15). MLD may provide some symptom relief and improve comfort.

Compression Therapy

Compression therapy for the palliative patient remains a critical part of management, but provision at a therapeutic level or dose may not be suitable even in the presence of lymphorrhoea. Lymphoedema compression in a reduced dose may be more suitable for comfort dependent on the extent and site of the lymphoedema.

Exercise is important to generate muscle activity to improve the propulsion of fluid through the lymphatic system. It helps avoid limb deconditioning by building muscle strength. It softens fibrosis and increases venous and lymphatic return. Deeper breathing activates the diaphragm to support lymphatic drainage. However, it is important to avoid overstraining in palliative patients, as trauma and inflammation worsen the symptoms of lymphoedema (International Lymphoedema Framework and Canadian International Lymphoedema Framework 2010, p. 14).

Skincare in palliative patients restores hydration, counteracting the mechanical stressors of compression therapy and maintaining hygiene (International Lymphoedema Framework and Canadian International Lymphoedema Framework 2010, p. 14). It is an opportunity to observe the skin for signs of infection and signs of risk factors such as cellulitis.

Summary

Lymphoedema has a significant prevalence within the population and has the potential to continue to increase further with the ageing population, the increase in obesity and the longer-term survivorship from cancer treatment. In addition, the correlation with lower limb wounds, venous insufficiency and decreased mobility demonstrates the need for a system-wide approach to management. Lymphoedema baseline education for all levels of healthcare professionals and increased awareness for the public are required to support early detection and management. Through early diagnosis and intervention, patient harm will be avoided and the risk of an increased economic burden will be reduced, alongside a reduction in the negative impact for those who live with lymphoedema. A tiered approach to management is required, allowing for early identification and screening, prompt assessment and management, and escalation to specialist services with the ability to take a multidisciplinary approach for the most complex cases.

LIPOEDEMA

What Is Lipoedema?

Lipoedema is a poorly understood long-term condition affecting adipose tissue. Commonly known as fat, adipose is a loose connective tissue consisting mainly of adipocytes (fat cells). Its primary function is for storing energy, but it is also involved in endocrine function through the release of hormones. In lipoedema, the adipocytes of the subcutaneous layer (under the skin) expand and replicate in an irregular way, leading to painful lumps beneath the skin. Lipoedema can be progressive and as progression occurs these lumps enlarge, leading to large overhanging fat pads and significant distortion of limb shape. In addition to causing pain, lipoedema restricts mobility, limits life choices and often has a profound impact on a patient's mental health. Lipoedema almost exclusively affects women, but some cases have been reported in men. Research from Germany estimates that 11% of women and post-pubertal girls are affected (Szél et al. 2014); however, the condition is under-recognised by health professionals, so the true percentage is almost certainly higher.

Outside of specialist services, lipoedema is generally not recognised and, since it appears at first glance similar to obesity or lymphoedema, it is often misdiagnosed. Lipoedema, lymphoedema and obesity are separate conditions with different pathologies, although it is possible to have them concurrently. For example, a patient with lipoedema may also have chronic secondary swelling (lymphoe-dema) or may still have obesity even if the abnormal lipoedema fat were not present. It is therefore essential that a holistic assessment is completed to ensure that advice is appropriate for the individual patient. Table 2.22 highlights key differences between lipoedema, lymphoedema and obesity.

How to Recognise Lipoedema in Practice

The frequent lack of recognition, particularly in primary care, often leads to patients being given unhelpful or harmful advice. Many patients report being dismissed as obese by their GP and end up pursuing a cycle of aggressive dieting, which will not address the lipoedema. One of the key features of lipoedema is that the affected adipose tissue does not respond in the same way to conventional dieting as normal body fat does, so little improvement is made and symptoms persist. The exact aetiology of lipoedema is not fully understood, but it is widely accepted that there are genetic, hormonal and inflammatory components to it. A family history of relatives with similar leg shapes is often noted, and the onset of the condition is typically seen around times of hormonal change such as puberty, childbirth or menopause (Al-Ghadban et al. 2021). Concurrent inflammatory conditions such as chronic bowel disorders and skin problems like acne and psoriasis are not uncommon for lipoedema patients. It is also estimated that around 40% of lipoedema patients have a thyroid disorder such as hypothyroidism or Hashimoto disease (Lukowicz et al. 2021).

In addition to an enlarged and distorted limb profile, the skin of lipoedematous areas often feels cool compared to unaffected areas. On palpation it also usually feels soft, floppy, and may have indentations and a texture like that of orange peel (also known as peau d'orange). In the early stages, a granular texture may be felt below the skin. Patients may report that the limbs feel tired, uncomfortable or tender to touch. Another common feature is being easily bruised. As lipoedema advances and the tissues expand, the size and shape of the limbs can change dramatically.

Visual examination is important because lipoedema can affect different parts of the body. Examples include full leg from buttocks to ankles (see Figures 2.4 and 2.5) or only around the hips and buttocks,

TABLE 2.22 Key differences between lipoedema, lymphoedema and obesity.

Characteristic	Lipoedema	Lymphoedema	Obesity
Sex of patient	Almost always women, rare in men	Men or women	Men or women
Age of onset	Times of hormonal change	Any age depending on the cause	Any age
Causes	Possibly genetic and/ or hormonal	Primary (genetic) or secondary (lifestyle, injury, cancer, etc.)	Usually lifestyle but sometimes triggered by other conditions (e.g. Cushing disease)
Familial history of the condition	Common	Yes if primary, coincidental if occurring via secondary causes	Common, but more to do with socioeconomic factors than genetics
Impact of weight loss	Very little, disproportionate if any	Beneficial, proportional weight loss across the body	Very beneficial, proportional weight loss
Body location	Legs, buttocks, hips and less frequently arms	Any body part	Any body part
Laterality	Bilateral	Unilateral or bilateral	Bilateral
Presence of pain	Usually painful	Not directly painful	Not directly painful but can impact other body parts (e.g. joint pain)

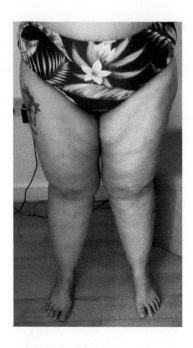

FIGURE 2.4 Type III, Stage 2 lipoedema, anterior view. Note the excess tissue around the inner aspect of the knees.

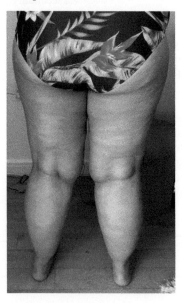

FIGURE 2.5 Same patient as in Figure 2.4, posterior view. Note the stance and position of the knees and ankles.

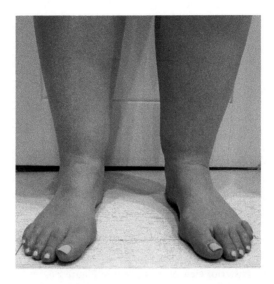

FIGURE 2.6 Close-up anterior view of ankles to demonstrate 'cuff' phenomenon in early stages. This becomes more prominent as the condition progresses.

but other presentations have been documented. The arms can also be affected, but lipoedema does not affect the feet or hands. If present below the knees it will stop suddenly at the ankles with a prominent 'cuff' effect, and the concave spaces behind the malleoli will be filled in (see Figures 2.6 and 2.7). Fat pads usually develop around the inner part of the knees, and these steadily become larger and more cumbersome as the condition progresses. Lipoedema presents bilaterally and the overall limb shape is usually symmetrical; however, one limb may be larger if there is secondary oedema. Figures 2.8, 2.9 and 2.10 show a more advanced case displaying many of the features described.

Venous disease is a common co-morbidity that occurs in patients who have lipoedema, with many patients displaying symptoms such as varicose veins and telangiectasia. Chapter 1 explores these and other venous conditions in more detail. Evidence suggests that lipoedema weakens connective tissue, including that of blood vessel walls, meaning that they are more susceptible to damage, which leads to venous disease (Allen et al. 2020). This could also explain

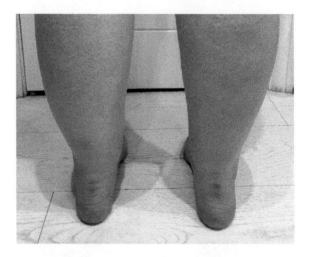

FIGURE 2.7   Posterior view of the patient in Figure 2.6.

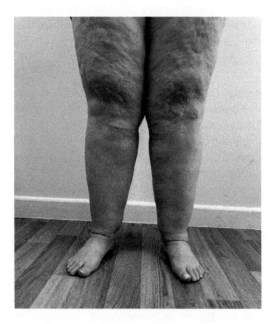

FIGURE 2.8   Type III late stage 2 with chronic oedema of lower legs and feet, anterior view. Note the more pronounced ankle 'cuff' and irregular texture of the skin.

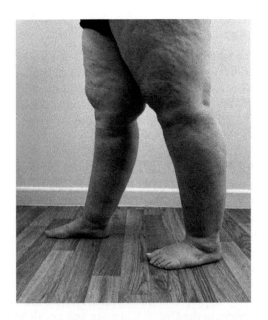

FIGURE 2.9 Same patient as figure 2.8, lateral view. The 'hood' of excess tissue over the knees becomes more pronounced as lipoedema progresses.

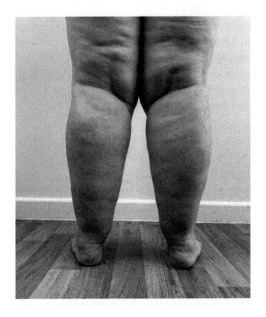

FIGURE 2.10 Same patient as figures 2.8 and 2.9, posterior view.

why lipoedema patients often report frequent and unexplained bruising. Hypermobility, where joints can extend beyond their normal range of motion, is also common among lipoedema patients and it is again thought that this is linked to weakened connective tissue. Hypermobility is discussed further in Chapter 4.

Diagnosing Lipoedema

There are currently no diagnostic tests for lipoedema and the condition is therefore diagnosed based on the patient's history and clinical examination. This is typically done by specialist services as it can be difficult to diagnose due to the similarities with obesity and lymphoedema. Lipoedema can be very unpredictable and patients do not all present with the same features. If lipoedema is suspected then referral to a specialist service should be arranged to confirm the diagnosis and ensure appropriate management. There are no dedicated lipoedema services in the United Kingdom and not all lymphoedema services will see lipoedema patients. Depending on the service, referrals may need to come from a doctor, so it is essential this is discussed with the patient's GP. Patients could also be signposted to groups such as Lipoedema UK.

A clear diagnosis should describe the location and progression of the condition, although it may be difficult to distinguish the true extent if there is lymphoedema or obesity present as well. Classification systems exist for both lipoedema location and severity. Tables 2.23 and 2.24 are collated in the Best Practice Statement (Wounds UK 2017) based on the work of multiple studies.

TABLE 2.23 Classification of lipoedema based on anatomy.

Type	Area affected
Type I	Pelvis, buttocks and hips
Type II	Buttocks to knees
Type III	Buttocks to ankles
Type IV	Arms
Type V	Lower legs

TABLE 2.24 Classification of lipoedema according to disease progression.

Stage	Description
Stage 1	Smooth appearance to the skin
	Small nodules or grainy texture felt beneath the skin
Stage 2	Skin has an irregular dimpled texture like orange peel
	Nodules beneath the skin can become fist sized
Stage 3	Skin texture becomes more irregular than in Stage 2.
	Fat deposits grow ever larger, particularly around the knees and thighs, significantly distorting limb shape
Stage 4	Lipoedema with lymphoedema
	Sometimes referred to as lipo-lymphoedema

Impact of Lipoedema

As explained earlier in the chapter, lipoedema fat does not reduce in the same way as normal body fat in response to dieting. This means that weight is lost mainly from areas unaffected by lipoedema, generally from the waist up, and patients sometimes describe themselves as 'pear-shaped' because of their disproportionate body shape. The pathophysiology behind this is not understood, but patients often report a long history of unsuccessful dieting before becoming aware of their lipoedema. Research has shown that weight loss in the affected areas through dietary means is not impossible, but cannot be expected to the same extent as for non-lipoedema fat. This common pattern of dieting with little or no improvement is understandably very upsetting for patients and can have a profound effect on their mental health. Due to the distorted limb shape, lipoedema patients also often report difficulty buying clothes and shoes, and many describe embarrassment and feeling that they need to hide their legs. This can lead to isolation and restricted social interaction, further feeding into the significant psychological impact that lipoedema can have.

Treatment and Management of Lipoedema

Current treatment for lipoedema is limited, but its management should always be holistic. Despite difficulty losing weight being a key feature, it is important that patients are supported to maintain their current weight as much as possible. This is because lipoedema deposition is exacerbated by further weight gain. There is increasing evidence that a ketogenic or anti-inflammatory diet can improve lipoedema symptoms (Jin et al. 2022). Such diets may not be appropriate for all patients, so referral to a dietitian for expert advice is sensible.

A focus on preserving and promoting mobility is also important as this often deteriorates as lipoedema progresses. Movement can be limited by pain caused by the inflamed fatty tissue, and if there are other factors such as venous disease or arthritis this will further exacerbate pain. Activity avoidance because of pain also contributes to the cycle of deteriorating mobility.

Genu valgum (knock knees) is common, as is degenerative knee pain, and this can lock a patient into a vicious cycle of deteriorating mobility and weight gain. It is felt that this structural weakness is partly due to the weakening of connective tissues in the joints. Another factor is the sheer size and weight of the excess limb bulk, which pulls joints out of alignment and affects gait, thus further restricting mobility. Lipoedema patients often develop a swaying gait, rocking from side to side as they walk, and this is caused in part simply by an involuntary attempt to avoid chafing of the thighs (Stutz and am Wald 2011). Support from therapy teams to optimise mobility is important, particularly if patients are felt to be at high risk of falls. Referral to podiatry, for biomechanical assessment and gait analysis, is also highly recommended, as supportive footwear and orthotics can better align the joints, leading to improved calf muscle pump function, optimised mobility and reduced pain.

As with most lower limb conditions, a core treatment for lipoedema is compression. For lymphoedema the aim of compression is to encourage the movement of fluid through the lymphatics to reduce swelling. Sadly, with lipoedema no amount of compression will reduce the affected fatty tissue and so the focus is to provide comfort and support, and thus a reduction of pain, to the affected limbs. The lymphatics will still be influenced, however, and so a well-fitting compression garment will help to reduce or prevent any secondary swelling that may occur.

Due to the shape distortion of lipoedema, custom-made flat-knit garments are often required, although off-the-shelf circular-knit garments can be appropriate in the early stages. Softer fabrics may be better tolerated because of the hypersensitivity some patients experience, but these are not always appropriate in terms of required support. If lipoedema extends above the knees into the hips or buttocks, then full-length garments such as leggings or tights should be considered. This may not be practical for some patients though, so a combination of below-knee stockings with Capri pants may be more appropriate. As with all compression, garments must be suited to what is therapeutic for the patient but also to what they can physically manage and are prepared to wear.

Non-cosmetic liposuction (NCL) can be performed to significantly reduce limb bulk and impressive results are possible. The procedure is not suitable in all cases and is not currently available on the NHS. There has been recent campaigning by patient groups, most notably Lipoedema UK, to obtain National Institute for Health and Care Excellence (NICE) approval for NCL for lipoedema. NICE acknowledged the debilitating impact on patients' lives that lipoedema can have, but concluded that the condition remains under-recognised and requires more research (NICE 2022).

SUMMARY

Lipoedema is poorly recognised and poorly understood creating distress for people who have this long term condition. Effective specialist assessment and management can dramatically improve a person's mobility and their quality of life.

REFERENCES

Alcorso, J. and Sherman, K.A. (2016). Factors associated with psychological distress in women with breast cancer-related lymphoedema. *Psycho-Oncology* 25 (7): 865–872. https://doi.org/10.1002/pon.4021.

Al-Ghadban, S., Teeler, M.L., and Bunnell, B.A. (2021). Estrogen as a contributing factor to the development of lipedema. In: *Hot Topics in Endocrinology and Metabolism* (ed. H.M. Heshmati), ch. 6. London: IntechOpen https://www.intechopen.com/online-first/estrogen-as-a-contributing-factor-to-the-development-of-lipedema.

Al-Kofahi, M., Yun, J.W., Minagar, A., and Alexander, J.S. (2017). Anatomy and roles of lymphatics in inflammatory diseases. *Clinical and Experimental Neuroimmunology* 8: 199–214.

Allen, M., Schwartz, M., and Herbst, K.L. (2020). Interstitial fluid in lipedema and control skin. *Women's Health Reports* 1 (1): 480–487. https://doi.org/10.1089/whr.2020.0086.

Appelen, D., van Loo, E., Prins, M.H. et al. (2017). Compression therapy for prevention of post-thrombotic syndrome. *Cochrane Database of Systematic Reviews* 9: CD004174. https://doi.org/10.1002/14651858.CD 004174.pub3.

Atkin, L. (2016). Cellulitis of the lower limbs: incidence, diagnosis and management. *Wounds UK* 12 (2): 38–41.

Atkin, L., Bullock, L., Chadwick, P. et al. (2021). Making legs matter: a case for system change and transformation in lower-limb management. *Journal of Wound Care* 30 (Sup11): S1. https://doi.org/10.12968/jowc.2021.30.Sup11.S1.

Azhar, S.H., Lim, H.Y., Tan, B.K., and Angeli, V. (2020). The unresolved pathophysiology of lymphedema. *Frontiers in Physiology* 17 (11): 137. https://doi.org/10.3389/fphys.2020.00137.

Baxter, G.D., Liu, L., Petrich, S. et al. (2017). Low level laser therapy (photobiomodulation therapy) for breast cancer-related lymphedema: a systematic review. *BMC Cancer* 17 (1): 833. https://doi.org/10.1186/s12885-017-3852-x.

Bazigou, E. and Makinen, T. (2013). Flow control in our vessels: vascular valves make sure there is no way back. *Cellular and Molecular Life Sciences* 70 (6): 1055–1066. https://doi.org/10.1007/s00018-012-1110-6.

Bowman, C., Piedalue, K.-A., Baydoun, M., and Carlson, L.E. (2020). The quality of life and psychosocial implications of cancer-related lower-extremity lymphedema: a systematic review of the literature. *Journal of Clinical Medicine* 9: 3200. https://doi.org/10.3390/jcm9103200.

British Lymphology Society (2016). Professional roles in the care of lymphoedema. https://www.thebls.com/public/uploads/documents/docu ment-25011520254971.pdf

British Lymphology Society (2020). What is lymphoedema? https://www.thebls.com/public/uploads/documents/document-78261580330781.pdf

British Lymphology Society (2021). Skin care for people with lymphoedema. https://www.thebls.com/search?query=skin%20care

British Lymphology Society (2022a) Self lymphatic drainage. https://www.thebls.com/search?query=self%20lymphatic

British Lymphology Society (2022b) Modern surgical options for lymphoedema. https://www.thebls.com/documents-library/lymph-facts-modern-surgical-options-for-lymphoedema

British Lymphology Society (BLS) (2022c). Guidelines on the management of cellulitis in lymphoedema. https://www.thebls.com/documents-library/guidelines-on-the-management-of-cellulitis-in-lymphoedema

British Lymphology Society (2023). Understanding and managing lymphor-rhoea in the community. https://www.thebls.com/search?query= understanding%20and%20managing

British Lymphology Society and Lymphoedema Support Network (2016). Consensus document on the management of cellulitis in lymphoedema. https://www.thebls.com/public/uploads/documents/document-75091530863967.pdf

Bromham, N., Schmidt-Hansen, M., Astin, M. et al. (2017). Axillary treatment for operable primary breast cancer. *Cochrane Database of Systematic Reviews* 1: CD004561. https://doi.org/10.1002/14651858.CD004561.pub3.

Brouillard, P., Witte, M.H., Erickson, R.P. et al. (2021). Primary lymphoe-dema. *Nature Reviews. Disease Primers* 7: 77. https://doi.org/10.1038/s41572-021-00309-7.

Burian, E.A., Karlsmark, T., Franks, P.J. et al. (2021). Cellulitis in chronic oedema of the lower leg: an international cross-sectional study. *British Journal of Dermatology* 185: 110–118. https://doi.org/10.1111/bjd.19803.

Campisi, C., Eretta, C., Pertile, D. et al. (2007). Microsurgery for treatment of peripheral lymphedema: long-term outcome and future perspectives. *Microsurgery* 27 (4): 333–338. https://doi.org/10.1002/micr.20346.

Chira, S. and Miller, L.G. (2010). Staphylococcus aureus is the most common identified cause of cellulitis: a systemic review. *Epidemiology and Infection* 138: 313–317.

Cobbe, S. (2021). Lymphoedema and oedema in palliative care patients. *British Journal of Community Nursing* 26 (Sup4): S6–S15. https://doi.org/10.12968/bjcn.2021.26.Sup4.S6.

Cox, N.H. (2009). Streptococcal cellulitis/erysipelas of the lower leg. In: *Evidence-Based Dermatology*, 2e: ch. 41 (ed. H. Williams, M. Bigby, T. Diepan, et al.). Oxford: Blackwell Publishing.

Dessources, K., Aviki, E., and Leitao, M.M. Jr. (2020). Lower extremity lymphedema in patients with gynecologic malignancies. *International Journal of Gynecological Cancer* 30 (2): 252–260. https://doi.org/10.1136/ijgc-2019-001032.

DiSipio, T., Rye, S., Newman, B., and Hayes, S. (2013). Incidence of unilateral arm lymphoedema after breast cancer: a systematic review and meta-analysis. *Lancet Oncology* 14 (6): 500–515. https://doi.org/10.1016/S1470-2045(13)70076-7.

Doherty, D.C., Morgan, P.A., and Moffatt, C.J. (2006). Role of hosiery in lower limb lymphoedema. In: *Compression Hosiery in Lymphoedema* (ed. L. MacGregor), 10–21. London: MEP.

Doherty, D. and Williams, A. (2004). The physiological effects of massage on individuals with lymphoedema/chronic oedema, and its role in the development of clinical techniques used in practice: a systematic review.

JBI Library of Systematic Reviews 2 (5): 1–17. https://doi.org/10.11124/jbisrir-2004-664.

Dunn, N., Williams, E.M., Dolan, G., and Davies, J.H. (2022). Intermittent pneumatic compression for the treatment of lower limb lymphedema: a pilot trial of sequencing to mimic manual lymphatic drainage versus traditional graduated sequential compression. *Lymphatic Research and Biology* 20 (5): 514–521. https://doi.org/10.1089/lrb.2021.0025.

Edwards, G., Freeman, K., Llewelyn, M.J., and Hayward, G. (2020). What diagnostic strategies can help differentiate cellulitis from other causes of red legs in primary care? *BMJ* 368: m54. https://doi.org/10.1136/bmj.m54.

Elwell R (2020). Red legs pathway. Lichfield: British Lymphology Society. https://www.thebls.com/public/uploads/documents/document-84341639738140.pdf

Fife, C.E., Farrow, W., Hebert, A.A. et al. (2017). Skin and wound care in lymphedema patients: a taxonomy, primer, and literature review. *Advances in Skin & Wound Care* 30 (7): 305–318. https://doi.org/10.1097/01.ASW.0000520501.23702.82.

Fu, M.R., Ridner, S.H., Hu, S.H. et al. (2013). Psychosocial impact of lymphedema: a systematic review of literature from 2004 to 2011. *Psychooncology* 22 (7): 1466–1484. https://doi.org/10.1002/pon.3201.

Gasparis, A.P., Kim, P.S., Dean, S.M. et al. (2020). Diagnostic approach to lower limb edema. *Phlebology* 35 (9): 650–655. https://doi.org/10.1177/0268355520938283.

Gordon, K. and Morgan, P.A. (2007). Lymphoedema: an underestimated health problem. *Journal of Lymphoedema* 2 (1): 3–10.

Gordon, S.J., Murray, S.G., Sutton, T. et al. (2019). LIMPRINT in Australia. *Lymphatic Research and Biology* 17 (2): 173–177. https://doi.org/10.1089/lrb.2018.0087.

Goswami, A.K., Khaja, M.S., Downing, T. et al. (2020). Lymphatic anatomy and physiology. *Seminars in Interventional Radiology* 37 (3): 227–236. https://doi.org/10.1055/s-0040-1713440.

Greene, A.K. and Goss, J.A. (2018). Vascular anomalies: from a clinicohistologic to a genetic framework. *Plastic and Reconstructive Surgery* 141 (5): 709e–717e. https://doi.org/10.1097/PRS.0000000000004294.

Hague, A., Bragg, T., Thomas, M. et al. (2020). Severe lower limb lymphoedema successfully treated with a two-stage debulking procedure: a case report. *Case Reports in Plastic Surgery and Hand Surgery* 7 (1): 38–42. https://doi.org/10.1080/23320885.2020.1736943.

Health Service Executive (Ireland) (2019). Lymphoedema and lipoedema treatment in Ireland: a model of care for Ireland. https://www.hse.ie/eng/services/publications/lymphoedema-model-of-care.pdf

Healthy London Partnership (2020). Commissioning guidance for lymphoedema services for adults living with and beyond cancer.

https://www.healthylondon.org/wp-content/uploads/2020/03/Lymphoedema-Commissioning-Guidance-2020.pdf

Ho, B., Gordon, K., and Mortimer, P.S. (2018). A genetic approach to the classification of primary lymphoedema and lymphatic malformations. *European Journal of Vascular and Endovascular Surgery* 56 (4): 465–466. https://doi.org/10.1016/j.ejvs.2018.07.001.

Houwen, F., Stemkens, J., de Schipper, P.J. et al. (2022). Estimates for assessment of lymphedema: reliability and validity of extremity measurements. *Lymphatic Research and Biology* 20 (1): 48–52. https://doi.org/10.1089/lrb.2019.0082.

International Lymphoedema Framework and Canadian Lymphoedema Framework (2010). The management of lymphoedema in advanced cancer and oedema at the end of life. https://www.lympho.org/uploads/files/files/Palliative-Document.pdf

International Society of Lymphology (2013). The diagnosis and treatment of peripheral lymphedema: 2013 consensus document of the International Society of Lymphology. *Lymphology* 46 (1): 1–11.

Jin, Y., Benzine, R., Dunford, L. et al. (2022). An investigation into the impact of diet and lifestyle on the management of lipoedema. *Current Developments in Nutrition* 6: 1064–1064. https://doi.org/10.1093/cdn/nzac070.023.

Kamijo, E., Ishizuka, K., Shikino, K. et al. (2021). Physical findings and tests useful for differentiating lymphedema. *Journal of General Family Medicine* 22: 227–228. https://doi.org/10.1002/jgf2.425.

Kataru, R.P., Wiser, I., Baik, J.E. et al. (2019). Fibrosis and secondary lymphedema: chicken or egg? *Translational Research* 209: 68–76.

Keast, D.H., Moffatt, C., and Janmohammad, A. (2019). Lymphedema impact and prevalence international study: the Canadian data. *Lymphatic Research and Biology* 17: 178–186.

Keeley, V., Crooks, S., Locke, J. et al. (2010). A quality of life measure for limb lymphoedema (LYMQOL). *Journal of Lymphoedema* 10 (5): 26–37.

Koshima, I., Nanba, Y., Tsutsui, T. et al. (2003). Long-term follow-up after lymphaticovenular anastomosis for lymphedema in the leg. *Journal of Reconstructive Microsurgery* 19 (4): 209–215. https://doi.org/10.1055/s-2003-40575.

Largeau, B., Cracowski, J.-L., Lengellé, C. et al. (2021). Drug-induced peripheral oedema: an aetiology-based review. *British Journal of Clinical Pharmacology* 87: 3043–3055. https://doi.org/10.1111/bcp.14752.

Levick, J.R. and Michel, C.C. (2010). Microvascular fluid exchange and the revised Starling principle. *Cardiovascular Research* 87 (2): 198–210. https://doi.org/10.1093/cvr/cvq062.

Lukowicz, D., Sauter, M., and Lipp, A. (2021). *All About Lipedema*. Kolinburg: Scout Medien.

Lymphoedema Framework (2006). *Best Practice for the Management of Lymphoedema: International Consensus.* London: MEP.

Mitchell, A. and Hill, B. (2020). Moisture-associated skin damage: an overview of its diagnosis and management. *British Journal of Community Nursing* 25(3):S12–S18. https://doi.org/10.12968/bjcn.2020.25.Sup3.S12.

Mortimer, P.S. (2000). Implications of the lymphatic system in CVI-associated edema. *Angiology* 51(1):3–7. https://doi.org/10.1177/000331970005100102.

Malicka, I., Rosseger, A., Hanuszkiewicz, J., and Woźniewski, M. (2014). Kinesiology taping reduces lymphedema of the upper extremity in women after breast cancer treatment: a pilot study. *Menopause Review* 13 (4): 221–226.

Margaris, K.N. and Black, R.A. (2012). Modelling the lymphatic system: challenges and opportunities. *Journal of the Royal Society Interface* 9 (69): 601–612. https://doi.org/10.1098/rsif.2011.0751.

Michel, C.C., Woodcock, T.E., and Curry, F.R.E. (2020). Understanding and extending the Starling principle. *Acta Anaesthesiologica Scandinavica* 64: 1032–1037. https://doi.org/10.1111/aas.13603.

Moffatt, C.J., Franks, P.J., Doherty, D.C. et al. (2003). Lymphoedema: an underestimated health problem. *QJM* 96 (10): 731–738. https://doi.org/10.1093/qjmed/hcg126.

Moffatt, C.J., Gaskin, R., Sykorova, M. et al. (2019). Prevalence and risk factors for chronic edema in U.K. community nursing services. *Lymphatic Research and Biology* 17(2):147–154. https://doi.org/10.1089/lrb.2018.0086.

Moffatt, C.J., Keeley, V., Franks, P.J. et al. (2017). Chronic oedema: a prevalent health care problem for UK health services. *International Wound Journal* 14 (5): 772–781. https://doi.org/10.1111/iwj.12694.

Morgan, P.A., Franks, P.J., and Moffatt, C.J. (2005). Health-related quality of life with lymphoedema: a review of the literature. *International Wound Journal* 2 (1): 47–62. https://doi.org/10.1111/j.1742-4801.2005.00066.x.

Mortimer, P.S. and Rockson, S.G. (2014). New developments in clinical aspects of lymphatic disease. *Journal of Clinical Investigation* 124 (3): 915–921. https://doi.org/10.1172/JCI71608.

National Cancer Control Programme (Ireland) (2015). Prevention of clinical lymphoedema after cancer treatment: early detection and risk reduction: a guide for health professionals. https://www.hse.ie/eng/services/list/5/cancer/patient/leaflets/prevention-of-clinical-lymphoedema-after-cancer-treatment.pdf

National Institute for Health and Care Excellence. (2022). Liposuction for chronic lipoedema. Interventional procedures guidance [IPG721]. https://www.nice.org.uk/guidance/ipg721

National Lymphoedema Partnership (2015). Consensus statement on the chronic oedema–lymphoedema interface. https://www.thebls.com/documents-library/chronic-oedema-lymphoedema-definitions

National Lymphoedema Partnership (2019). Commissioning guidance for lymphoedema services for adults in the United Kingdom. https://www. lymphoedema.org/wp-content/uploads/2020/01/nlp_commissioning_ guidance_march_2019.pdf

Negrini, D. and Moriondo, A. (2011). Lymphatic anatomy and biomechanics. *Journal of Physiology* 589 (Pt 12): 2927–2934. https://doi.org/10.1113/ jphysiol.2011.206672.

Nørregaard, S., Bermark, S., Karlsmark, T. et al. (2019). LIMPRINT: prevalence of chronic edema in health Services in Copenhagen, Denmark. *Lymphatic Research and Biology* 17 (2): 187–194. https://doi.org/10.1089/lrb.2019.0019.

Osti M (2018). Lipodermatosclerosis. DermNet NZ. https://dermnetnz. org/topics/lipodermatosclerosis

Ostby, P.L., Armer, J.M., Smith, K., and Stewart, B.R. (2018). Patient perceptions of barriers to self-management of breast cancer-related lymphedema. *Western Journal of Nursing Research* 40 (12): 1800–1817. https://doi.org/10.1177/0193945917744351.

Pajero Otero, V., García Delgado, E., Martín Cortijo, C. et al. (2019). Kinesio taping versus compression garments for treating breast cancer-related lymphedema: a randomized, cross-over, controlled trial. *Clinical Rehabilitation* 33 (12): 1887–1897. https://doi.org/10.1177/0269215519874107.

Pal, S., Rahman, J., Mu, S. et al. (2022). Drug-related lymphedema: mysteries, mechanisms, and potential therapies. *Frontiers in Pharmacology* 4 (13): 850586. https://doi.org/10.3389/fphar.2022.850586.

Paskett, E.D., Dean, J.A., Oliveri, J.M., and Harrop, J.P. (2012). Cancer-related lymphedema risk factors, diagnosis, treatment, and impact: a review. *Journal of Clinical Oncology* 30 (30): 3726–3733. https://doi.org/10.1200/ JCO.2012.41.8574.

Patel, M., Lee, S.I., Thomas, K.S., and Kai, J. (2019). The red leg dilemma: a scoping review of the challenges of diagnosing lower-limb cellulitis. *British Journal of Dermatology* 180 (5): 993–1000. https://doi.org/10.1111/ bjd.17415.

Quéré, I., Palmier, S., Noerregaard, S. et al. (2019). LIMPRINT: estimation of the prevalence of lymphoedema/chronic oedema in acute Hospital in in-patients. *Lymphatic Research and Biology* 17 (2): 135–140. https://doi. org/10.1089/lrb.2019.0024.

Real, S., Cobbe, S., and Slattery, S. (2016). Palliative care edema: patient population, causal factors, and types of edema referred to a specialist palliative care edema service. *Journal of Palliative Medicine* 19 (7): 771–777. https://doi.org/10.1089/jpm.2015.0337.

Ridner, S.H., Dietrich, M.S., and Kidd, N. (2011). Breast cancer treatment-related lymphedema self-care: education, practices, symptoms, and quality of life. *Support Care Cancer* 19 (5): 631–637. https://doi.org/ 10.1007/s00520-010-0870-5.

Schaverien, M.V., Moeller, J.A., and Cleveland, S.D. (2018). Nonoperative treatment of lymphedema. *Seminars in Plastic Surgery* 32 (1): 17–21. https://doi.org/10.1055/s-0038-1635119.

Shah, C., Arthur, D.W., Wazer, D. et al. (2016). The impact of early detection and intervention of breast cancer-related lymphedema: a systematic review. *Cancer Medicine* 5 (6): 1154–1162. https://doi.org/10.1002/cam4.691.

Sherry, K.L. and McAuley, G. (2004). Symptom prevalence and the use of systematic symptom assessment. *Palliative Medicine* 18 (1): 75–76. https://doi.org/10.1177/026921630401800118.

Singh, A. and Zahra, F. (2023). Chronic venous insufficiency. In: *StatPearls*. Treasure Island, FL: StatPearls Publishing https://www.ncbi.nlm.nih.gov/books/NBK587341.

Stutz, J.J. and am Wald, S. (2011). Liposuction in lipedema to prevent later joint complications. *Vasomed* 23: 6.

Szél, E., Kemény, L., Groma, G., and Szolnoky, G. (2014). Pathophysiological dilemmas of lipedema. *Medical Hypotheses* 83 (5): 599–606.

Thomas, M.J. and Morgan, K. (2017). The development of Lymphoedema Network Wales to improve care. *British Journal of Nursing* 26 (13): 740–750. https://doi.org/10.12968/bjon.2017.26.13.740.

Tranmer, J.E., Heyland, D., Dudgeon, D. et al. (2003). Measuring the symptom experience of seriously ill cancer and noncancer hospitalised patients near the end of life with the memorial symptom assessment scale. *Journal of Pain and Symptom Management* 25 (5): 420–429. https://doi.org/10.1016/s0885-3924(03)00074-5.

Urner, S., Kelly-Goss, M., Peirce, S.M., and Lammert, E. (2018). Mechanotransduction in blood and lymphatic vascular development and disease. In: *Vascular Pharmacology: Cytoskeleton and Extracellular Matrix* (ed. R.A. Khalil), 155–208. Cambridge, MA: Academic Press. doi: https://doi.org/10.1016/bs.apha.2017.08.009.

Vignes, S., Poizeau, F., and Dupuy, A. (2022). Cellulitis risk factors for patients with primary or secondary lymphedema. *Journal of Vascular Surgery. Venous and Lymphatic Disorders* 10 (1): 179–185.e1. https://doi.org/10.1016/j.jvsv.2021.04.009.

Webb, E., Neeman, T., Gaida, J. et al. (2019). Impact of compression therapy on cellulitis (ICTOC) in adults with chronic oedema: a randomised controlled trial protocol. *BMJ Open* 9 (8): e029225. https://doi.org/10.1136/bmjopen-2019-029225.

Woodcock, T.E. and Woodcock, T.M. (2012). Revised Starling equation and the glycocalyx model of transvascular fluid exchange: an improved paradigm for prescribing intravenous fluid therapy. *British Journal of Anaesthesia* 108 (3): 384–394. https://doi.org/10.1093/bja/aer515.

Wound Care People (2019). Chronic oedema: best practice in the community. https://www.woundcare-today.com/uploads/files/files/66774-Best-Practice-Statement.PDF

Wounds UK (2021). Best Practice Statement: Addressing skin tone bias in wound care: assessing signs and symptoms in people with dark skin tones. Wounds UK, London.

Wounds, U.K. (2017). *Best Practice Guidelines: The Management of Lipoedema*. London: Wounds UK.

Young, T., Chadwick, P., Fletcher, J. et al. (2021). *The Benefits of Intermittent Pneumatic Compression and How to Use WoundExpressTM in Practice*. London: Wounds UK.

Zaleska, M., Olszewski, W.L., and Durlik, M. (2014). The effectiveness of intermittent pneumatic compression in long-term therapy of lymphedema of lower limbs. *Lymphatic Research and Biology* 12 (2): 103–109. https://doi.org/10.1089/lrb.2013.0033.

CHAPTER 3

Atypical Causes of Leg Ulceration

SARAH BRADBURY AND KIRSTEN MAHONEY

Most leg ulcers will typically come under the diagnosis of either venous, arterial, mixed aetiology (venous and arterial), lymphoedema or diabetic foot ulcers (National Wound Care Strategy Programme [NWCSP] 2023). A small proportion of lower leg wounds, however, may be caused by less common aetiologies that are often associated with, or caused by, inflammation, infection, malignancy, chronic illness or genetic disorders (Isoherranen et al. 2019). These types of leg ulcers are usually referred to as *atypical wounds*. One of the most important aspects to consider when treating a patient with an atypical ulcer is the correct identification and management of the underlying systemic condition that is contributing to or causing the ulceration (Falanga 2007).

The diagnosis of an atypical leg ulcer is often challenging in clinical practice, and treatment regimens can be complex, requiring a multidisciplinary approach from specialist teams that may include dermatology, rheumatology, vascular, haematology, oncology and psychology. This list is not exhaustive and is dependent on the diagnosis and local availability of services. It is often the significant delay in diagnosis that contributes to inappropriate

Lower Limb and Leg Ulcer Assessment and Management, First Edition.
Edited by Aby Mitchell, Georgina Ritchie, and Alison Hopkins.
© 2024 John Wiley & Sons Ltd. Published 2024 by John Wiley & Sons Ltd.

management and higher mortality rates for this cohort of patients (Isoherranen et al. 2019).

Early identification and referral to an appropriate specialist team for a patient suspected of having an atypical leg ulcer are essential and can assist in preventing unnecessary wound deterioration, managing the symptoms effectively, decreasing the risk of complications and improving the quality of life for the individual. Healthcare professionals (HCPs) therefore are required to have the appropriate skills and knowledge to undertake a structured holistic wound assessment (see Chapter 5) to assist in identifying the aetiology of the wound and potential barriers that may impact the healing process (Wounds UK 2018).

The HEIDI (History, Examination, Investigations, Diagnosis, Interventions) framework offers a unified and systematic approach to wound assessment that is particularly useful for identifying atypical aetiologies (Harding et al. 2007). It encapsulates identification of the co-morbidities, environmental and local wound factors that contribute to wound complexity and are essential criteria for making a definitive diagnosis and an effective multidisciplinary management plan.

Factors that may lead to the suspicion of an atypical leg ulcer diagnosis include (Isoherranen et al. 2019):

- Abnormal presentation/location.
- High levels of pain for the size of the wound.
- Non-healing after 4–12 weeks of evidence-based care.

It is important for HCPs to be aware of these factors to aid in the diagnosis, treatment and management of atypical ulcers.

INFLAMMATORY/AUTOIMMUNE DISORDERS

Pyoderma Gangrenosum

Pyoderma gangrenosum (PG) is a rare autoinflammatory skin condition characterised by neutrophilic infiltration of the dermis (neutrophilic dermatosis). Although the condition can occur on any part of the body and at any age, it is more commonly found in the lower limb and in women over the age of 50 (Binus et al. 2011). The exact aetiology and pathophysiology of the disease are unknown and possibly multifactorial. However, it has been recognised that there are characteristically abnormal neutrophils and high levels of inflammatory mediators present within the wound environment (George et al. 2019).

There are five main subtypes of PG: classic ulcerative, bullous, vegetative, pustular and peristomal. The most common subtype that is usually seen on the lower leg is classic ulcerative PG, which accounts for 85% of cases (Fletcher et al. 2019). Classic ulcerative PG is most commonly seen on the lower extremities, although it occasionally appears on the trunk, abdomen and genital area.

History

The dermatological presentation of PG often manifests as a result of systemic inflammatory disease and can be associated with other inflammatory or haematological conditions, such as rheumatoid arthritis (RA), inflammatory bowel disease or leukaemia, or pro-inflammatory genetic syndromes (e.g. PAPA – pyogenic arthritis, PG and acne; or PASH – PG, acne and suppurative hidradenitis) (Fletcher et al. 2019; Patel and Piguet 2022). It has been suggested that 50% of patients with PG have underlying associated diseases (George et al. 2019), therefore consideration of associated co-morbidities should be an essential part of history taking and may assist in establishing a diagnosis.

Patient history may indicate that the wound started as an erythematous nodule or pustule, which developed quickly into a painful deep ulcer within days. PG ulcers also sometimes occur and deteriorate rapidly following trauma, biopsy or surgery – this is known as pathergy (George et al. 2019).

PG ulcers typically are extremely painful; assessment of pain levels should be conducted at each dressing change and following the commencement of any treatment using an appropriate validated pain assessment tool, such as the Visual Analogue Scale (VAS) (Scott-Thomas et al. 2017).

Examination

Individuals may present with up to three ulcers (Fletcher et al. 2019). Features that are commonly seen in PG are a purple discoloration to the edge of the wound, known as a violaceous border (Figure 3.1), and the surrounding skin may have the appearance of 'wrinkled

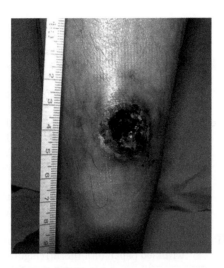

FIGURE 3.1 Typical presentation of PG with violaceous (purple border).
Source: Used with permission from Cardiff & Vale University Health Board.

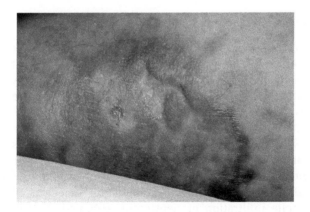

FIGURE 3.2 Cribriform scar.
Source: Used with permission from Cardiff & Vale University Health Board.

paper' over the sites of previously healed ulcers, which is referred to as cribriform scarring (Figure 3.2) (Fletcher et al. 2019). Examination of the lower limb should follow the principles of TIMES as outlined in Chapter 5 (see Table 3.1).

TABLE 3.1   Typical clinical presentation of pyoderma gangrenosum (PG).

Tissue within the wound bed	The wound bed may be variable. There may be friable granulation and necrosis, and soft slough may also be evident
Infection/ inflammation	Inflamed peri-wound skin. Secondary infection may be present
Moisture balance	Exudate levels may be variable and could range from minimal to moderate depending on the amount of non-viable tissue, the presence of infection and the amount of oedema present in the lower limb
Edge	The appearance of the wound edge is often seen as dark purple in colour (typically referred to as a violaceous border). The edge may also appear ragged or scalloped
Surrounding skin	Previous scars from PG often have the appearance of 'wrinkled paper' (cribriform) (Figure 3.2)

Source: Adapted from George et al. (2019) and Rice (2007).

Investigations

There is currently no clinical criterion or laboratory test to confirm the presence of PG (George et al. 2019) and it is often described as a diagnosis by exclusion (Isoherranen et al. 2019). A biopsy of the active ulcer edge may be required to exclude other possible causes such as malignancy or infection. However, one of the classic manifestations of PG is the exaggerated response to trauma or minor skin injury (known as pathergy), therefore biopsies are undertaken with caution as they may cause deterioration and enlargement of the ulcer and worsening of symptoms (George et al. 2019). With PG, typically biopsies of the ulcer edge will demonstrate infiltration of neutrophils (Maverakis et al. 2018). Infiltration of neutrophils has an important role in inflammation and can contribute to tissue damage, it is often present in autoinflammatory skin conditions as a response to underlying systemic disease. To exclude arterial disease, measurement of an ankle brachial pressure index (ABPI) should be undertaken as part of the lower limb assessment (Todhunter 2019). It may however not be possible to undertake an ABPI measurement in patients with PG who are experiencing uncontrolled pain or if the limb size is outside the ankle cuff range (Wounds UK 2019). Toe pressures, or a toe brachial pressure index (TBPI), should therefore be considered if the ankle cuff cannot be applied or if calcification of the arteries is suspected (Wounds UK 2016).

Diagnosis

There are currently no national or international criteria for the diagnosis of PG and not all PG ulcers present with the characteristic violaceous border or cribriform scarring, which can make diagnosis more challenging in clinical practice (Fletcher et al. 2019). Misdiagnosis, however, can lead to inappropriate treatments such as debridement, which potentially could contribute to a significant deterioration in the ulcer due to pathergy (George et al. 2019).

A diagnosis is typically made using clinical indicators such as ulcer presentation, and clinical history and exclusion of other possible causes such as malignancy and infection (Fletcher et al. 2019). Maverakis et al. (2018) proposed a diagnostic tool (Table 3.2) to assist in reducing the probability of an inaccurate diagnosis. Within the diagnostic tool, patients would need to display one major criterion and four minor criteria.

TABLE 3.2   Diagnostic tool for pyoderma gangrenosum.

Major criteria	Biopsy of ulcer edge that shows neutrophil infiltrate
Minor criteria	Exclusion of infection
	Pathergy
	History of inflammatory bowel disease or inflammatory arthritis
	Papule or pustule that ulcerates within four days of appearance
	Peripheral erythema, undermining border and pain at the ulcer site
	Multiple ulcerations, at least one on the lower leg
	Cribriform scarring
	Responds to treatment with immunosuppressive medications

Source: Adapted from Maverakis et al. (2018) and George et al. (2019).

Intervention

The management of PG is often challenging due to a lack of recognised clinical guidelines and is usually based on disease severity and the extent of PG (George et al. 2019; Fletcher et al. 2019). Early identification of PG is essential to ensure that prompt referral to an appropriate speciality such as dermatology is undertaken, and that treatment with systemic therapies is instigated in a timely manner (George et al. 2019). Treatment options must be patient centred and consider patient preferences, location and size of the wound, underlying systemic disease and possible side effects of interventions (Fletcher et al. 2019). Delays in appropriate interventions may result in delayed healing and have a significant impact on an individual's quality of life, which may include pain, low self-esteem and scarring.

Treatment for PG is described in the following sections.

Reducing Systematic Inflammation

Local topical therapy with potent corticosteroids or tacrolimus ointment to the wound and affected surrounding skin can be instigated as an adjunct to systemic treatment. Topical therapy alone is not usually sufficient to manage PG (George et al. 2019).

The first line of systemic treatment is oral corticosteroids. These can be used on their own or in conjunction with immunosuppressants such as cyclosporine. More recently there has been growing evidence to support the use of biologics such as infliximab to improve healing and remission rates (George et al. 2019). Biologics assist in promoting a pro-inflammatory environment and act as a chemoattractant for neutrophils, and have been useful for patients who have been unresponsive to corticosteroids and immunosuppressant therapies (Maronese et al. 2022). Due to the many possible side effects and contraindications, systemic therapies are usually commenced and monitored by a dermatologist throughout the treatment.

Optimising the Local Wound Environment

Local wound management goals should address the outcomes of the wound assessment using the TIMES framework and the principles of moist wound healing. Dressings selected should manage exudate appropriately while allowing atraumatic removal. Mechanical or surgical debridement to devitalised tissue within the wound bed would only be considered if the PG was responding to systemic treatment and should be carried out by a trained HCP due to the risk of wound enlargement (Isoherranen et al. 2019). Less traumatic methods of debridement can be considered, such as utilising dressings that support autolytic debridement or larvae therapy (Isoherranen et al. 2019). Wound bed preparation and methods of debridement are discussed fully in Chapter 5.

Corticosteroids and immunosuppressant agents are known to suppress the activity of the immune system, which results in an increased risk of developing an infection for patients who have these prescribed to manage their PG (Youseff et al. 2016). Wound infection is discussed in Chapter 5. HCPs should familiarise themselves with the signs and symptoms of infection and be particularly vigilant in this patient group. If infection is suspected, antimicrobials should be initiated accordingly (International Institute of Wound Infection 2022). For example, topical antimicrobials should be commenced if local wound infection is suspected. Systemic antibiotics should be prescribed if spreading infection/sepsis or systemic infection is present. Prescribing of any antimicrobial must follow local prescribing policy and guidance (see Chapter 5).

Compression therapy is advocated if oedema is present to support adjunctive therapies and the wound healing environment (Fletcher et al. 2019). The importance of compression therapy to aid healing in PG is undecided, but expert opinion is that compression therapy is beneficial for all patients with lower extremity wounds (Isoherranen et al. 2019). Compression to counteract the impact of gravity remains a cornerstone of treatment (Partsch and Mortimer 2015).

Compression can be instigated safely after an assessment of vascular status (see Chapter 5). Due to the pain experienced in patients with PG, it may not be possible to instigate full compression at 40 mmHg and therefore it may be more acceptable for the patient to start at a lower compression of 20 mmHg (Isoherranen et al. 2019). Wrap systems and hosiery are available in reduced compression formats, bandage systems can also be adapted to provide reduced compression and familiarity with compression products is an important part of treating and managing any patient with leg ulceration. Types of compression therapy are discussed in full in Chapter 8.

Appropriate Management of Pain

Patients with PG often present with high levels of uncontrolled pain. Appropriate pain management is therefore an important part of the patient's treatment pathway and should be guided by the type, duration and severity of the pain, as identified within the patient's pain assessment. The type of pain experienced may be a significant influence in the choice of analgesia (Brown 2015). For example, neuropathic pain, which is usually associated with nerve damage, is often described by the patient as tingling, shooting pain, burning, stabbing or pins and needles (Brown 2015). Conversely, nociceptive pain is associated with damaged tissue and can be described as aching or throbbing (Brown 2015). Various resources are available to guide decision-making around analgesia prescribing, as outlined in Chapter 6. Should neuropathic pain be present, certain neuropathic medications may be helpful such as antidepressants or anticonvulsants, including amitriptyline or gabapentin (Anekar and Cascella 2023). As with any analgesia, the effectiveness should be monitored and reassessed at each dressing change using a personalised approach; see Chapter 6 for more exploration.

Vasculitis

Cutaneous vasculitis is an inflammatory event that causes inflammation and damage to the walls of the blood vessels (Rayner et al. 2009). The condition can affect any blood vessel or any organ and is usually classified by the size of the vessels that are involved. Large vessel vasculitis affects the large and medium-sized arteries, while small vessel vasculitis affects the small arteries, arterioles, capillaries and small veins (Isoherranen et al. 2019). The resulting ischaemia due to vessel damage often leads to skin necrosis and ulceration (Isoherranen et al. 2019). Cutaneous vasculitis has several manifestations (Table 3.3). The severity of symptoms and whether there is organ involvement dictate treatment choice (Micheletti 2022). Vasculitis can be triggered by reactants such as infection, malignancy, medications and connective tissue diseases (Weinstien et al. 2012).

History

The patient may have a history of general malaise, joint pain, fever and raised inflammatory markers. Vasculitis may also be associated with autoimmune disorders such as RA, scleroderma or lupus

TABLE 3.3   Some common forms of vasculitis.

Examples of cutaneous vasculitis	Vessels involved	Clinical features
Takayasu arteritis Giant cell arteritis	Large vessel vasculitis	Usually affect large arteries such as aorta Skin manifestations are rare Occasionally necrosis is observed if the extracutaneous arteries that feed the skin are affected
Polyarteritis nodosa cutanea (cutaneous arteritis)	Medium vessel	Often localised to the lower leg May be associated with infection (e.g. hepatitis B, hepatitis C or *Streptococci*), but can also be drug induced Palpable subcutaneous nodules are often seen Deep ulceration may occur
Microscopic polyarteritis Granulomatosis with polyarteritis Leucocytoclastic vasculitis Churg Strauss syndrome Cutaneous immunoglobulin (Ig)M/IgG	Small vessel	Palpable round and inflammatory purpura Livedo (a network-like pattern of reddish-blue skin discoloration) Haemorrhagic nodules
Vasculitis associated with systemic disease (e.g. rheumatoid vasculitis)	Small vessel disease	Palpable round inflammatory purpura Livedo Haemorrhagic necrosis

Source: Adapted from Isoherranen et al. (2019) and Micheletti (2022).

(Todhunter 2019). Other factors that can contribute to vasculitis are infection and some medications, for example anticoagulants, penicillin and sulphonamides (Rayner et al. 2009).

Examination

The appearance of vasculitis differs according to the size of the blood vessel that is affected (Weinstien et al. 2012). Vasculitis affecting the

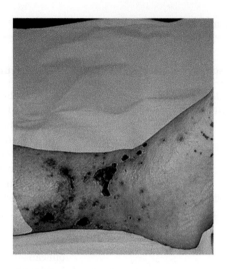

FIGURE 3.3 Typical presentation of vasculitis.
Source: Used with permission from Cardiff & Vale University Health Board.

small vessels, such as leucocytoclastic vasculitis, often presents with regular lesions and ulcers on the skin, while large or medium vessel vasculitis, such as polyarteritis nodosa, may present with irregular widespread purpura, necrosis and ulceration (see Table 3.3) (Falanga 2007; Weinstien et al. 2012).

The typical clinical presentation of vasculitis includes (Figure 3.3):

- Rash
- Purpura
- Necrosis
- Painful wounds

Investigations

The most common investigation to confirm the diagnosis of vasculitis is a tissue biopsy for histological examination (Isoherranen et al. 2019). Tissue biopsies are only helpful if performed as early as possible after the presentation of symptoms. Biopsies performed later in the disease process may not be able to adequately detect the inflammatory cells and their by-products that are usually present in vasculitis lesions (Weinstien et al. 2012). Biopsies may reveal inflammation within the blood vessels and can be used to assist in diagnosis. Blood tests such as erythrocyte sedimentation rate (ESR) or C-reactive protein can reveal the presence of inflammation, or antineutrophil cytoplastic antibody (ANCA) is a blood test used to identify specific proteins that are associated with vasculitis (Isoherranen et al. 2019).

Diagnosis

Diagnosis of vasculitis will primarily be based on the observable criteria seen on examination, such as palpable purpura and necrosis, although it can mimic other disorders. Test investigations that may assist in diagnosing vasculitis are a raised ESR or C-reactive protein, a positive ANCA result, along with a biopsy that may indicate inflammation within the blood vessels.

Intervention

The main objective in managing patients with vasculitis is to establish and treat the causative factor (Falanga 2007), Treatment will also be guided by the severity of the disease and whether there is internal organ involvement (Micheletti 2022). A multidisciplinary approach may be required to assist in management due to the lack of robust evidence to indicate the most effective treatment and the complexities that may accompany the disease (Micheletti 2022). Reduction of inflammation is usually a priority for treatment and drugs that can reduce inflammation and are commonly used. First-line considerations are corticosteroids, dapsone or colochine (Micheletti 2022). Topical steroids can be used if the surrounding skin becomes itchy and oral non-steroidal anti-inflammatory drugs (NSAIDs) can be helpful to reduce inflammation locally (Micheletti 2022). For systemic or severe vasculitis, immunosuppressants may be considered (e.g. methotrexate, azathioprine). For vasculitides that are unresponsive, treatment with biologics may be considered (Micheletti 2022). Due to the lack of robust clinical studies into the treatment of vasculitis and the fact that management is often variable and based on expert opinion, further studies in this area are needed to support implementation practice (Micheletti 2022).

Local wound management should follow the principles of TIMES as outlined in Chapter 5. If oedema is present, elevation of the limb can be helpful to reduce swelling (Micheletti 2022).

Rheumatoid Arthritis

RA is a chronic systemic inflammatory disease that is thought to affect about 1% of the population (NICE 2020). Leg ulceration develops in approximately 10% of patients with RA (Chakrabarty and Phillips 2003). These wounds often have poor outcomes, such as non-healing, and have been linked to an increased risk of amputation and a higher incidence of mortality (Jebakumar et al. 2014). Table 3.4 lists the co-morbidities and risk factors that are associated with leg ulcers in RA, highlighting the multifactorial nature of ulcer development that can be attributed to several different aetiologies.

RA is also a well-documented co-morbidity in patients who develop PG and vasculitic ulceration, therefore assessment of the underlying cause is important, as the disease may occur concurrently and require additional treatment approaches.

The treatment for RA can make clinical management of any associated leg ulceration challenging due to the inflammatory nature of the disease process, which needs to be brought under control. RA is often treated with steroid therapy and immunosuppressive treatments, such as disease-modifying anti-rheumatic drugs (DMARDs) and tumour necrosis factor (TNF) inhibitors (e.g. infliximab), which have

TABLE 3.4 Co-morbidities and risk factors for leg ulceration in rheumatoid arthritis (RA).

Severity and duration of RA	Venous disease
Age	Arterial disease
Medication to treat RA (e.g. oral corticosteroids and immunosuppressant agents)	Mixed vessel disease
Diabetes and/or neuropathy	Venous thromboembolism
Cardiovascular disease	Limited ankle movement and reduced calf muscle pump function
Pressure damage	Vasculitis

Source: Adapted from Isoherranen et al. (2019); Jebakumar et al. (2014); NICE (2020).

a known link with delayed wound healing (Bootan 2013). Immunosuppressive treatments reduce the production and/or proliferation of the inflammatory mediator cells that are required to regulate the normal wound healing process (Bootan 2013). Anti-TNF treatment can have an adverse effect on the immune system overall, and as a consequence patients can be more susceptible to wound infection (Firth and Critchley 2011). Corticosteroids can also adversely affect the inflammatory, proliferative and maturation stages of wound healing, preventing normal cell division, which leads to delayed epithelialisation and fragile, thinned skin, and causing vasoconstriction, which reduces blood supply to the tissues (Firth 2005).

History

Patients will present with a history of RA that is often long-standing, as the risk of ulceration increases with the duration of the disease (Rayner et al. 2009). Patients will also often have a concurrent history of venous and/or arterial disease, with suggestions that peripheral arterial disease (PAD) occurs concurrently with RA in approximately a third of patients, and venous insufficiency in approximately half of patients (Hafner et al. 2010; Seitz et al. 2010). Rates of macrovascular disease are higher than expected in patients with RA due to a proposed link between the pathology of RA, endothelial cell dysfunction and the formation of atheroma (Firth 2005). Immobility and reduced ankle movement due to fixed ankle joints can lead to calf muscle pump failure, contributing to reduced venous return (Jebakumar et al. 2014); an increased risk of venous thromboembolism has also been identified in association with RA (Conforti et al. 2021). In addition, patients may experience peripheral neuropathy as a result of nerve damage from joint deformity (Firth 2005).

There can be evidence of foot deformities and rheumatoid nodules. Nodules usually occur over bony prominences, such as the elbows, ankles and heels, and can vary in size. Prominent nodules can mean that there is increased pressure and friction on the skin from external factors, such as footwear and mobilising, which can lead to skin breakdown and ulceration (Firth 2005). Joint destruction and joint displacement affecting the muscles in the foot from RA cause various foot deformities, such as claw and hammer toes, hallux valgus (bunion), flattening of the arch of the foot and valgus heel deformities (Firth 2005). All these issues also contribute to increased pressure, friction and potential for trauma to the skin of the foot and ankle, which can result in ulceration (Figure 3.4), particularly if associated with a loss of protective sensation due to neuropathy.

Due to the multifactorial causes of leg ulcers in patients with RA, there can be confusion or inconsistencies around what to classify as the ulcer aetiology – as pressure is a frequent contributing factor in ulcer development, it can be difficult to decide if the ulcer is a pressure ulcer or a rheumatoid ulcer. The same debate has raised its head for many years around the classification of diabetic foot ulcers and pressure ulcers, particularly to the heel (Greenwood 2021; Ousey et al. 2011). There is some suggestion that if the ulcer occurs on a bony prominence, such as the posterior aspect of the heel, in an immobile or bedbound patient, then the most likely cause is pressure; if it occurs in an area of the foot or ankle affected by ill-fitting footwear, for example, in a mobile patient, then the underlying disease could be considered the primary cause (Greenwood 2021). Ultimately, regardless of the label given to the wound, the common denominator is the reduction of pressure where this is deemed to be

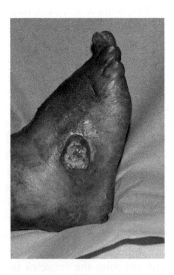

FIGURE 3.4 Punched-out ulceration to the foot with visible foot deformity due to rheumatoid arthritis.
Source: Used with permission from Cardiff & Vale University Health Board.

a contributory factor, and also holistic assessment and management of the patient (Ousey et al. 2011). Consideration should always be given to the effect that the underlying disease, in this case RA, is having on the potential for delayed wound healing and increased risk of wound complications to ensure that an appropriate management plan is devised that covers all aspects that are contributing to the wound development and progression.

Examination

Leg ulceration related to RA will typically present on the lower gaiter, ankle and foot and can be associated with high levels of pain. Lesions may include nodules, purple non-blanching papules, plaques, bruising and signs of ischaemic involvement to the lower limb, such as pale or discoloured, hairless, shiny skin and pain on elevation (Chakrabarty and Phillips 2003). Wound beds are often sloughy with clear demarcation of the wound edge, often appearing punched out in the same way as arterial ulceration (Figure 3.4).

Mobility status should be assessed during the examination to decide if immobility, footwear or other potential sources of pressure are contributing to the ulcer.

Investigations

A vascular assessment is recommended due to the known link with venous and arterial disease. Testing for neuropathy is useful to determine if loss of protective sensation is a potential causative factor for the development of the ulcer and should be considered as part of the management plan.

A skin biopsy can help to determine any co-existing pathology, such as vasculitis or PG, and to rule out other causes, such as malignancy and atypical infections.

Diagnosis

A diagnosis of rheumatoid ulceration is made in the first instance based on the patient's history and examination, namely a diagnosis of RA and signs of disease progression, such as foot and joint deformity, rheumatoid nodules and neuropathy. The diagnosis is often multifactorial and considered in relation to signs and symptoms of associated vascular disease and the results of a vascular assessment. Ulcer appearance and location can be indicative of the underlying inflammatory disorder as described earlier, and of the potential impact of pressure and friction. All of these factors can be combined with the results of a skin biopsy if one is performed to make a diagnosis.

Intervention

A multidisciplinary approach involving the rheumatologist is important to successfully manage rheumatoid ulcers. Due to the link between the systemic treatments for RA and wound healing, advice from the rheumatologist with regard to the therapies being used to manage RA is paramount. Reduction of the dose of immunosuppressant medication or temporary discontinuation until wound healing has been achieved may be advocated in some cases (Bootan 2013), or suggestions around switching to a different type of DMARD or anti-TNF treatment may be made. Such discussions will assist in balancing control of the underlying RA, prevention of disease progression and minimising the impact of RA symptoms on a patient's quality of life with maximising the wound healing potential of associated ulceration.

Podiatrist and/or orthotist input can also be useful to manage and offload any foot deformities contributing to existing ulceration, and also for prevention of further wounds. Input from a physiotherapist and occupational therapist can help with improving mobility, functional activity and education on protecting the joints (Firth 2011).

Management of the wound bed and exudate levels using appropriate primary and secondary dressings is important – gentle autolytic debridement of sloughy tissue is recommended as opposed to less conservative methods to reduce the risk of infection in immunocompromised patients. Good skincare using cleansing and emollients will help to maintain skin integrity, particularly if the skin is thin and fragile as a consequence of corticosteroid use. This should also be a consideration when choosing appropriate dressings. If using an adhesive dressing, gentle silicone dressings are advised, and a silicone medical adhesive remover can also be useful to reduce the risk of skin trauma and any dressing-related pain (Young 2019). Topical antimicrobial dressings may be required if the wound is displaying any signs of local infection.

Compression therapy following vascular assessment is a useful adjunct when managing rheumatoid ulcers to address any venous insufficiency and dependent oedema once significant arterial disease has been ruled out. While peripheral neuropathy is not an absolute contraindication to compression therapy, clinicians should be mindful of the loss of protective sensation experienced by these patients. Patients may not detect any pain or discomfort associated with compression therapy that is too tight or that may have inadvertently caused trauma to the skin from pressure damage (Dissemond et al. 2016). It is recommended that compression therapy instigated in patients with peripheral neuropathy is reviewed more frequently for signs of complications from compression, particularly in the early stages after commencing treatment, and a reduced level of compression therapy (see Chapter 8) may be indicated where there are concerns over the patient's ability to detect increasing pain or complications (Australian Wound Management Association and New Zealand Wound Care Society 2011; Todhunter 2019). Compression bandaging may be the most appropriate option for therapy in view of the likelihood of reduced dexterity and limb deformity making the application of compression hosiery or adjustable compression wraps difficult. Also, the requirement for adequate padding over bony prominences, nodules and fragile areas susceptible to high pressure may be more easily achieved with the use of sub-bandage wadding underneath compression bandages.

Systemic Scleroderma

Systemic scleroderma or sclerosis is a rare autoimmune disorder that results in damage to connective tissue to the skin and internal organs, and functional and structural abnormalities of small blood vessels (Volkmann et al. 2023). Scleroderma is a long-term condition for which there is no cure. It is associated with life-threatening conditions and has a high mortality rate (Tate et al. 2019). Scleroderma occurs due to an overproduction of collagen that is deposited in the skin, blood vessels and internal organs, resulting in scarring and fibrosis in affected areas (Rayner et al. 2009). Immune dysfunction and microvascular abnormalities are also common features (Tate et al. 2019).

There are two main clinical forms of systemic scleroderma – diffuse, which primarily affects the upper arms, thighs and trunk; and limited, which involves the lower arms and legs (Rayner et al. 2009).

History

Patients with scleroderma may present with a known history of systemic scleroderma, thus making the association with leg ulceration and a subsequent diagnosis of the underlying aetiology a more obvious consideration for the assessing clinician. Scleroderma can be difficult to diagnose, particularly in the earlier stages of the disease, so patients may present with cutaneous symptoms and wounds before a formal diagnosis of the disease has been made (Volkmann et al. 2023). Skin changes become more apparent as the disease progresses over time, with skin thickening of the fingers being the primary diagnostic criterion. Patients may present with overlapping symptoms of other autoimmune diseases, such as RA and Sjögren syndrome, which can co-exist with systemic scleroderma (Volkmann et al. 2023). Positive family history is also the strongest identified risk factor for systemic scleroderma (Arnett et al. 2001).

Raynaud's phenomenon is commonly associated with scleroderma and is often the first reported symptom along with swelling and inflammation of the hands and feet (Volkmann et al. 2023). Patients may present with the typical symptoms of Raynaud's: pain, numbness, white skin and pins and needles to the fingers and toes caused by reduced blood flow from vasoconstriction. Raynaud's may be quite severe when it occurs alongside scleroderma, with ulceration occurring to the digits in up to 50% of cases (Khimdas et al. 2011).

Patients may report some difficulties with swallowing because of scleroderma and consequently have a reduced nutritional intake, which can affect wound healing (Tate et al. 2019). Malnutrition, particularly protein deficiency, adversely affects the formation of new blood vessels and the synthesis of collagen, which are essential for rebuilding the extracellular matrix during the proliferative phase of wound healing (Ghaly et al. 2021). Micronutrients (e.g. amino acids) and key vitamins also play important roles in the inflammatory phase for collagen synthesis. Wound healing requires significant amounts of energy that would normally be provided by the body's natural energy stores, but these are significantly depleted when nutritional intake is poor (Ghaly et al. 2021).

Examination

Known skin-related symptoms of systemic sclerosis are thickened skin, finger ulcerations, joint contractures, skin pigmentation changes and itching (Hudson et al. 2009; Tate et al. 2019). Patients may also present with dry, scaly skin (Figure 3.5).

Calcium deposits may be visible or palpable within the wound bed (Figure 3.6) – calcinosis cutis, a deposition of insoluble calcium salts in the skin and/or subcutaneous tissues that can occur in damaged, inflamed, neoplastic or necrotic skin (Ngan 2005), is a common feature with systemic sclerosis (Tate et al. 2019), and ulceration can occur secondary to the calcinosis in some places. Calcium deposits can contribute to a prolonged inflammatory response within the wound as they are perceived as a foreign body; thus they can delay healing and increase the risk of infection. They can also cause pain and strongly adhere to the wound bed, making removal difficult.

Ulcers related to scleroderma are often very painful due to the ischaemia caused by Raynaud's, and in more severe cases gangrene may be evident.

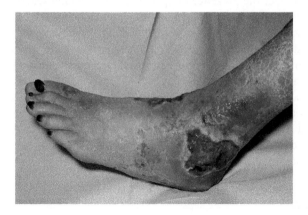

FIGURE 3.5 Ulceration associated with systemic scleroderma with visible skin fibrosis.
Source: Used with permission from Cardiff & Vale University Health Board.

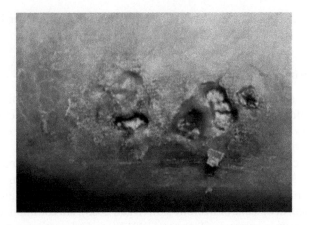

FIGURE 3.6   Calcium deposits in the wound bed related to calcinosis cutis and scleroderma.
Source: Chave et al. (2001) / John Wiley & Sons. Reproduced with permission.

Investigation

If systemic scleroderma is suspected but not yet diagnosed, blood tests to detect the presence of specific autoantibodies can aid in the diagnostic process, as can skin biopsy. The involvement of the heart, lungs, kidneys and gastrointestinal system would also need to be assessed (Tate et al. 2019). Referral to a specialist team for diagnosis and management of both scleroderma and any associated ulceration is recommended (Tate et al. 2019).

Vascular assessment is advised to identify any concomitant venous and/or arterial disease in the lower limb, with appropriate onward referral to vascular for intervention as indicated. An X-ray may be ordered if calcinosis is present to check the extent of calcium deposition in and around the wound.

Diagnosis

Diagnosis of systemic scleroderma itself is usually based on the classification criteria stipulated by the American College of Rheumatology and European League Against Rheumatism collaborative

(Table 3.5; van den Hoogen et al. 2013). Early identification is key and referral to appropriate specialists will aid in timely diagnosis and management.

Diagnosis of leg ulcers associated with scleroderma will primarily be based on the medical history and patient examination. Skin biopsy can indicate the blocking of the small vessels and the presence of inflammatory mediators (Shanmugam et al. 2010).

TABLE 3.5 The American College of Rheumatology and European League Against Rheumatism collaborative criteria for classification of systemic sclerosis[a].

Item	Sub-item(s)	Weight/score[b]
Skin thickening of the fingers of both hands extending proximal to the metacarpophalangeal joints *(sufficient criterion)*	—	9
Skin thickening of the fingers *(only count the higher score)*	Puffy fingers;	2
	Sclerodactyly of the fingers (distal to the metacarpophalangeal joints but proximal to the proximal interphalangeal joints)	4
Fingertip lesions *(only count the higher score)*	Digital tip ulcers	2
	Fingertip pitting scars	3
Telangiectasia	—	2
Abnormal nailfold capillaries	—	2
Pulmonary arterial hypertension and/or interstitial lung disease *(maximum score is 2)*	Pulmonary arterial hypertension	2
	Interstitial lung disease	2
Raynaud's phenomenon	—	3

(Continued)

TABLE 3.5   (Continued)

Item	Sub-item(s)	Weight/score[b]
SSc-related autoantibodies (anticentromere, anti–topoisomerase I [anti–Scl-70], anti–RNA polymerase III) *(maximum score is 3)*	Anticentromere Anti–topoisomerase I Anti–RNA polymerase III	3

[a] These criteria are applicable to any patient considered for inclusion in a systemic sclerosis study. The criteria are not applicable to patients with skin thickening sparing the fingers or to patients who have a scleroderma-like disorder that better explains that manifestation (e.g. nephrogenic sclerosing fibrosis, generalised morphea, eosinophilic fasciitis, scleredema diabeticorum, scleromyxedema, erythromyalgia, porphyria, lichen sclerosis, graft-versus-host disease, diabetic cheiroarthrophy).
[b] The total score is determined by adding the maximum weight (score) in each category. Patients with a total score of ≥9 are classified as having definite systemic sclerosis. SSc, systemic sclerosis.
Source: van den Hoogen et al. (2013) / BMJ Publishing Group. Reproduced by permission.

Implementation

Pharmacological management of systemic scleroderma usually involves some form of immunosuppressant agent, such as rituximab or cyclophosphamide, which can exert anti-inflammatory and/or anti-fibrotic properties to manage the underlying fibrosis and vasculopathy at a cellular level (Volkmann et al. 2023).

As well as the potential for these types of drugs to affect the wound healing process, they can diminish the immune response to the extent that there is a higher risk of opportunistic infection, particularly if malnutrition is also involved (Volkmann et al. 2023). Calcinosis in the wound bed also increases the risk of infection. Overt and covert signs of local and spreading wound infection should be closely observed and treated appropriately (see Chapter 5). Patients should also undergo regular nutritional screening using validated tools as per local policy, and a referral made to a dietician for nutritional support as recommended by local pathways.

Treatment of leg ulcers related to scleroderma focuses on the management of symptoms and prevention of deterioration. Pain management is an important part of symptom control due to the severe pain that can be experienced both from the scleroderma generally and from the scleroderma-related leg ulceration, which can affect the patient's quality of life. Appropriate pain assessment should be conducted and documented and local pain management algorithms followed; referral should be made to pain management specialists as required (see Chapter 6). Pain from the reduced blood flow associated with the Raynaud's component of the disease is often treated with systemic vasodilators, such as sildenafil or nifedipine, or prostacyclins (e.g. iloprost), alongside traditional analgesia such as paracetamol and NSAIDs. Other recommendations for preventing and managing Raynaud's attacks include avoiding the cold where possible; wearing warm mittens and hand and foot warmers can be useful (Pope 2022). Treating Raynaud's phenomenon is also important from a calcinosis perspective, as underlying ischaemia is known to worsen calcinosis, which tends to form in areas of local trauma (Pope 2022).

Skincare is another key component of the management of skin thickening from scleroderma and for maintaining the integrity of peri-wound skin. Patients are also prone to pruritic rashes, which can be uncomfortable and bothersome. Regular use of skin emollients to promote adequately moisturised skin is essential; joint guidelines from the British Society of Rheumatology (BSR) and British Health Professionals in Rheumatology (BHPR) recommend the use of lanolin-based moisturisers specifically (Denton et al. 2016). Antihistamines are useful to help reduce skin itch alongside moisturisation; other practical recommendations include limiting time in hot baths and showers and avoiding harsh soaps and fragranced moisturisers (Volkmann et al. 2023).

In terms of local wound care, competent practitioners may choose to remove superficial and loose pieces of calcium where possible and as tolerated by the patient; this in essence removes the perceived foreign body to promote healing and reduce infection risk. Surgical intervention is usually only considered if the calcinosis is severe and affects the patient's ability to function and their quality of life (Tate et al. 2019). Dressing choice should be guided by the TIMES assessment of the wound environment, with consideration given to minimising wound pain at dressing change and managing infection. Exudate management can be supported through the use of compression, often at a reduced dose unless accompanied by significant venous disease.

Sickle Cell Disease

Sickle cell disease (SCD) is an umbrella term for various genotypes that all present with sickle-shaped blood cells. It is an inherited haematological disorder where a mutation in the βb globin genes in the bone marrow produces red blood cells with defective haemoglobin HbS. Where both parents carry the gene there is a one in four chance of a child having the disease. The HbS produces blood dyscrasia affecting multiple organs and related systems, with sickle cell anaemia occurring when there are two abnormal HbSS genes from two parents. Variants present where genes from one parent combine with another haemoglobin variant as with thalassaemia, which reduces the concentration of haemoglobin. Sickle cell anaemia and thalassaemia variant are the most severe forms of SCD. Sickle cell trait occurs where there are genes from one parent only, resulting in the child being a carrier of the disease but asymptomatic.

The genetic presence of the disease has been linked to areas where malaria occurs, commonly in Africa and among people of African origin, but also in the Caribbean, South and Central America, the Eastern Mediterranean and Asia. The highest prevalence is found in populations from sub-Saharan Africa. In the United Kingdom SCD affects 15 000 people with almost 300 babies born each year. Children with SCD are at an increased risk of stroke, the highest risk being between 2 and 16 years of age (www.sicklecellsociety.org). The median UK survival is 66/67 years (DeBaun et al. 2019; Gardner et al. 2016).

History

The sickle shape is caused by long rigid polymer chains forming within the red blood cell once it has become deoxygenated. This distinguishes it from normal red blood cells and has multiple effects. The sickle cell has a shorter lifespan (normal 90–120 days; sickle 10–20 days) and is less able to travel through the circulation due to its shape. It is dehydrated, rigid and sticky with a weakened cell membrane, which along with its shape makes it vulnerable to adhesion and aggregation. As a result, it is easily trapped in smaller vessels leading to impaired blood flow preventing oxygen delivery to the tissues, ischaemia and tissue death. This produces an acute crisis with chronic damage. Narrowing and occlusion of larger vessels produce chronic sheer damage and adherence of red blood cells to the endothelium alongside vasoconstriction and nitric oxide deficiency. This leads to pulmonary hypertension and stroke.

Examination

The severity of the disease varies from mild to severe, including being life limiting. Different areas of the body may be affected, and the consequences include lung and cardiopulmonary disease, central nervous system complications including infarcts, retinopathy and blindness, renal disease and hip necrosis. Symptoms therefore vary between individuals, with chronic anaemia and severe intermittent pain being the most common clinical manifestations. Chronic daily pain has been found to increase with age, affecting 30–40% of adults and adolescents (Brandow and Liem 2022). Painful acute episodes are triggered by the inflammatory process and when the red blood cell changes shape after oxygen has been released. A sickle cell crisis is severely painful and occurs in one isolated site or multiple locations including pelvis, ribs, spine and sternum. Chronic pain develops with the sensitisation of the central and/or peripheral nervous system. It may be diffuse and have neuropathic elements (see Chapter 7).

Sickle cell leg ulceration is one of the clinical presentations of this disease and is associated with low haemoglobin concentrations combined with a high rate of intravascular haemolysis (Koshy et al. 1989). Minniti and Kato (2016) imaged, measured and examined the effect of SCD and found that ulcerated sites contained a high blood flow with evidence of chronic inflammation, cutaneous vasodilation, venostasis and thrombosis, and that leg ulcers were an end-organ complication.

Minniti and Kato (2016) outline three different presentations of ulceration: the one-time ulcer, the stuttering ulcer that comes and goes, and the chronic recurrent disabling ulcer. Common sites of ulceration are the medial and lateral malleolus, the foot and the Achilles' tendon (Figure 3.7). The clinical appearance is similar to ischaemic ulceration with wounds being heavily colonised, presenting with slough and necrosis. The presence of biofilms with episodes of wound infection is common. The severe pain of the ulceration is unrelated to size and is against a background of sickle cell pain from the disease process itself (see Chapter 6) and other organ complications. Ulceration may be slow and difficult to heal, with management often being challenging and complex because of the disease pathology and progression, the site of the ulcer(s) and the management challenges of SCD. Wound infection and associated pain may precipitate a sickle cell crisis that in turn has adverse impacts on wound healing.

(a)

(b)

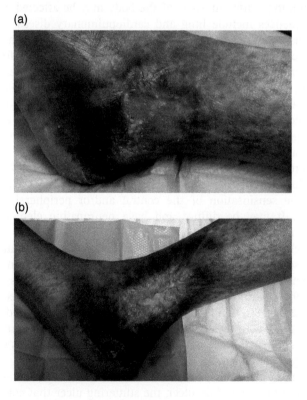

FIGURE 3.7 (a, b) Sickle cell ulceration.

Commonly observed biomechanical changes in those with lower limb sickle cell ulceration include leg length discrepancy, calf muscle atrophy, loss of ankle range of motion and the foot fixed into a position of pronation or supination. Hip necrosis may offer further complications in terms of pain and biomechanical changes (see Chapter 4). Reduced ankle function is common in those with SCD ulceration due to the pain experienced; pain causes the person to adapt their gait and walk on the ball of their foot to reduce the pain and any pull of dressings (Farrelly 2018). While biomechanical changes are common in those suffering from leg ulceration, Farrelly (2018) states that those with SCD present these changes in the extreme. Thus, obtaining biomechanical advice is essential for this cohort. All these factors add to the complexity of management and healing outcomes; healing of ulceration may be up to 16 times slower compared to purely venous disease ulceration (Trent and Kirsner 2004).

Management

Sickle cell management is complex and presents with various care challenges. The underlying pathology needs to be determined and medically managed by haematology. Medical management is ongoing and relates to medication and care of sickle cell crisis episodes, which will often involve acute admissions. Regular blood transfusions are appropriate and helpful for some but not all sickle cell patients. Due to the diverse range of symptoms and the different areas of the body that are affected, care is multidisciplinary and will involve both acute and community nursing. Besides haematology, it is common for people to be supported by vascular and specialist SCD teams, tissue viability, pain teams, social care agencies and more. Cohesive communication between the different professions is foundational to delivering effective and therapeutic care.

Management will draw on the principles of good leg ulcer management:

- Wound management and regular debridement. See Chapter 8 on clinical management.
- Compression therapy remains a cornerstone of clinical management due to the presence of venous disease or ineffective

calf muscle pump resulting from reduced ankle range of movement. It is critical to recognise that ulceration over the forefoot or behind the malleolus in the presence of rigid ankles will reduce the efficacy of a standard compression regime. Non-healing will exacerbate pain and referral will be required to a specialist practitioner who may need to provide a more bespoke compression regime that will optimise compression at the ulcer bed.

- Prevention of recurrence can be supported with hosiery, often flat-knit, and supportive or corrective footwear. See Chapter 4 on biomechanical assessment and Chapter 9 on lifelong management.
- Principles of management for the SCD leg or foot ulcer will be similar to other leg ulcers.

Together with standard clinical management, it is critical to provide validation of the person's pain, their likely struggles working with a less than perfect healthcare system and, because they are often of working age, their need to manage all these conflicting priorities alongside their day job. Personalised care (see Chapter 7) alongside a deep understanding of pain management and the patient's own triggers is vital for people with sickle cell ulceration.

METABOLIC DISORDERS

Necrobiosis Lipoidica

Necrobiosis lipoidica (NL) is a rare non-infectious inflammatory condition of the skin, predominantly affecting the subcutaneous tissue (Isoherranen et al. 2019; Mistry et al. 2017). Although NL-like lesions can be found alongside conditions such as thyroid disease, RA, sarcoidosis, inflammatory bowel disease and even in otherwise healthy patients (Murray and Miller 1997; Reid et al. 2013), it is most associated with diabetes mellitus (DM). For this reason, it is also often referred to as necrobiosis lipoidica diabeticorum. Approximately 50–80% of patients with NL will have diabetes or go on to develop it, although NL only affects about 0.7% of the diabetic population (Feily and Mehraban 2015; Rayner et al. 2009).

The underlying aetiology of NL is largely unknown, but is thought to relate to reduced blood flow in the microcirculation linked to diabetes, combined with an immune system/inflammatory response and abnormal collagen degradation (Bonura et al. 2014; Rayner et al. 2009).

History

NL is three times more common in females than males, and onset usually occurs in young to middle age (Reid et al. 2013). Patients will normally present with a history of DM, although if this is not the case then close monitoring for the onset of DM should take place, as it has been documented as a precursor to the disease (Paron and Lambert 2000).

If presenting with existing ulceration/lesion, patients will normally have experienced initial signs of demarcated reddened papules and non-scaly plaques to the skin of the lower leg, most commonly to the pretibial area (Duff et al. 2015). NL can occur in other areas of the body, such as the hands, face and abdomen, but this is more unusual (Reid et al. 2013). Patients may report the presence of plaques for many months or years before lesions develop (Dissemond et al. 2018), with ulceration of the inflammatory plaques affecting approximately 35% of patients (Nelzen et al. 1994). Ulceration can arise spontaneously, but often occurs following localised trauma.

Examination

On examination, NL may present in different phases of the condition. In the initial stages, papules or nodules are normally present with raised, reddened and sometimes hardened, fibrous edges that can then slowly coalesce into large, reddened plaques (Figure 3.8). The centre of the lesions usually begins as red/brown colour evolving into a yellow/brown discoloration that can take on a waxy appearance (Reid et al. 2013). The skin here is often atrophied – shiny, thin and fragile – with visible fine blood vessels. Lesions should be closely examined for signs of ulceration or potential breakdown; these should be monitored on initial examination and on follow-up for any signs of malignant changes as the evolution of squamous cell

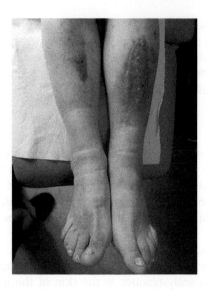

FIGURE 3.8   Reddened plaques to the pretibial region associated with necrobiosis lipoidica.
Source: Used with permission from Cardiff & Vale University Health Board.

carcinoma (SCC) has been identified in long-standing lesions (Santos-Juanes et al. 2004).

NL lesions are normally present as multiple, painless lesions affecting both lower limbs. The lesions can become very painful if an ulcer develops (Figure 3.9) (Lacroix et al. 2008).

Investigations

Clinical presentation and patient history are the key components to making a diagnosis of NL, although skin biopsies can be taken to confirm the diagnosis. Blood tests for diabetes may be taken where NL is suspected in patients who are not known to be diabetic (British Association of Dermatologists 2019).

A vascular assessment is recommended due to the increased risk of PAD present in diabetic patients (Jeffcoate et al. 2006). This can help to guide appropriate vascular interventions and compression therapy following diagnosis if required.

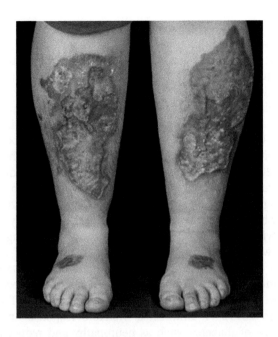

FIGURE 3.9   Ulcerated necrobiosis lipoidica.
Source: Dissemond et al. (2018) / John Wiley & Sons. Reproduced with permission.

Diagnosis

Clinical diagnosis is usually made based on the identifiable skin changes seen on examination and on the evolution of these skin changes as described by the patient. If a skin biopsy has been taken to confirm a diagnosis, the histological examination would indicate granulomas and inflammatory reaction around destroyed collagen, and thickening of blood vessel walls (Oakley 2021). This aligns with the disease processes thought to cause the development of NL as described earlier, namely reduced blood flow, immune response and abnormal collagen degradation.

Intervention

Treatment for NL can be challenging and inconsistent due to a lack of substantial evidence to support various treatment options. If associated with diabetes, improved diabetes management and glycaemic control can contribute to the improvement and eventual healing of any ulcerations, although this is not always the case (Mistry et al. 2017). The condition can be self-limiting, spontaneously resolving in up to 17% of cases (British Association of Dermatologists 2019).

The mainstay of treatment for NL is often topical or intralesional steroid therapy, with the occasional need for oral steroids (Duff et al. 2015). Topical steroids should be applied to the active borders of lesions, avoiding the thin and fragile atrophic areas in the centre (Reid et al. 2013). Other topical treatments and systemic medications, such as tacrolimus, pentoxifylline and phototherapy, have been used with varying results (Feily and Mehraban 2015; Reid et al. 2013) and would only be commenced following specialist dermatology advice.

Identifying and managing infection can be challenging but important with diabetic patients. The disease process of diabetes leads to an altered local and systemic inflammatory and immune response, meaning that the incidence and severity of infection are increased in diabetic patients and innate defence is poor (Edmonds and Sumpio 2019). A diminished systemic response and other complications of diabetes, such as neuropathy and reduced blood supply to the lower limb, can lead to classic signs and symptoms of infection being lesser or absent, thus diagnosis can be delayed and progression more rapid than normal (Edmonds and Sumpio 2019). Poorly controlled diabetes is also associated with an increased risk of wound infection (IWII 2022). This, along with the altered response to infection with diabetes, leads to wounds being classed as at high risk of infection and so judicious prophylactic use of topical antimicrobials may be appropriate in these cases (IWII 2022).

While there is no conclusive evidence on the benefits of compression therapy with NL, particularly as a first-line treatment, anecdotal evidence and expert opinion have recommended it for treatment and prevention if there are no other contraindications, due to the clinical benefits associated with reduced oedema and inflammatory cytokines and improved microcirculation that are achieved with compression therapy (Erfurt-Berge et al. 2015; Isoherranen et al. 2019; Zhang and McMullin 2022). Padding of the lesions using simple gauze pads, absorbent pads or soft cotton wadding is also recommended to reduce the risk of injury and ulceration. These can be applied directly over the area of ulceration to provide protection of fragile skin and plaques, or in the case of soft cotton wadding used underneath compression therapy, applied to the lower leg as recommended by the manufacturer of the specific compression system used.

Martorell's Ulcers

Martorell's ulcers, sometimes referred to as Martorell hypertensive ischaemic leg ulcers (HYTILU) or due to ischaemic arteriolosclerosis, are a rare condition that can occur in patients with prolonged, severe or sub-optimally controlled hypertension (Graves et al. 2001; Mansour and Alavi 2019). The effect of prolonged hypertension is to cause localised tissue ischaemia and skin infarction due to the increased resistance in blood vessels and narrowing of the arterioles (Isoherranen et al. 2019).

History

Martorell's ulcers were originally more common in females than males, particularly between the ages of 55 and 65 years, although in more recent studies males and females can be equally affected (Hafner et al. 2010; Mansour and Alavi 2019). Approximately 60% of patients will also have type 2 DM and 50% will have PAD (Hafner et al. 2010).

Examination

Martorell's ulcers often manifest as lower leg ulcers above or around the ankle, to the outer posterior region or over the Achilles' tendon that gradually worsen, contain dry, necrotic tissue and are disproportionally painful to the size of the wound (Figure 3.10). Initially Martorell's ulcers can present as dusky, painful plaques with a mottled appearance to the surrounding skin.

Investigations

Alongside assessment of the clinical presentation, a tissue biopsy is a key investigation if there is a suspicion of arteriolosclerosis linked to hypertension being the underlying cause of the ulceration. Biopsy

(a) (b)

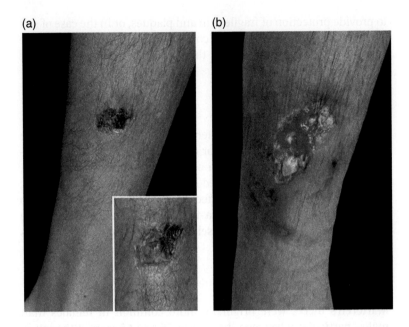

FIGURE 3.10 (a) Martorell's ulceration to the lower limb with typical dry necrotic tissue and (b) progressing to an ulcer with a livid edge and satellite lesions.
Source: King et al. (2017) / John Wiley & Sons. Reproduced with permission.

findings would show thickening of the small–medium arterial walls and narrowing of the vessels.

A vascular assessment is also recommended due to the high incidence of PAD with Martorell's ulcers to determine the need for vascular intervention, such as angioplasty (Isoherranen et al. 2019).

Diagnosis

The diagnosis of Martorell's ulcers must primarily be differentiated from calciphylaxis and PG. Martorell's ulcers are most misdiagnosed for these conditions, which can adversely affect outcomes. Treatments for each condition are significantly different, and if incorrect treatments are given wounds can be exacerbated rather than improved. Thus, it is important to identify the correct aetiology before treatment plans are formulated. Once other typical causes of ulceration have been excluded and the histopathology results of the biopsy are supportive (usually indicated by the thickening of some layers of the arterial walls), a diagnosis of Martorell's can be made.

Intervention

A key area of the treatment plan for this aetiology to promote wound healing involves a multidisciplinary approach to optimise anti-hypertensive medication and pain control, and to assess the need for early surgical intervention. A multidisciplinary approach to engaging with the patient will also be important if there are lifestyle issues, such as poor diet and smoking, and other co-morbidities, particularly poorly controlled diabetes, that are contributing to the challenge of controlling hypertension and increasing cardiovascular risk.

Early surgical intervention has been suggested to give the best outcomes, particularly for larger areas of ulceration, and may take the form of surgical debridement, application of negative-pressure wound therapy and, in some cases, use of split-thickness skin grafting (Dagregario and Guillet 2006; Hafner et al. 2010). While pain reduction is usually experienced quite quickly following surgical treatment, appropriate analgesia will be required up to this point and beyond as clinically indicated.

Electrostimulation, achieved through commercially available medical devices that deliver a low-voltage electrical current via a dressing electrode on intact skin, has also been shown to have some success in those patients unsuitable for surgical intervention (Leloup et al. 2015). Electrostimulation is thought to encourage wound healing by promoting new blood vessels within the wound, wound debridement and increasing granulation tissue by restoring the skin's natural electrical field. It has also been found to be beneficial for wound pain in some cases (Leloup et al. 2015).

Calciphylaxis

Calciphylaxis is a rare and complex condition that is mostly associated with end-stage renal failure (ESRF) in patients usually receiving haemodialysis (Nigwekar et al. 2018). It occurs due to excessive accumulation of calcium in the small blood vessels within the skin and subcutaneous fatty tissue (Baby et al. 2019), usually as a consequence of problems with calcium and phosphorous metabolism. The more common areas for calciphylaxis to develop are those with larger amounts of adipose tissue, such as the lower limb and abdomen (Isoherranen et al. 2019). It can also be associated with hyperparathyroidism (the parathyroid glands in the neck are responsible for regulation of blood calcium levels) (Roncada et al. 2012).

Calciphylaxis is a life-threatening condition with a very poor prognosis, even if detected in its early stages; the one-year mortality rate has been calculated at between 45% and 80% (Bliss 2002; Roncada et al. 2012) and it is closely associated with septicaemia.

History

An existing history of ESRF will be a key marker when assessing for potential calciphylaxis. There is a documented link between the development of calciphylaxis and the length of time for which patients require dialysis, with the risk increasing after two years of treatment (Nigwekar et al. 2018).

Some of the risk factors associated with calciphylaxis include hypertension, diabetes, obesity, certain medications including warfarin, and coagulation disorders (Nigwekar et al. 2018). Suggestions for why calciphylaxis is at higher risk of developing alongside these factors include their link to chronic renal disease, dialysis and a potential role of autoimmunity, although for many risk factors the cause is unknown (Nigwekar et al. 2018). It is also more prevalent in females (Kuypers 2009).

Examination

Calciphylaxis in the early stages is characterised by the presence of dusky and mottled skin that is usually extremely painful (Figure 3.11), which can progress to necrotic lesions and non-healing areas of ulceration (Figure 3.12), often within a few days (Kodumudi et al. 2020; Nigwekar et al. 2018). Areas of necrosis are irregular and typically have inflamed and undermining borders (Isoherranen et al. 2019).

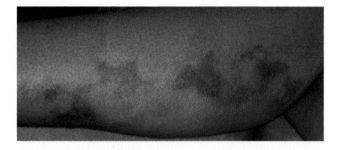

FIGURE 3.11 Dusky, mottled skin seen in early stages of calciphylaxis. *Source:* Ng and Peng 2011 / John Wiley & Sons. Reproduced with permission.

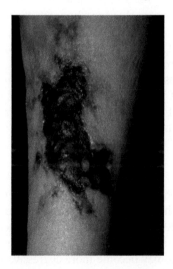

FIGURE 3.12 Necrotic lesion from calciphylaxis. *Source:* Dissemond et al. 2018 / John Wiley & Sons. Reproduced with permission.

Investigations

The investigations include blood tests to identify high levels of calcium and phosphate and parathyroid hormone abnormalities. An X-ray and bone scan can also be useful adjuncts to detect calcification.

A skin biopsy may be performed to rule out other conditions that can present similarly, although there is some debate over whether additional skin trauma may worsen the progression of the disease (Chang 2019).

Diagnosis

Diagnosis of calciphylaxis can be challenging due to the other conditions that can present with similar symptoms, such as cellulitis, vasculitis and warfarin-induced skin necrosis (Nigwekar et al. 2018). Calciphylaxis also shares common clinical patterns with Martorell's ulcers (Isoherranen et al. 2019). Key indicators present in the medical history, such as ESRF, need to be considered; blood tests and X-ray results can often be inconclusive (Chang 2019). A multidisciplinary approach to diagnosis can be useful to reach an agreement due to the multiple differential diagnoses for the condition and the complexities associated with co-morbidities.

Investigation results, such as high calcium and phosphate blood levels, may support the diagnosis, as evidence of clear calcification seen on the X-ray. If a biopsy is taken, usual findings include calcification of vessel walls, thrombosis and infarction (Oakley 2016).

Intervention

Treatment for calciphylaxis begins with the management of any known risk factors, such as hypertension, diabetes and associated medications (Isoherranen et al. 2019). Patients may also be treated with medication such as intravenous sodium thiosulfate during their dialysis sessions, and dialysis regimes may become more aggressive to ensure that calcium and phosphate levels are managed (Nigwekar et al. 2018).

Smaller ulcers are usually managed conservatively or with minor debridement, but larger areas may be treated with skin grafts (Isoherranen et al. 2019). Antibiotics are often required since the risk of developing a wound infection increases as necrosis progresses.

Patients typically experience acute ischaemic pain with calciphylaxis, due to the damage to tissues from ischaemia and infarction as small vessels are occluded. Some patients also experience neuropathic pain with this condition. The pain can vary from patient to patient, such as a constant background pain that is exacerbated on movement or during procedures, or breakthrough pain that is unprovoked (Chinnadurai et al. 2020). First-line treatment for pain usually involves opioid-based analgesia, with paracetamol and anti-seizure drugs, such as gabapentin, used as adjuvants and for managing nerve pain. Consideration needs to be given to impaired renal function in those patients with calciphylaxis associated with renal failure and the potential for medication toxicity. With the level of pain usually experienced by patients with calciphylaxis, input from a pain management specialist is recommended.

The primary management aim is the removal of necrotic tissue, following a specialist and multidisciplinary review. Dietitian advice should be sought to support optimisation of nutritional needs (helpful for promoting wound healing) and the control of calcium and phosphorous intake by limiting certain foods in the diet (Hess 2002). Local wound care measures, exudate and odour management and decontamination using local antimicrobial cleansers and treatments should form part of the wound management plan. The use and tolerance of compression therapy will be dependent on the presence of oedema and the need to control exudate.

MALIGNANT/NEOPLASTIC WOUNDS

As with other unusual aetiologies, lower limb wounds that are unresponsive to standard treatments should raise suspicion of an atypical cause, which can include malignancy/skin cancer. There is also the potential that the wound has undergone a malignant transformation from an otherwise benign aetiology. Clinicians managing leg ulcers need to be familiar with the normal characteristics of common leg ulcer aetiologies to be able to identify abnormalities such as malignancy. Primary skin cancers that ulcerate when located on the leg are often misdiagnosed as chronic leg ulcers (Senet 2014).

Neoplastic or malignant ulcers can be classified as primary skin cancers or as metastatic secondary skin cancers. Primary cancers result from the direct extension of a tumour to the skin surface, initially presenting as an inflamed and indurated area with pain, tenderness and sometimes an 'orange peel' appearance. This area can go on to ulcerate and proliferate as the tumour grows, becoming commonly referred to as fungating wounds.

Metastatic tumours occur when detached cells from the initial site travel to other organs, including the skin (Rayner et al. 2009). Between 5% and 15% of patients with metastatic cancer will develop a fungating wound (Stringer et al. 2014).

Research suggests that around 2–4% of leg ulcers are found to be malignant (Misciali et al. 2013), although one study indicated a prevalence as high as 10.4% (Senet et al. 2012). Their appearance can range from completely innocent-looking lesions typical of a chronic leg ulcer to more overt growths. When mimicking a chronic leg ulcer, the malignancy will often present as a single area of ulceration with indurated or pigmented edges (Senet 2014). It is suggested that abnormal excessive granulation tissue, particularly at the wound edges, can be highly indicative of a malignant leg ulcer, as can abnormal bleeding (Senet et al. 2012). It should be remembered that not all malignant lesions will ulcerate, so anything atypical in appearance should be investigated further – early diagnosis can reduce the risk of metastases developing and of a simpler and potentially less complex and disfiguring treatment (Hayes and Dodds 2003). Also, it should not be assumed that multiple ulcers to the same limb are of the same aetiology.

Basal Cell Carcinoma, Squamous Cell Carcinoma, Malignant Melanoma and Marjolin's Ulcers

The most common types of primary skin cancers that occur on the lower limb are basal cell carcinoma (BCC), SCC and malignant melanoma (MM) (Table 3.6). BCCs and SCCs are sometimes referred to as 'non-melanoma skin cancers' or keratinocyte carcinomas as they arise from the keratinocyte cells in the skin (Karimkhani et al. 2015), whereas melanomas arise from melanocytes.

BCCs are sometimes referred to as 'rodent ulcers', a traditional term coined because the ulcerated area may look like a tiny rodent bite on the skin. Some SCCs may be referred to as Bowen's disease, or squamous cell carcinoma in situ, indicating a precursor to SCC before the development of any invasive malignancy (Shimizu et al. 2011). These typically present as multiple, superficial, scaly, irregular plaques most commonly to the legs, and can be treated with a variety of options following a diagnostic biopsy, including excision, cryotherapy and photodynamic therapy (Tillman 2004).

TABLE 3.6 Key risk factors and presentation of basal cell carcinoma (BCC), squamous cell carcinoma (SCC) and malignant melanoma (MM).

	BCC	SCC	MM
Risk factors/history	All of these skin cancers are more common in people with pale skin and light hair (blond/red) and light eye colour and in areas of sun-exposed skin		
	Twice as common in men than women		**No sex-associated risk globally**
	Intermittent intense sun exposure	Cumulative pattern of sun exposure Smoking (Diepgen and Maher 2002)	Varying patterns of sun exposure High number of moles on the skin – 80% arise as new moles rather than changes in an existing mole Family or personal history of melanoma

(*Continued*)

TABLE 3.6 (Continued)

	BCC	SCC	MM
Typical presentation/ examination	Tend to be superficial Can be cystic, nodular or keratotic (crusting) Start as a red, dome-shaped nodule with visible capillaries that may be pigmented Can develop necrosis and ulceration with a rolled edge as they grow If ulcerated – often have well-defined borders with a 'pearly' appearance to the wound edge	Firm, nodular, crusted lesions Can ulcerate as they grow and have a propensity to develop secondary infections Often have rolled and/or raised edges and hyper-granulation tissue in the wound bed	Pigmented lesion/mole that has changed in shape, size and/or colour – can have uneven pigmentation, irregular borders and be slightly raised from the skin surface Most commonly presents on the legs in women and trunk/back in men Some types are associated with nail beds and the soles of feet and are more common with Asian skin Can become amelanotic (non-pigmented) – skin-coloured, pink, red or purple Some types are associated with spontaneous bleeding, and if ulcerate often have darkly pigmented borders and peri-ulcer skin
Development	Localised, slow growing over years, minimally invasive and rarely metastasise	Locally invasive, grow noticeably in months and with potential to metastasise	Aggressive development with high risk of metastasising, particularly if diagnosis is delayed

Source: Adapted from Freak (2005); Rayner et al. (2009); Senet (2014). Photos from Price et al. (2022) / John Wiley & Sons. Reproduced with permission.

Other types of malignant leg ulcers or lesions are Marjolin's ulcers (which usually evolve from SCCs), Kaposi's sarcoma and cutaneous presentations of lymphoma that can result in leg ulcers (Senet 2014). Classic Kaposi's sarcoma, which is unrelated to human immunodeficiency virus (HIV), usually presents as multiple dark blue macules (flat, distinct, discoloured areas of skin) that progress to larger plaques and tumours/lesions (Senet 2014). They are usually confined to the lower limb and frequently appear on both legs.

Marjolin's ulcers are malignant transformations that occur over many years in chronic wounds of another aetiology, including chronic leg ulcers. They were named after the French Physicist Jean-Nicolas Marjolin, who first described them in 1827 (Senet, 2014). Marjolin's ulcers are very rare, estimated to occur in 1.7% of chronic wounds, and typically consisting of SCCs, although other types of skin cancers have been identified more rarely (Trent and Kirsner 2003). These ulcers have been shown to be more aggressive and metastasise more often than if a new SCC was to develop directly on the skin (Senet 2014). Marjolin's ulcers are often overlooked or misdiagnosed, leading to a poor prognosis and mortality rate of around 21% (Saaiq and Ashraf 2014). Their underlying cause is largely unknown, although suggestions include occurrence due to constantly dividing skin cells trying to resurface a chronic wound (Menendez and Warriner 2006) and chronic inflammation from chronic venous insufficiency (CVI) as contributing factors (Isoherranen et al. 2019).

History

The incidence of primary skin cancer can relate to age, with rates rising significantly in the over 50s and peaking in the over 75s, although a quarter of melanomas are diagnosed in the under 50 age group (Jones et al. 2020). Over 60 is also the age group when venous insufficiency and/or PAD are most frequent, hence the potential for misdiagnosis. Table 3.3 outlines some of the key risk factors to look for in a patient's history that can be indicative of BCC, SCC or MM, of which sun exposure is common to all.

Marjolin's ulcers can have a very long latent time over which they transform, usually over 10 years and often much longer (Combemale et al. 2007). The long duration of a pre-existing ulcer is one of the key factors for diagnosing this type of malignant leg wound. They are also associated with sites of previously healed burns, traumatic injury and osteomyelitis (Menendez and Warriner 2006). Suspicion should be raised if the patient is reporting sudden or unexpected changes in a long-standing wound, such as new pain, foul-smelling discharge, increased volume of exudate or change in nodular appearance to the wound bed (Choa et al. 2015).

Examination

Ulcers on the calf are unusual when of vascular origin or diabetes related, so the location of a wound in this area is worth investigating for an atypical cause, usually either malignancy, infection or vasculitis (White 1999).

The presence of apparent granulation tissue that is nodular (like a cauliflower), raised, budding, exuberant, translucent, shiny or rolling over the wound edge should raise suspicion of malignancy (Harris et al. 1993; Poccia et al. 2014; Tchanque-Fossuo et al. 2018) (Figures 3.13 and 3.14). Other key signs suggestive of malignancy include (Harris et al. 1993; Poccia et al. 2014):

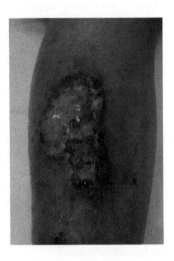

FIGURE 3.13   Basal cell carcinoma presenting as a leg ulcer – note the raised granulation tissue with raised borders. The ulcer was unresponsive to standard treatment.
Source: Misciali et al. (2013) / John Wiley & Sons. Reproduced with permission.

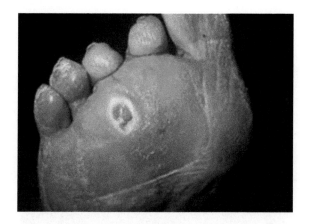

FIGURE 3.14   Amelanotic malignant melanoma disguised as a diabetic foot ulcer – note exuberant granulation tissue.
Source: Gregson and Allain (2004) / John Wiley & Sons. Reproduced with permission.

- Islands of epithelium (new skin produced within the wound bed) that form but do not continue to produce healed tissue and often break down again.
- Firm indurated surrounding skin unrelated to venous skin changes.
- Unusual pain or bleeding.

Necrosis may be evident as the malignancy progresses, and large volumes of exudate are associated with the invasion of the lymphatic system by malignant cells (Adderley and Holt 2014).

Marjolin's ulcers may not always exhibit classical malignant changes such as an abnormal wound edge, raised crusty growths or bleeding, but are more likely to have an irregular wound bed and hyper-granulation (Choa et al. 2015) (Figure 3.15). The key sign for Marjolin's ulcers along with their long duration is an increase in size despite appropriate treatment.

A clinical knowledge summary from the National Institute for Health and Care Excellence (NICE 2022a) on melanoma recommends that suspicious skin lesions should be assessed using a weighted seven-point checklist (Table 3.7) (Mackie 1990), with any lesion

(a)

(b)

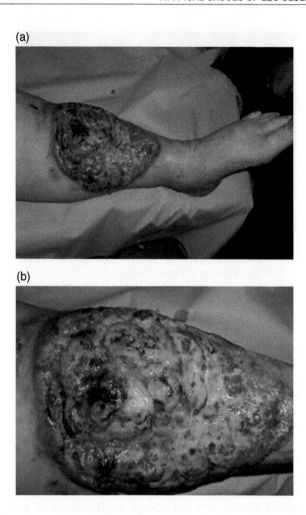

FIGURE 3.15 (a, b) Marjolin's ulcer – SCC transformation in a leg ulcer originally diagnosed as of venous aetiology. Note the raised edges rolling outward and exuberant protruding tissue to the wound bed with necrotic tissue and excess greyish slough.
Source: Enoch et al. (2004) / John Wiley & Sons. Reproduced with permission.

scoring ≥3 being referred via an urgent suspected cancer pathway (NICE 2022a); these lesions are at higher risk of being an MM.

NICE (2022a) recommends that the following should also be referred through an urgent suspected cancer pathway: nail changes including a

TABLE 3.7 Weighted seven-point checklist.

Major features (2 points)	Minor features (1 point)
Change in size of the lesion	Inflammation
Change in colour/irregular pigmentation	Itch or altered sensation
Change in shape/irregular border	Larger than other lesions (diameter > 7 mm)
	Oozing/crusting of the lesion

Source: Adapted from Mackie (1990).

new pigmented line or lesion under the nail; or any persistent or slowly evolving skin lesion, especially if growing, pigmented or vascular in appearance, that is unresponsive and with an uncertain diagnosis.

Investigations

Skin biopsy by the dermatology service is the primary investigation required for any wound showing suspicion of malignancy. The best practice document on chronic wounds published by the European Wound Management Association (EWMA) suggests that a biopsy should be performed on any presumed chronic vascular leg ulcer if there has been no response to standard treatment after 4–12 weeks (Isoherranen et al. 2019). At least two biopsies taken from the wound and the wound edge are recommended to ensure that abnormalities are detected (Senet et al. 2012).

Some trained clinicians, such as dermatology specialists and general practitioners, may undertake dermoscopy in the clinical setting to check the appearance of lesions more thoroughly. Dermoscopy involves microscopic examination of the skin surface, allowing trained clinicians to more closely examine the colour and structure of skin pigmentation. This can help detect melanomas more easily and differentiate them from other skin lesions (Oakley and Stevens 2023).

A wound swab should be taken if there are clinical signs of spreading infection to guide appropriate antibiotic therapy.

Diagnosis

Diagnosis of malignancy in leg ulcers can be identified by examining the patient history, presence of risk factors, atypical presentation of the skin, lesion or ulcer and histology reports from a skin biopsy. It is recommended to perform at least two biopsies that include the wound edge and the wound bed to decrease the risk of a false-negative result from a single biopsy (Isoherranen et al. 2019). Sequentially repeated biopsies may be required to make some formal diagnoses, especially if previous biopsy results have been negative but the wound continues to look or behave suspiciously (Isoherranen et al. 2019).

Staging examinations, such as ultrasound, computed tomography (CT) or magnetic resonance imaging (MRI) scans, may be performed following diagnosis to detect any spread of cancer to the lymph nodes or other organs. Results will then be used to guide required treatment, such as local resection or radiotherapy, or if there is a need for systemic treatments or chemotherapy (Isoherranen et al. 2019).

Intervention

Following referral to dermatology, the usual first course of action is surgical excision of the malignant area. Depending on the extent of the excision required, some areas may require skin grafting to treat the residual wound.

Also depending on location and depth and if the malignancy has been identified as having become metastatic or at high risk of spread, such as with an ulcerated MM, patients may be offered treatment in the form of radiotherapy and/or chemotherapy (Rice 2007). In rare cases, if the malignancy is especially large or has bony involvement, major amputation may be required (Trent and Kirsner 2003).

With regard to local wound management and pre- and post-excision of any area of malignancy, key considerations will be the use of non-adherent primary dressings to ensure atraumatic removal and primary and secondary dressings with sufficient levels of absorption for the wound exudate levels; compression therapy is required for exudate management and any accompanying venous hypertension. Symptom management for issues such as malodour and pain may also be required.

If linked to the presence of necrotic or sloughy tissue, malodour may be decreased through safe autolytic debridement, although overtly moist debridement should be avoided if exudate levels are high. Autolytic debridement may also result in increased exudate, which can be unsatisfactory to the patient if it is excessive and difficult to manage and leads to leakage, skin excoriation and discomfort (Tandler and Stephen-Haynes 2017). Other options can include topical treatments, such as metronidazole gel or charcoal dressings in conjunction with antimicrobial dressings. Metronidazole has been shown to be effective in reducing wound odour, particularly if the odour is related to an increased bioburden as it has broad-spectrum activity. It is particularly effective against anaerobic bacteria that cause odour (Kavitha et al. 2014; Paul and Pieper 2008). Charcoal dressings work by absorbing bacteria and locally released toxins and chemicals responsible for wound odour (Wounds International 2012). Consideration should also be given to the frequency of dressing changes required to manage malodour and exudate.

Some malignant wounds will be prone to bleeding; management with a dressing with haemostatic properties, such as calcium alginate, may be required. There is also a potential for infection with malignant leg ulcers. Gentle cleansing with normal saline or water is advised, particularly if there is a risk of bleeding, and treatment with a topical antimicrobial dressing as clinically indicated. Some patients may benefit from compression bandaging to reduce oedema following excision (Todhunter 2019).

Tailored patient education on the risks of continued sun exposure will form part of the individual intervention for patients diagnosed with any form of malignant leg ulcer as a means of preventing recurrence (NICE 2016). Patients should be educated on how to check their skin and have regular follow-up appointments to assess for further development, spread or recurrence. Consideration should also be given to the provision of psychosocial support to patients diagnosed with malignancy.

DRUG-INDUCED LEG ULCERS

Medication-Related Ulceration

Adverse drug reactions are always a potential complication to be considered when prescribing any medication. This is particularly pertinent with the current ageing population who have complex co-morbidities that require polypharmacy to manage their long-term conditions (Ramadan 2023). Cutaneous reactions may vary in appearance from a simple urticaria-type rash to vasculitis and skin necrosis (Table 3.8). Early identification of the severity of the skin damage and medication that is contributing to the cutaneous drug

TABLE 3.8 Common drugs that may cause cutaneous atypical wounds and considerations to observe when undertaking assessment.

Drug	Considerations to note when undertaking examination and history
Hydroxycarbamide	Commonly seen on the lower limb of the malleolus area as a small, defined, painful ulcer
	Seen in 10% of patients with myelodysplastic disorders
	May still present after years of hydroxyurea use
	Usually resolves after discontinuing the drug
Methotrexate	May present as erythematous eruptions, blisters or epidermal necrosis
	Most seen in psoriasis patients with pre-existing psoriatic plaques
	May indicate early signs of methotrexate toxicity
	Drugs may require discontinuation or adjustment of dose
Warfarin and heparin	Start as erythematous plaques that evolve into necrotic lesions
	Usually appear between days 3 and 10 of treatment
	Usually very painful and can be fatal
	Treatment involves discontinuation of the drug; patient may also require initiation of vitamin K
Nicorandil	Used for the treatment of angina
	Most ulceration occurs in mucosal membranes, but 60% have been reported in the lower limb
	Can be seen from day 2 up to 19 years after commencing nicorandil
	Most episodes of ulceration will resolve following discontinuation of the medication

Source: Adapted from Nickles et al. (2022); Isoherranen et al. (2019); Babic et al. (2018).

reaction is of paramount importance and may prevent the onset of more serious reactions that could be life-threatening (Ramadan 2023).

Diagnosis of an ulcer that is potentially related to medication often occurs once other systemic diseases have been excluded, raising awareness and allowing identification of medication that could potentially be causing the skin damage.

Treatment of medication-induced ulcers may require a multidisciplinary approach and can include stopping the medication and prescribing antihistamines to reduce side effects such as itching and corticosteroids to reduce inflammation (Ramadan 2023). Wounds usually resolve once the medication has stopped (Isoherranen et al. 2019). Local wound management should follow the principles of moist wound healing and address the requirements of the local wound environment (see Chapter 5). A more in-depth exploration of mediations known to cause ulceration is offered in Chapter 8.

Leg Ulceration in People Who Inject Drugs

Drug use in the United Kingdom is estimated to be the highest in Europe, with people who inject drugs (PWIDs) having far poorer health outcomes than the general population (UKHSA 2023). It is thought that approximately 87 000 people aged 15–64 in England are PWIDs (Hay et al. 2017), with the most commonly used drug for injection being heroin (UKHSA 2022), closely followed by crack cocaine. Crack cocaine is associated with high incidences of skin and soft tissue infections and is linked to risk factors such as sharing equipment, groin injecting, higher frequency of injecting, unsterile injection practices, poor wound care and late presentations of symptoms (UKHSA 2023; Edmundson et al. 2021). Injection-related wounds are common in PWIDs and early detection and treatment can assist in reducing the possibility of serious complications that can be life-threatening, such as infection (Sanchez et al. 2021). However often, there is often a reluctance for PWIDs to seek medical assistance when a wound occurs and maintaining consistency and concordance can be challenging. This behaviour often leads to patients being marginalised within society (Geraghty 2021); understanding the lived experience is critical to awareness and management of their conditions.

History

When assessing and treating a person who has a leg ulcer that may be associated with drug injecting, gaining the individual's trust and presenting a non-judgemental approach are of paramount importance. Very often the lack of engagement of PWIDs with HCPs is due to the stigma and discrimination that are often associated with drug injecting and the lack of knowledge and skills that HCPs may have surrounding drug-injecting issues (Lang et al. 2013). An understanding of how injecting can cause a wound, complications that may occur following injecting, along with social and mental health aspects that may affect the individual is an important part of the knowledge and skill set needed by HCPs treating and managing PWIDs with wounds.

- Wounds in PWIDS can occur due to many aspects, which include injecting frequently into the same site. Repeated injection into the veins, especially the femoral vein, can result in significant damage to the venous system, leading to CVI, deep vein thrombosis (DVT) development and venous leg ulceration (Doran et al. 2022). Frequent injecting also increases the risk of infection (Sanchez et al. 2021).
- Products injected can put the user at higher risk of skin damage and infection. Certain contaminants in cocaine (e.g. levamisole) have been linked to vasculitis and skin necrosis (Nickles et al. 2022). Some mixing agents and contaminants found in heroin preparations have also been linked to a higher risk of infection (Sanchez et al. 2021) and acidifiers such as citric acid have been associated with an increased risk of DVT development (Doran et al. 2022). Neuropathy, nerve damage and muscle fibrosis have been associated with the toxicity of the substance injected and the frequency of injecting (Sanchez et al. 2021).
- Poor injection techniques may also play a role. Injecting drugs into the skin rather than into a vein is known as skin popping and usually is performed when venous access has become difficult. This technique increases the risk of microvascular and lymphatic occlusion as well as infection and skin necrosis (Nickles et al. 2022). Attempts to inject into a vein may result in a 'missed hit', where the substance is inadvertently injected intramuscularly or into the subcutaneous tissue, which increases the risk of infection (Sanchez et al. 2021).

As with any other wound, a full patient history should be obtained as outlined in Chapter 5. However, there may be specific questions that may be helpful to gain a better understanding of the

TABLE 3.9 Aspects of drug-taking history that can be included in the assessment of people who inject drugs (PWIDs).

- Substance injected (if known).
- Any other recreational drugs that are taken.
- Frequency of injecting.
- Sites used for injection.
- Any previous history of deep vein thrombosis.
- Any previous history of wounds associated with injecting sites.
- If the patient participates in needle sharing, does the patient have access to a needle exchange site?
- Is the patient under a drug and alcohol team or mental health services?
- Is the patient homeless?
- Does the patient have access to clean conditions to undertake injections (this may be particularly relevant if the patient is homeless or lives in unsanitary conditions)?
- Has the patient been screened for human immunodeficiency virus (HIV), hepatitis B and hepatitis C? PWIDs have a high risk of contracting these infections due to needle sharing (UKHSA 2023).

patient's injecting habits, social circumstances and mental health, and these may be relevant when implementing a treatment plan. Table 3.9 outlines some questions that may be helpful to consider during the assessment.

Examination

PWIDs have a high prevalence of venous ulceration due to CVI (Doran et al. 2022). Signs and symptoms of venous disease as outlined in Chapter 5 may be identified through examination. Ulcer presentation can often differ from that of standard venous ulceration; ulceration is typically multiple sites above the ankle to the knee, including the tibial crest region. The patient should also be assessed for nerve or muscle damage, impaired calf muscle and ankle joint function, which may be compromised by frequent injecting into the lower limb (Sanchez et al. 2021).

PWIDs have a high incidence of infection, which increases significantly the mortality and morbidity of this population (Sanchez et al. 2021). Serious complications identified in PWIDs associated with infection include sepsis, gangrene, amputation and death

(Sanchez et al. 2021). Bacterial infections that are commonly associated with poor injecting practices are *Staphylococcus aureus*, group A *Streptococcus* (GAS) and methicillin-sensitive and -resistant *Staphylococcus aureus* (UKHSA 2023). There is also a smaller potential for toxin-producing bacteria such as botulism, tetanus and anthrax, which are found in the environment and can contaminate drugs at any point (UKHSA 2023). Vigilance in observing for infection is therefore of paramount importance in this at-risk group. The signs and symptoms of infection can be found in Chapter 5.

Other symptoms that are often present in PWIDs' wounds that have been associated with causing depression and anxiety are high levels of pain and exudate and malodour (Sanchez et al. 2021). A large proportion of PWIDs have been identified as being nutritionally deficient, which will have a detrimental effect on the healing process, therefore a nutritional assessment should be considered an important part of the holistic assessment.

Investigations

Vascular assessment should be undertaken to identify any concomitant venous and/or arterial disease in the lower limb, with appropriate onward referral to vascular for intervention as indicated.

A wound swab may be helpful if wound infection is suspected (as per local policy) and is not responding to antimicrobial therapy.

Diagnosis

PWIDs have a high prevalence of CVI and therefore are more at risk of developing a venous ulcer. However, diagnosis can only be made using the information obtained from the patient's history, the clinical appearance of the wound and the vascular assessment.

Intervention

Management in PWIDs can be complex, as drug-using habits may be unpredictable and many PWIDs have other health and social issues such as poverty, homelessness, difficulty in getting to venues for wound dressings and also the stigma and discrimination that they are often subjected to within the healthcare system (Doran et al. 2022).

A non-judgemental approach, multidisciplinary working and patient collaboration are all important parts of the patient's journey. The main role of the HCP is to reduce or prevent further harm by signposting individuals to agencies or services that may be helpful, such as needle exchange sites, homeless and outreach services and drug and alcohol support services, as well as discussing aspects of safe injecting such as not sharing needles.

Local wound management and treatment plans will address aspects of TIMES as identified within the wound assessment, and what the patient is identifying as important to them; very often this is pain and malodour (Sanchez et al. 2021). For the HCP early detection and treatment of infection are imperative and may require treatment in secondary care if spreading or systemic infection is suspected (see Chapter 5 on infection).

Many PWIDs wish to participate in self-care for convenience, and the HCP is instrumental in supporting this by ensuring that they are provided with appropriate dressings, given advice on how to redress the wound to reduce the possibility of infection, how to identify infection and when to seek help and whom to go to if a problem occurs. If compression therapy is appropriate, and the patient is deemed able to cooperate, compression hosiery kits and compression wraps are products that assist in self-management (see Chapter 8). Even if they are self-caring, patients should always be encouraged to attend regularly for reassessments with whoever provides their local wound care management (e.g. practice nurse), to monitor the progress of the wound and to support the patient with any ongoing wound issues.

EROSIVE PUSTULAR DERMATOSIS

Erosive pustular dermatosis (EPD) is a condition that is not widely recognised outside of dermatology. It is rarely discussed within the nursing leg ulcer literature, yet is not uncommon within community leg ulcer management. EPD is challenging to treat and manage (Duffus-Grovell 2021).

EPD is a rare chronic inflammatory skin condition that occurs most commonly on the scalp and lower limbs (British Association of Dermatologists 2022). The presentation of EPD is often poorly

TABLE 3.10   Possible differential diagnoses of erosive pustular dermatosis.

Allergic contact dermatitis
Varicose eczema
Bacterial folliculitis
Pustular psoriasis
Pyoderma gangrenosum
Bullous pemphigoid
Malignancy
Cellulitis
Venous ulceration

Source: Adapted from Conde (2015) and Nichol et al. (2017).

recognised and can be confused with other lower limb conditions, as indicated in Table 3.10 (Duffus-Grovell 2021; Conde 2015), therefore the exact incidence and prevalence of EPD are unknown (Conde 2015). EPD is thought to be most commonly seen in individuals who are elderly, female and have a history of chronic venous insufficiency (Lee et al. 2020; British Association of Dermatologists 2022).

The exact cause of EPD is unclear, but it is thought to be triggered by sun damage or as a result of skin injury (e.g. previous surgery or trauma). On the leg, EPD is often accompanied by venous stasis or atrophy and is not uncommon in those having long-term compression therapy (Dawn et al. 2003). It can be confused with cellulitis (Zhou et al. 2015) but has unique characteristics that determine its management. Nicol et al. (2017) indicated that there is a strong association between the development of EPD and the chronic inflammation that is associated with venous insufficiency. Other proposed causative factors are neutrophil dysfunction, zinc deficiency and occlusion with compression bandaging (Conde 2015; Di Altobrando et al. 2020).

Examination

EPD usually occurs on the gaiter region of the limb and can be unilateral or bilateral. The condition typically presents with superficial crusted erosions and multiple pustules with sterile pus to surrounding skin (Figure 3.16); the removal of the crusts reveals

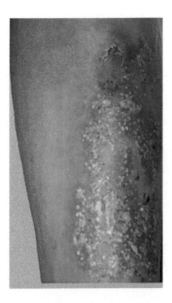

FIGURE 3.16   Pustules and crusted areas to surrounding skin.
Source: Erdmann et al. (2009) / John Wiley & Sons. Reproduced
with permission.

shiny granulation tissue (Nichol et al. 2017; Di Altobrando et al. 2020)
after the removal of the frank pus.

Left untreated, areas of EPD simply increase and join up to form
larger, shallow erosive lesions; the condition has been described as
having 'pustular lakes' (Bull and Mortimer 1995). On the leg, it is not
uncommon to find circumferential patches of crusty fragile scabs or
ragged erosive areas from ankle to knee. When scabs are absent the
clinical features have similarities to cellulitis. Large erosive areas are
often wrongly described as ulceration.

Investigations

Histology from a biopsy of the lesions is often non-specific and may
reveal infiltration of polynuclear neutrophils in the dermis (Nichol
et al. 2017; Reschke et al. 2021). Reschke et al. (2021) proposed that
the presence of these inflammatory cells (possibly attributed to
trauma in the area) contributes to exacerbating the cycle of

inflammation, resulting in poor healing. A biopsy of the area may also be helpful to exclude other possible wound aetiologies (Conde 2015).

Wound swabs are not usually indicated and can be misleading in the treatment of EPD. The swab results often reveal secondary colonisation with bacteria and fungi such as *Staphylococcus aureus* and *Candida albicans* rather than a primary cause of infection (Zhou et al. 2015; Nichol et al. 2017). A study by Dawn et al. (2003) found 54% of patients to have laboratory evidence of fungal infection that cleared after antifungal treatment. The remaining participants achieved clearance with topical steroids and interestingly a change in management from multilayered 'four-layer' compression to a long-stretch regime.

Arterial status should be established using a Doppler ultrasound to calculate the ABPI and will assist in guiding suitability for compression therapy (Wounds UK 2016).

Diagnosis

There are currently no specific clinical criteria for the diagnosis of EPD and presenting clinical features may be similar to other aetiologies, thus reaching an accurate diagnosis can be challenging (Nichol et al. 2017). Table 3.10 indicates possible differential diagnoses to be considered. Diagnosis of EPD is often made following exclusion of other possible aetiologies and failure to respond to previous management such as dressings, compression and antimicrobials (Conde 2015).

EPD is most commonly misdiagnosed as cellulitis, since the clinical features such as pustules, suppurative exudate with crusts and erosions, as well as a positive swab result, can be present in both aetiologies (Zhou et al. 2015). EPD therefore should be considered as a differential diagnosis of exclusion for patients who have not responded to local or systemic antibiotics for the treatment of suspected cellulitis (Zhou et al. 2015).

Intervention

The evidence to support best practice in treating EPD is currently lacking and further research to support clinical pathways is needed in this area. There is currently no cure for this condition and treatment will depend on accurate and early diagnosis (British Association of Dermatologists 2022). Involvement in the appropriate clinical team such as dermatology can assist in devising an appropriate treatment plan (British Association of Dermatologists 2022).

Clinical management is aimed at removing the crusts, treating the erosions with topical therapy and allowing them to dry out and heal (British Association of Dermatologists 2022). Removal of the crusts can be done by using a skin cleansing cloth, debridement pad or simple lifting of the scab with forceps. It should not create any pain for the patient. The removal of the scab will release the tell-tale sign of pus and then the erosion needs to be cleansed. The erosive area can be friable and thus the patient can be positioned forward so as not to cause alarm; any bleeding should stop swiftly and extra care must be taken not to create any skin tears in the atrophied skin. The next step is the application of the topical treatment; this can be problematic on wet erosions, so the practitioner or patient may find it useful to apply the ointments to the non-adherent dressing first and then to the limb.

Topical Treatments

- High-potency topical steroids have been found to be one of the most effective treatments (British Association of Dermatologists 2022; Nichol et al. 2017; Zhou et al. 2015).
- Topical tacrolimus 0.1% does not cause skin atrophy, unlike corticosteroids, and is often used in conjunction with corticosteroids or prophylactically to prevent recurrence (Conde 2015).

Oral Treatments

Retinoids or zinc supplements can be used (British Association of Dermatologists 2022).

Local Wound Care

Initially gentle removal of the crusts and daily dressings with a non-adherent dressing are advised (British Association of Dermatologists 2022; Conde 2015).

Compression Therapy

Compression therapy is recommended to manage the venous insufficiency (Wounds UK 2016) that is commonly present in EPD. However, it was surmised by Dawn et al. (2003) that continuous use of compression therapy with four-layer bandaging could contribute to a potential risk of developing a fungal infection and poor progress of wound healing. Dawn et al. further suggested that patients responded better when intermittent short-stretch bandaging was used as opposed to continuous four-layer bandaging. It has to be recognised, however, that their study is from 2003 and the types of compression therapy available today are more extensive and may not have the same outcomes should a similar study be conducted (refer to Chapter 7 for the types of compression available). Indeed, the suggestion was not supported by a more recent study by Nichol et al. (2017), who concluded that compression hosiery was not a contributory factor to poor healing in EPD patients once treatment with topical corticosteroids had been commenced. Nevertheless, careful consideration should be given to the type of compression, as the topical treatments and removal of crusts will initially be required to be undertaken daily and compression bandaging may not be the best option, especially if the patient is willing and able to perform self-care.

Patient Self-Care

It is critical to recognise that EPD is often a life-long skin disorder and can be experienced as a recalcitrant condition on the lower leg (Brouard et al. 2002), thus it is imperative that a self-management schedule is instigated as soon as an effective treatment regime is identified. It is unlikely that an effective regime will follow a linear pattern or achieve complete resolution. Therefore, enabling and empowering the patient to manage their care and condition if they are able are important aspects of treating EPD due to its often life-long and recurring nature. Treatment regimens are also required daily both in the early stages of treatment and for prevention of recurrence. Thus visiting a healthcare establishment or waiting for community nursing visits can become arduous and affect the individual's quality of life.

Some considerations and advice for patients with EPD are:

- Ensure the patient has an understanding of EPD and treatment options that are available.
- Assess the patient for their willingness and ability to undertake self-care.
- Develop an appropriate treatment plan in collaboration with the patient (see Box 3.1).
- Identify red flags and who to contact in the event of any concerns.
- Organise a follow-up appointment for review with whoever is overseeing the care of the patient. This should include dermatology.
- Once the condition has healed, patients should be given advice on maintenance of the skin and prevention of recurrence. This may be short term using tacrolimus 0.1% twice a week, emollients

Box 3.1   Self-management of EPD

Skin care should be carried out using debridement cloths or similar to remove scabs and cleanse the erosive areas. Bathing with an emollient should be encouraged.

Help the patient understand what they are experiencing and provide resources such as the British Association of Dermatologists information leaflet. This will give the patient confidence in their self-management of the scabs and treatment of the erosions and surrounding skin with the prescribed topical treatments and emollients. They will learn how to respond to any flare-ups of the condition.

If oedema is significant, then use compression bandages, but for a limited period only in order to reduce the oedema:

- A moderate dose of compression is often therapeutic for these conditions.
- A nurse-led bandage regime can promote dependency; the nurse will be providing the skin care and application and in this often recalcitrant condition it can prove difficult to break this pattern of treatment.

A self-management regime is focused on:

- Maintaining a skin care regime and removal of scabs.
- Use of a zinc oxide–impregnated stocking under a compression liner sock.
- A hosiery garment at the prescribed dose of compression.
- Protection from further sun damage.
- Self-management of relapses, but swift access to medical support when required.

and compression hosiery to manage venous insufficiency and protecting the skin from further sun damage (British Association of Dermatologists 2022; Conde 2015).

Factitious/Artefactual Ulcers and Self-Harm Wounds

Factitious ulcers, artefactual ulcers or self-harm wounds have been described as 'The deliberate and conscious production of self-inflicted lesions to satisfy an unconscious psychological or emotional need' (Isoherranen et al. 2019). These wounds can also be referred to as dermatitis artefacta.

These types of wounds can occur on any part of the body that is easily accessible to the patient. Diagnosis is often difficult, as the patient's history can be vague and may not always fit with the appearance of the wound itself (Isoherranen et al. 2019). The motivation for patients to cause wounds to themselves can be complex and may be triggered by deep psychological stress. Triggers may include trauma, psychological disorders and sexual or physical abuse (Hunt 2017).

History

It can be difficult to obtain an accurate history from the patient, who may be vague about the way the wound occurred (Kilroy-Findley and Bateman 2016). A previous history of multiple attendances to the hospital's emergency department, and a history of mental illness or psychological trauma, may raise suspicion that the wound is due to self-harm (Hunt 2017). If possible, the method of how the wound was caused should be established.

Examination

The more typical features of how self-harm wounds may present clinically are as follows:

- The wounds may be in areas that are easy for the patient to reach and uniform in shape.
- The appearance of the wound may vary depending on the method of injury (Figure 3.17 indicates continual gouging or scratching of the area).
- Infection may be suspected if an unclean implement was used to cause the injury.
- There may be scarring or evidence of previous historical wounds to surrounding skin.

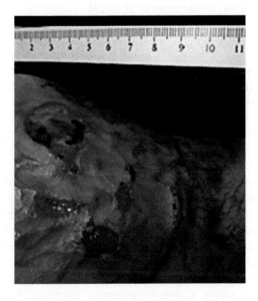

FIGURE 3.17   Leg wounds due to self-harm with continual gouging/ scratching of the area.

Investigations

Investigations are not usually required for this type of wound, especially at first presentation. However, wound infection is a common occurrence of a factitious wound (Kilroy-Findley and Bateman 2016). The development of wound infection may be linked with how the injury was caused, for instance by unclean instruments or dirty fingernails, environmental factors, or specific patient risk factors for infection, such as diabetes (see Chapter 5 on infection). A wound swab may therefore be helpful to identify the pathogen responsible if the wound is unresponsive to topical antimicrobials or if spreading infection is suspected, as per local guidelines.

Diagnosis

Diagnosis can be challenging, especially if the patient withholds key information on how the wound occurred and their past medical history. Diagnosis is therefore often made after exclusion of other wound aetiologies (Isoherranen et al. 2019).

Intervention

A patient's mental state may influence their ability to engage with treatment options (Kilroy-Findley and Bateman 2016). NICE (2022b) suggests that HCPs dealing with patients who self-harm should be familiar with and able to apply the principles of the Mental Capacity Act 2005, Mental Health Act 2007, Care Act 2014 and local safeguarding procedures, should the patient be deemed to be a risk to themselves or others (NICE 2022b).

It is important to recognise that a factitious wound is often a sign that an individual is experiencing psychological distress (NHS Choices 2015). The treatment will involve understanding triggers for self-harm and providing a referral for support and guidance. This may be to the local mental health team or one of the many third-sector agencies available, such as Mind (NHS Choices 2015). A patient who self-harms will require the HCP to have empathy and understanding using a non-judgemental approach to gain the patient's trust (Hunt 2017). An understanding of underlying issues that have triggered the self-harm is essential, as the patient will need the correct psychological support to help prevent reoccurrence.

NICE (2022b) suggests that an important part of assisting a patient who self-harms is ensuring that appropriate support and guidance are given and recommends that information giving should be:

- Tailored to individual needs and circumstances, taking into account, for example, whether this is a first presentation or repeated self-harm, the severity and type of self-harm, and if the person has any co-existing health conditions, neurodevelopmental conditions or a learning disability.
- Provided throughout their care.
- Sensitive and empathetic.
- Supportive and respectful.
- Consistent with their care plan, if there is one in place.
- Conveyed in the spirit of hope and optimism.

It may not be possible to stop an individual from self-harming, therefore management should be centred around reducing harm (Kilroy-Findley and Bateman 2016). This may be achieved by providing patient education in the following areas:

- How to reduce the potential for a wound to get infected should the individual feel the need to undertake self-harm, e.g. by using a clean instrument during the process and ensuring that it is performed in a clean environment where possible.
- How to recognise the signs of infection and what to do if an infection is suspected.
- How to avoid areas where major blood vessels are present, reducing the risk of a major bleed.
- What to do if a major bleed occurs.
- Whom to contact when if the individual has any concerns.
- How to access local mental health services and mental health support groups.
- How to redress the wounds appropriately.

A recommended approach to dressing selection is to follow the principles of moist wound healing with dressings that are acceptable to the patient, and in many cases allow the individual to self-care if they need to self-harm (Hunt 2017). Covering wounds with occlusive

TABLE 3.11   Suggested contents of self-harm rescue pack.

All dressing products in the pack should be in accordance with
   local formulary

- Cleansing solution (water or saline) – an individual can use tap water if potable tap water is available
- Non-adherent wound contact layer
- Secondary dressing (e.g. sterile gauze/adhesive or non-adhesive foam) – this will depend on exudate levels
- Tubular bandage (may assist in securing dressings on a limb)
- Wound leaflet that includes how to undertake dressing changes and red flags – when to seek help for, e.g., excessive bleeding, or signs and symptoms of infection
- Information on where to seek help for self-harming

Source: Adapted from Hunt (2017).

dressings or making them inaccessible to the patient may not be helpful and may encourage the individual to self-harm on other areas of the body (Amr et al. 2017). Hunt (2017) has suggested providing the patient with a 'rescue pack' containing dressings that are easy for the individual to use and would assist in empowering the patient to manage their injuries safely while reducing the potential for infection (Table 3.11).

INFECTIVE CONDITIONS

Lower limb wounds can have various infective causes, including bacterial, viral, parasitic and fungal, resulting from infective conditions such as leishmaniasis, ecthyma and Hansen disease. While historically these types of conditions were associated with 'tropical' diseases and/or developing countries, they are increasingly being seen in developed countries as international travel and migration increase. As such, any patient who presents with an unusual ulcer and has recently returned from Asia, Africa, South America or Australia should consider a possible infective cause. Diagnosis will be predominantly through wound swabbing and a wide biopsy for tissue cultures would be indicated if considering an infective aetiology to a leg ulcer to identify the atypical organism to be treated (Shelling et al. 2010). Occasionally blood cultures may be required and a tissue biopsy for histology. Management should involve a specialist in infectious diseases to guide appropriate antibiotic or antifungal therapy, treatment strategies and localised wound care, dependent on the presentation and following wound assessment.

Ecthyma

Ecthyma is one of the more common infective causes of leg ulcers and develops from a bacterial skin infection – it is sometimes associated with deep impetigo. It is mainly caused by group A beta-haemolytic *Streptococci*, but is also often linked to *Pseudomonas aeruginosa* (sometimes referred to as ecthyma gangrenosum) and can also be caused by other common bacteria, such as *Staphylococcus aureus, Escherichia coli* and *Klebsiella pneumoniae* in some cases (Isoherranen et al. 2019). Ecthyma normally occurs when the skin is in poor condition, for example due to poor hygiene and malnutrition, or following an insect bite or sting, which is often the case when seen in a recent international traveller (Isoherranen et al. 2019).

Ecthyma usually begins as a yellowish pustule, typically to the lower limb, which can quickly ulcerate and develop a necrotic base with a purple/red border (Isoherranen et al. 2019) (Figure 3.18). There can be multiple lesions present and they often leave residual scarring. Ecthyma can be difficult to diagnose as it has numerous differential diagnoses, including leishmaniasis, Buruli ulcer, calciphylaxis, pyoderma gangrenosum and vasculitis (Vaiman et al. 2015).

Leishmaniasis

Cutaneous leishmaniasis (more commonly seen in developed countries) is caused by a parasitic infection transmitted through sandfly bites (Rice 2007). Approximately 20% of leishmaniasis lesions occur on the lower limbs (Ather et al. 2006).

Cutaneous leishmaniasis presents as an ulcerated lesion with raised, reddened edges and a crusty covering (Figure 3.19). Some lesions will heal spontaneously over a relatively long period of 4–15 months and can lead to severe scarring (Rice 2007).

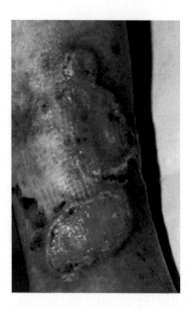

FIGURE 3.18 Ecthyma gangrenosum on the lower leg with multiple, painful ulcers with areas of necrosis and a purple/red edge.
Source: Kim et al. (2010) / John Wiley & Sons. Reproduced with permission.

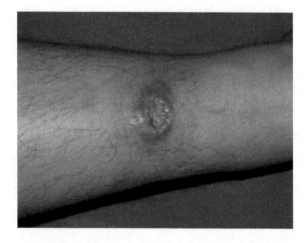

FIGURE 3.19 Cutaneous leishmaniasis.
Source: Neuber 2008 / John Wiley & Sons. Reproduced with permission.

Hansen Disease/Leprosy

Hansen disease or leprosy is caused by a bacterial organism called *Mycobacterium leprae,* transmitted through respiratory droplets. It mainly affects the skin and peripheral nerves; therefore patients may present with altered sensation and neuropathic ulcers to the legs and feet. Skin changes indicative of Hansen disease are thickened, cracked skin that is prone to ulceration, with possible papules or nodules and pale areas of skin that has lost its pigmentation (Walker and Lockwood 2007) (Figure 3.20).

Buruli Ulcers

Buruli ulcers are caused by a different *Mycobacterium* to Hansen disease, *Mycobacterium ulcerans,* and can be associated with mosquito bites, animal transmission and poor rural living conditions (Hartley 2014). These ulcers tend to present on the lower limbs as painless nodules or larger, hardened plaques that slowly develop into ulcers with undermined borders and necrosis over approximately

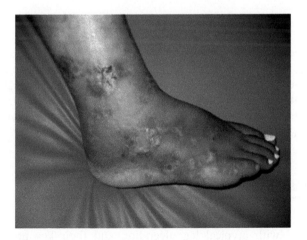

FIGURE 3.20 Leg ulcer associated with Hansen disease – note the areas of uneven pigmentation.
Source: Da Costa Nery et al. (2009) / John Wiley & Sons. Reproduced with permission.

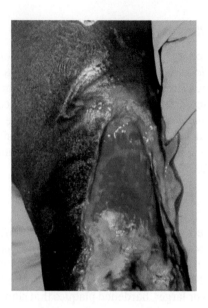

FIGURE 3.21 Buruli ulcer with typical necrosis and undermining edge. *Source:* Evans et al. (2003) / John Wiley & Sons. Reproduced with permission.

four weeks (Franco-Paredes et al. 2018) (Figure 3.21). Extensive swelling to the whole limb may occur and can be misdiagnosed as unresolved cellulitis or possibly related to a spider bite (Rice 2007).

Treatment can involve surgery and antibiotics, and local wound management may need to address the debridement of devitalised tissue and large volumes of thick exudate.

CONCLUSION

This chapter has highlighted some of the conditions that may be associated with atypical leg ulceration and their key presenting features and more typical patient histories. While the diagnosis of atypical leg ulcers will continue to be clinically challenging, an important focus should remain on making as early a diagnosis of the underlying aetiology as possible. Continuous reassessment of leg ulcers that are non-healing and unresponsive to standard therapies or with abnormal features is vital for detecting the more uncommon causes and allowing for more timely intervention. The HEIDI assessment framework can be used to guide the need for reassessment when wound progression is not as expected.

A multidisciplinary approach is key to the successful diagnosis and management of atypical leg ulcers. Aim to make prompt and appropriate referrals to relevant specialities as soon as suspicion is raised that an uncommon cause may be present.

Local wound care and skincare remain important considerations, as with other leg ulcer aetiologies, utilising the principles of wound bed preparation and the TIMES assessment to guide appropriate dressing selection and timely identification of infection. Pain assessment using a validated scale is of high importance for patients with atypical causes of leg ulcers; uncontrolled pain is a common presenting feature requiring an effective pain management plan and specialist advice. The judicious use of compression therapy in lower extremity wounds is considered beneficial for all leg wounds.

REFERENCES

Adderley, U.J. and Holt, I.G.S. (2014). Topical agents and dressings for fungating wounds. *Cochrane Database of Systematic Reviews* 15 (5): CD003948. https://doi.org/10.1002/14651858.CD003948.pub3.

Amr, A., Schmitt, C., Kuipers, T. et al. (2017). Identifying and managing patients with factitious wounds. *Advances in Skin & Wound Care* 30 (12): 1–7.

Anekar, A.A. and Cascella, M. (2023). WHO analgesic ladder. In: *StatPearls*. Treasure Island, FL: StatPearls Publishing https://www.ncbi.nlm.nih.gov/books/NBK554435.

Arnett, F.C., Cho, M., Chatterjee, S. et al. (2001). Familial occurrence frequencies and relative risks for systemic sclerosis (scleroderma) in 3 United States cohorts. *Arthritis and Rheumatism* 44 (6): 1359–1362.

Ather, S., Chan, D.S.Y., Leaper, D.J., and Harding, K.G. (2006). Case report and literature review of leishmaniasis as a cause of leg ulceration in the United Kingdom. *Journal of Wound Care* 15 (9): 389–391.

Australian Wound Management Association and New Zealand Wound Care Society (2011). Australian and New Zealand clinical practice guideline for prevention and management of venous leg ulcers. www.awma.com.au/files/publications/2011_awma_vlu_guideline_abridged.pdf

Babic, V., Petitpain, N., Guy, C. et al. (2018). Nicorandil-induced ulcerations: a 10-year observational study of all cases spontaneously reported to the French pharmacovigilance network. *International Wound Journal* 15 (4): 508–519.

Baby, D., Upadhyay, M., Joseph, M.D. et al. (2019). Calciphylaxis and its diagnosis: a review. *Journal of Family Medicine and Primary Care* 8 (9): 2763–2767.

Binus, A.M., Qureshi, A.A., Li, V.W. et al. (2011). Pyoderma gangrenosum: a retrospective review of patient characteristics, comorbidities and therapy in 103 patients. *British Journal of Dermatology* 165: 1244–1250.

Bliss, D.E. (2002). Calciphylaxis: what nurses need to know. *Nephrology Nursing Journal* 29 (5): 433–438.

Bonura, C., Frontino, G., Rigamonti, A. et al. (2014). Necrobiosis lipoidica diabeticorum: a pediatric case report. *Dermato-Endocrinology* 6 (1): e983683-1–e983683-3.

Bootan, R. (2013). Effects of immunosuppressive therapy on wound healing. *International Wound Journal* 10 (1): 98–104.

Brandow, A.M. and Liem, R.I. (2022). Advances in the diagnosis and treatment of sickle cell disease. *Journal of Haematology and Oncology* 15: 20. https://doi.org/10.1186/s13045-022-01237-z.

British Association of Dermatologists (2019). Patient information leaflet: Necrobiosis lipoidica. https://www.bad.org.uk/pils/necrobiosis-lipoidica.

British Association of Dermatologists (2022). Patient information leaflet: Erosive pustular dermatosis. https://badmainstage.wpengine.com/wp-content/uploads/2021/11/Erosive-pustular-dermatosis-PIL-16-Nov-2022.pdf

Brouard, M.C., Prins, C., Chavaz, P. et al. (2002). Erosive pustular dermatosis of the leg: report of three cases. *British Journal of Dermatology* 147 (4): 765–769.

Brown, A. (2015). The assessment and treatment of wound pain. *Nursing Times* 111 (47): 15–17.

Bull, R.H. and Mortimer, P.S. (1995). Erosive pustular dermatosis of the leg. *British Journal of Dermatology* 132 (2): 279–282.

Chakrabarty, A. and Phillips, T. (2003). Leg ulcers of unusual causes. *International Journal of Lower Extremity Wounds* 2 (4): 207–216.

Chang, J.J. (2019). Calciphylaxis: diagnosis, pathogenesis, and treatment. *Advances in Skin & Wound Care* 32 (5): 205–215.

Chave, T.A., Varma, S., and Knight, A.G. (2001). Dystrophic calcinosis cutis in venous ulcers: a cause of treatment failure. *British Journal of Dermatology* 145: 364–365.

Chinnadurai, R., Sinha, S., Lowney, A.C. et al. (2020). Pain management in patients with end-stage renal disease and calciphylaxis – a survey of clinical practices among physicians. *BMC Nephrology* 21: 403–411.

Choa, R., Rayatt, S., and Mahtani, K. (2015). Marjolin's ulcer. *BMJ* 351: h3997.

Combemale, P., Bousquet, M., Kanitakis, J. et al. (2007). Malignant transformation of leg ulcers: a retrospective study of 85 cases. *Journal of the European Academy of Dermatology and Venereology* 21 (7): 935–941.

Conde, E. (2015). Pustular and erosive leg dermatosis: you may have seen a case without knowing it. https://www.elenaconde.com/en/pustular-and-erosive-leg-dermatosis-you-may-have-seen-a-case-without-knowing-it

Conforti, A., Berardicurti, O., Pavlych, V. et al. (2021). Incidence of venous thromboembolism in rheumatoid arthritis, results from a 'real-life' cohort and an appraisal of available literature. *Medicine* 100 (33): e26953.

Da Costa Nery, J., Schreuder, P., Teixeira, C. et al. (2009). Hansen's disease in a general hospital: uncommon presentations and delay in diagnosis. *Journal of the European Academy of Dermatology and Venereology* 23: 150–156.

Dagregario, G. and Guillet, G. (2006). A retrospective review of 20 hypertensive leg ulcers treated with mesh skin grafts. *Journal of the European Academy of Dermatology and Venereology* 20 (2): 166–169.

Dawn, G., Loney, M., Zamiri, M. et al. (2003). Erosive pustular dermatosis of the leg associated with compression bandaging and fungal infection. *British Journal of Dermatology* 148 (3): 489–492.

DeBaun, M.R., Ghafuri, D.L., Rodeghier, M. et al. (2019). Decreased median survival of adults with sickle cell disease after adjusting for left truncation bias: a pooled analysis. *Blood* 133 (6): 615–617.

Denton, C.P., Hughes, M., and Gak, N. (2016). The BSR and BHPR guideline for scleroderma: what does it mean for patients? https://www.sruk.co.uk/about-us/news/bsrbhpr-guideline-scleroderma-what-does-it-mean

Di Altobrando, A., Patrizi, A., Vara, G. et al. (2020). Topical zinc oxide: an effective treatment option for erosive pustular dermatosis of the leg. *British Journal of Dermatology* 182 (2): 483–516.

Diepgen, T.L. and Maher, V. (2002). The epidemiology of skin cancer. *British Journal of Dermatology* 146 (s61): 1–6.

Dissemond, J., Assenheimer, B., Bultemann, A. et al. (2016). Compression therapy in venous leg ulcers. *Journal of the German Society of Dermatology* 14 (11): 1055–1200.

Dissemond, J., Erfurt-Berge, C., Goerge, T. et al. (2018). Systemic therapies for leg ulcers. *Journal of the German Society of Dermatology* 16 (7): 873–890.

Doran, J., Hope, V., Wright, T. et al. (2022). Prevalence and factors associated with chronic venous insufficiency, leg ulceration and deep-vein thrombosis among people who inject drugs. *Drug and Alcohol Review* 41: 677–685.

Duff, M., Demidova, O., Blackburn, S., and Shubrook, J. (2015). Cutaneous manifestations of diabetes mellitus. *Clinical Diabetes* 33 (1): 40–48.

Duffus-Grovell, D. (2021). Erosive pustular dermatosis: a complication in chronic venous leg ulcers. *Journal of Community Nursing* 35 (3): 42–48.

Edmonds, M. and Sumpio, B.E. (2019). *Limb Salvage of the Diabetic Foot: An Interdisciplinary Approach*. Cham: Springer Nature.

Edmundson, C., Croxford, S., Emanuel, E. et al. (2021). Increases in crack injection and associated risk factors among people who inject psychoactive drugs in England and Wales. International Network on Health and Hepatitis in Substance Users (INHSU) conference, 13 October. https://www.inhsu.org/resource/vp06-increases-in-crack-injection-and-associated-risk-factors-among-people-who-inject-psychoactive-drugs-pwid-in-england-and-wales

Enoch, S., Miller, D.R., Price, P.E., and Harding, K.G. (2004). Early diagnosis is vital in the management of squamous cell carcinomas associated with chronic non healing ulcers: a case series and review of the literature. *International Wound Journal* 1: 165–175.

Erdmann, M., Kiesewetter, F., Schuler, G., and Schultz, E. (2009). Erosive pustular dermatosis of the leg in a patient with ankylosing spondylitis: neutrophilic dysfunction as a common etiological factor? *International Journal of Dermatology* 48: 513–515. https://doi.org/10.1111/j.1365-4632.2009.03312.x.

Erfurt-Berge, C., Dissemond, J., Schwede, K. et al. (2015). Updated results of 100 patients on clinical features and therapeutic options in necrobiosis lipoidica in a retrospective multicentre study. *European Journal of Dermatology* 25 (6): 595–601.

Evans, M.R.W., Mawdsley, J., Bull, R. et al. (2003). Buruli ulcer in a visitor to London. *British Journal of Dermatology* 149: 907–909.

Falanga, V. (2007). Inflammatory ulcers. In: *Leg Ulcers A Problem-Based Learning Approach* (ed. M. Morison, C. Moffatt, and P. Franks), 341. Beijing: Mosby Elsevier.

Farrelly, I. (2018). The adversarial relationship between wounds and biomechanics in the lower limb. *Wounds UK* 14 (5): 70–76.

Feily, A. and Mehraban, S. (2015). Treatment modalities of necrobiosis lipoidica: a concise systematic review. *Dermatology Reports* 7 (2): 5749.

Firth, J. (2005). Tissue viability in rheumatoid arthritis. *Journal of Tissue Viability* 15 (3): 12–18.

Firth, J. (2011). Rheuamtoid arthritis: diagnosis and multi-disciplinary management. *British Journal of Nursing* 20 (19): 240–245.

Firth, J. and Critchley, S. (2011). Treating to target in rheumatoid arthritis: biologic therapies. *British Journal of Nursing* 20 (20): 1284–1291.

Fletcher, J., Alhusayen, R., and Alavi, A. (2019). Recent advances in managing and understanding pyoderma gangrenosum [version 1; peer review:

2 approved]. *F1000Research* 8:2092. https://doi.org/10.12688/f1000 research.19909.1

Franco-Paredes, C., Marcos, L.A., Henao-Martínez, A.F. et al. (2018). Cutaneous mycobacterial infections. *Clinical Microbiology Reviews* 32 (1): e00069-18.

Freak, J. (2005). Identification of skin cancers 2: malignant lesions. *British Journal of Community Nursing* 10 (2): 58–64.

Gardner, K., Douiri, A., Drasar, E. et al. (2016). Survival in adults with sickle cell disease in a high income setting. *Blood* 128 (10): 1436–1438.

George, C., Deroide, F., and Rustin, M. (2019). Pyoderma gangrenosum – a guide to diagnosis and management. *Clinical Medicine* 19 (3): 224–228.

Geraghty, J. (2021). Marginalised voices in wound care: experiences of people who inject drugs living with leg ulceration *"the gutter, the Nick or a box!!"*. *Journal of Tissue Viability* 30 (4): 499–504.

Ghaly, P., Illiopoulos, J., and Ahmad, M. (2021). The role of nutrition in wound healing: an overview. *British Journal of Nursing* 30 (5): S38–S42.

Graves, J.W., Morris, J.C., and Sheps, S.G. (2001). Matorell's hypertensive leg ulcer: case report and concise review of the literature. *Journal of Human Hypertension* 15 (4): 279–283.

Greenwood, C. (2021). Heel pressure ulcers: understanding why they develop and how to prevent them. *Nursing Standard* 37 (2): 60–66.

Gregson, C.L. and Allain, T.J. (2004). Amelanotic malignant melanoma disguised as a diabetic foot ulcer. *Diabetic Medicine* 21: 924–927.

Hafner, J., Nobbe, S., Partsch, H. et al. (2010). Martorell hypertensive ischaemic leg ulcer: a model of ischaemic subcutaneous arteriolosclerosis. *Archives of Dermatology* 146 (9): 961–968.

Harding, K.G., Gray, D., Timmons, J. et al. (2007). Evolution or revolution? Adapting to complexity in wound management. *International Wound Journal* 4 (s2): 1–12.

Harris, B., Eaglstein, W.H., and Falanga, V. (1993). Basal cell carcinoma arising in venous ulcers and mimicking granulation tissue. *Journal of Dermatologic Surgery and Oncology* 19 (2): 150–152.

Hartley, M. (2014). Buruli ulcer. *DermNetNZ*. https://dermnetnz.org/topics/buruli-ulcer.

Hay, G., Rael dos Santos, A., Reed, H., and Hope, V. (2017). *Estimates of opiate and crack cocaine use prevalence: 2016 to 2017*. Liverpool: Liverpool John Moores University https://www.ljmu.ac.uk/~/media/phi-reports/pdf/2017_09_estimates_of_the_prevalence_of_opiate_use_andor_crack_cocaine_use_201415_sweep_11_.pdf.

Hayes, S. and Dodds, S.R. (2003). The identification and diagnosis of malignant leg ulcers. *Nursing Times* 99 (31): 50–52.

Hess, C.T (2002). Calciphylaxis: identification and wound management. *Advances in Skin & Wound Care* 15 (2): 64.

van den Hoogen, F., Khanna, D., Fransen, J. et al. (2013). 2013 classification criteria for systemic sclerosis: an American College of Rheumatology/European League Against Rheumatism collaborative initiative. *Annals of the Rheumatic Diseases* 65 (11): 2737–2747.

Hudson, M., Thombs, B., Steele, R. et al. (2009). Health-related quality of life in systemic sclerosis: a systematic review. *Arthritis and Rheumatism* 61 (8): 111201120.

Hunt, S. (2017). Top tips: skin and tissue trauma caused by self-harm. *Wounds International* 8 (4): 12–17.

International Wound Infection Institute (IWII) (2022) Wound Infection in Clinical Practice. https://woundinfection-institute.com/wp-content/uploads/IWII-CD-2022-web-1.pdf

Isoherranen, K., Jordan O'Brien, J., Barker, J. et al. (2019). Atypical wounds: best clinical practice and challenges. EWMA document. *Journal of Wound Care* 28 (6): S1–S92.

Jebakumar, A., Udayakumar, D., Crowson, C. et al. (2014). Occurrence and impact of lower extremity ulcer in rheumatoid arthritis – a population based study. *Journal of Rheumatology* 41 (3): 437–443.

Jeffcoate, W.J., Chipchase, S.Y., Ince, P. et al. (2006). Assessing the outcome of the management of diabetic foot ulcers using ulcer-related and person-related measures. *Diabetes Care* 29: 1784–1787.

Jones, O.T., Ranmuthu, C.K.I., Hall, P.N. et al. (2020). Recognising skin cancer in primary care. *Advances in Therapy* 37: 603–616.

Karimkhani, C., Boyers, L.N., Dellavalle, R.P., and Weinstock, M.A. (2015). It's time for 'keratinocyte carcinoma' to replace the term 'nonmelanoma skin cancer'. *Journal of the American Academy of Dermatology* 72 (1): 186–187.

Kavitha, K.V., Tiwari, S., Purandare, V.B. et al. (2014). Choice of wound care in diabetic foot ulcer: a practical approach. *World Journal of Diabetes* 5 (4): 554–556.

Khimdas, S., Harding, S., Bonner, A. et al. (2011). Associations with digital ulcers in a large cohort of systemic sclerosis: results from the Canadian scleroderma research group registry. *Arthritis Care and Research* 63: 142–149.

Kilroy-Findley, A. and Bateman, S. (2016). Case studies: Octenilin wound irrigation solution and Octenisan wash in self-harm wounds. *Wounds UK* 12 (4): 88–94.

Kim, H.S., Lee, J.S.S., and Tand, M.B.Y. (2010). Localized ecthyma gangrenosum in patients with diabetes mellitus: diagnosis and management. *Journal of Dermatology* 37: 758–761.

King, T., Carr, R.A., and Sharma, M. (2017). A painful leg ulcer. *Clinical and Experimental Dermatology* 42: 106–108.

Kodumudi, V., Jeha, G.M., Mydlo, N., and Kaye, A.D. (2020). Management of cutaneous calciphylaxis. *Advances in Therapy* 37 (12): 4797–4807.

Koshy, M., Entuah, R., Koranda, A. et al. (1989). Leg ulcers in patients with sickle cell disease. *Blood* 74 (4): 1403–1408.

Kuypers, D.R.J. (2009). Skin problems in chronic kidney disease. *Nature Clinical Practice. Nephrology* 5 (3): 157–170.

Lacroix, R., Kalisiak, M., and Rao, J. (2008). Can you identify this condition? *Canadian Family Physician* 54 (6): 857–867.

Lang, K., Neil, J., Wright, J. et al. (2013). Qualitative investigation of barriers to accessing care by people who inject drugs in Saskatoon, Canada: perspectives of service providers. *Substance Abuse Treatment, Prevention, and Policy* 8: 35.

Lee, K., Carley, S., Kraus, C., and Mesinkovska, N.A. (2020). Treatment of erosive pustular dermatosis: a systematic review of the literature. *International Journal of Dermatology* 59 (7): 770–786.

Leloup, P., Toussaint, P., Lembelembe, J.P. et al. (2015). The analgesic effect of electrostimulation (WoundEL) in the treatment of leg ulcers. *International Wound Journal* 12: 706–709.

Mackie, R.M. (1990). Clinical recognition of early invasive malignant melanoma. *BMJ* 301 (6759): 1005–1006.

Mansour, M. and Alavi, A. (2019). Martorell ulcer: chronic wound management and rehabilitation. *Chronic Wound Care Management Research* 6: 83–88.

Maronese, C., Pimentel, M., Li, M. et al. (2022). Pyoderma gangrenosum: an updated literature review on established and emerging pharmacological treatment. *American Journal of Clinical Dermatology* 23: 615–634.

Maverakis, E., Ma, C., Shinkai, K. et al. (2018). Diagnostic criteria of ulcerative pyoderma gangrenosum. A Delphi consensus of international experts. *JAMA Dermatology* 154: 461–466.

Menendez, M. and Warriner, R.A. (2006). Marjolin's ulcer: report of 2 cases. *Wounds* 18 (3): 65–70.

Micheletti, R.G. (2022). Treatment of cutaneous vasculitis. *Frontiers in Medicine (Lausanne)* 9: 1059612.

Minniti, C.P. and Kato, G. (2016). How we treat sickle patients with leg ulcers. *American Journal of Hematology* 91 (1): 22–30.

Misciali, C., Dika, E., Fanti, P.A. et al. (2013). Frequency of malignant neoplasms in 257 chronic leg ulcers. *Dermatologic Surgery* 39 (6): 849–854.

Mistry, B.D., Alavi, A., Ali, S., and Mistry, N. (2017). A systematic review of the relationship between glycaemic control and necrobiosis lipoidica diabeticorum in patients with diabetes mellitus. *International Journal of Dermatology* 56: 1319–1327.

Murray, C.A. and Miller, R.A. (1997). Necrobiosis lipoidica diabeticorum and thyroid disease. *International Journal of Dermatology* 36: 799.

National Institute for Health and Care Excellence (NICE) (2016). Sunlight exposure: risks and benefits. NICE guideline [NG34]. https://www.nice.org.uk/guidance/ng34

National Institute for Health and Care Excellence (NICE) (2020). Clinical knowledge summary: Rheumatoid arthritis – how common is it? https://cks.nice.org.uk/topics/rheumatoid-arthritis/background-information/prevalence-incidence

National Institute for Health and Care Excellence (NICE) (2022a). Melanoma clinical knowledge summary. https://cks.nice.org.uk/topics/melanoma.

National Institute for Health and Care Excellence (NICE) (2022b). Self harm – assessment, management and preventing reccurrence. NICE guideline [NG225]. www.nice.org.uk/guidance/ng225

National Wound Care Strategy Programme (2023). Recommendations for lower limb ulcer. https://www.nationalwoundcarestrategy.net/wp-content/uploads/2023/08/NWCSP-Leg-Ulcer-Recommendations-1.8.2023.pdf

Nelzen, O., Bergqvist, D., and Lindhagen, A. (1994). Venous and non-venous leg ulcers: clinical history and appearance in a population study. *British Journal of Surgery* 81 (2): 182–187.

Neuber, H. (2008). Leishmaniasis. *Journal der Deutschen Dermatologischen Gesellschaft* 6: 754–765.

Ng, A.T. and Peng, D.H. (2011). Calciphylaxis. *Dermatologic Therapy* 24: 256–262.

Ngan, V. (2005). Calcinosis cutis. *DermNetNZ*. https://dermnetnz.org/topics/calcinosis-cutis

NHS Choices (2015) Self-harm. https://www.nhs.uk/mental-health/feelings-symptoms-behaviours/behaviours/self-harm

Nichol, P., Perceau, G., Barbe, C., and Bernard, P. (2017). Erosive pustular dermatosis of the leg: a prospective, multicentre, observational study of 36 cases. *Annales de Dermatologie et de Venereologie* 144 (10): 582–588.

Nickles, M., Tsoukas, M., Sweiss, N. et al. (2022). Atypical ulcers: a stepwise approach for clinicians. *Wounds* 34 (10): 236–244.

Nigwekar, S.U., Thadhani, R., and Brandenburg, V.M. (2018). Calciphylaxis. *New England Journal of Medicine* 378 (18): 1704–1714.

Oakley, A. (2016). Differential diagnosis of leg ulcer. https://dermnetnz.org/topics/differential-diagnosis-of-leg-ulcer

Oakley, A. (2021). Necrobiosis lipoidica. *DermNetNZ*. https://dermnetnz.org/topics/necrobiosis-lipoidica

Oakley, A. and Stevens, T. (2023). Dermoscopy. *DermNetNZ*. https://dermnetnz.org/topics/dermoscopy

Ousey, K., Chadwick, P., and Cook, L. (2011). Diabetic foot or pressure ulcer on the foot? *Wounds UK* 7 (3): 105–108.

Paron, N.G. and Lambert, P.W. (2000). Cutaneous manifestations of diabetes mellitus. *Primary Care* 27: 371–383.

Partsch, H. and Mortimer, P. (2015). Compression for leg wounds. *British Journal of Dermatology* 173: 359–369.

Patel, G. and Piguet, V. (2022). Uncommon causes of ulceration. In: *ABC of Wound Healing*, 2e (ed. A. Price, J. Grey, G. Patel, and K. Harding), 49. Oxford: Wiley-Blackwell.

Paul, J.C. and Pieper, B.A. (2008). Topical metronidazole for the treatment of wound odour: a review of the literature. *Ostomy/Wound Management* 54 (3): 18–27.

Poccia, I., Persichetti, P., Marangi, G.F. et al. (2014). Basal cell carcinoma arising in a chronic venous leg ulcer: two cases and a review of the literature. *Wounds* 26 (4): E30–E35.

Pope, J.E. (2022). Limited cutaneous systemic sclerosis. *BMJ Best Practice*. https://bestpractice.bmj.com/topics/en-gb/593/pdf/593/Limited%20 cutaneous%20systemic%20sclerosis.pdf

Price, A., Grey, J., Patel, G., and Harding, K. (ed.) (2022). *ABC of Wound Healing*, 2e. Oxford: Wiley-Blackwell.

Ramadan, F. (2023). Adverse cutaneous drug reactions: manifestations, diagnosis and management. *British Journal of Community Nursing* 28 (2): 72–76.

Rayner, R., Carville, K., Keaton, J. et al. (2009). Leg ulcers: atypical presentations and associated comorbidities. *Wound Practice and Research* 17 (4): 168–185.

Reid, S.D., Ladizinski, B., Lee, K. et al. (2013). Update on necrobiosis lipoidica: a review of etiology, diagnosis, and treatment options. *Journal of the American Academy of Dermatology* 69: 783–791.

Reschke, R., Grunewald, S., Paasch, U. et al. (2021). Erosive pustular dermatosis of the scalp: clinicopathological correlation leading to a definition. *Wounds* 33 (6): 143–146.

Rice, J. (2007). Unusual leg ulcers: a global phenomenon. *Primary Intention* 15 (4): 165–175.

Roncada, E.V., Abreu, M.A., Pereira, M.F. et al. (2012). Calciphylaxis, a diagnostic and therapeutic challenge: report of a successful case. *Anais Brasileiros de Dermatologia* 87 (5): 752–755.

Saaiq, M. and Ashraf, B. (2014). Marjolin's ulcers in the post-burned lesions and scars. *World Journal of Clinical Cases* 2 (10): 507–514.

Sanchez, D.P., Tookes, H., Pastar, I., and Lev-Tov, H. (2021). Wounds and skin and soft tissue infections in people who inject drugs and the utility of syringe service programs in their management. *Advances in Wound Care* 10 (10): 571–582.

Santos-Juanes, J., Galache, C., Curto, J.R. et al. (2004). Squamous cell carcinoma arising in long-standing necrobiosis lipoidica. *Journal of the European Academy of Dermatology and Venereology* 18 (2): 199–200.

Scott-Thomas, J., Hayes, C., Ling, J. et al. (2017). A practice guide to systematic wound assessment to meet the 2017–19 CQUIN target. *Journal of Community Nursing* 31 (5): 30–34.

Seitz, C.A., Berens, N., Brocker, E.-B. et al. (2010). Leg ulceration in rheumatoid arthritis--an underreported multicausal complication with considerable morbidity: analysis of thirty-six patients and review of the literature. *Dermatology* 220 (3): 268–273.

Senet, P. (2014). Cutaneous cancers and chronic leg ulcers. *Phlebolymphology* 21 (2): 75–80.

Senet, P., Combemale, P., Combemale, P. et al. (2012). Malignancy and chronic leg ulcers: the value of systematic wound biopsies: a prospective, multicenter, cross-sectional study. *Archives of Dermatology* 148 (6): 704–708.

Shanmugam, V.K., Price, P., Attinger, C.E. et al. (2010). Lower extremity ulcers in systemic sclerosis: features and response to therapy. *International Journal of Rheumatology* 2010: 747946.

Shelling, M.L., Federman, D.G., and Kirsner, R.S. (2010). Clinical approach to atypical wounds with a new model for understanding hypertensive ulcers. *Archives of Dermatology* 146 (9): 1026–1029.

Shimizu, I., Cruz, A., Chang, K.H., and Dufresne, R.G. (2011). Treatment of squamous cell carcinoma in situ: a review. *Dermatologic Surgery* 37 (10): 1394–1411.

Stringer, J., Donald, G., Knowles, R., and Warn, P. (2014). The symptom management of fungating malignant wounds using a novel essential oil cream. *Wounds UK* 10 (3): 54–59.

Tandler, S. and Stephen-Haynes, J. (2017). Fungating wounds: management and treatment options. *British Journal of Nursing* 26 (12): S6–S14.

Tate, S., Price, A., and Harding, K. (2019). Cutaneous wounds in systemic sclerosis. *Wounds UK* 15 (1): 44–47.

Tchanque-Fossuo, C.N., Millsop, J.W., Johnson, M.A. et al. (2018). Ulcerated basal cell carcinomas masquerading as venous leg ulcers. *Advances in Skin & Wound Care* 31 (3): 130–134.

Tillman, D. (2004). Uncommon causes of leg ulceration and lesions not to be missed. *British Journal of Community Nursing* 2004 (Suppl 5): S23–S28.

Todhunter, J. (2019). Understanding the differential diagnosis of leg ulcers: focus on atypical leg ulcers. *Journal of Community Nursing* 33 (1): 29–37.

Trent, J.T. and Kirsner, R.S. (2003). Wounds and malignancy. *Advances in Skin & Wound Care* 16 (1): 31–34.

Trent, J.T. and Kirsner, R.S. (2004). Leg ulcers in sickle cell disease. *Advances in Skin Wound Care* 17: 410–416.

UK Health Security Agency (UKHSA) (2022). People who inject drugs: HIV and viral hepatitis monitoring. https://www.gov.uk/government/publications/people-who-inject-drugs-hiv-and-viral-hepatitis-monitoring

UK Health Security Agency, Public Health Agency Northern Ireland, Public Health Scotland and Public Health Wales (UKHSA) (2023). Shooting up: infections and other injecting-related harms among people who inject drugs in the UK. Data to end of 2021. London: UK Health Security Agency. https://www.gov.uk/government/publications/shooting-up-infections-among-people-who-inject-drugs-in-the-uk

Vaiman, M., Lazarovitch, T., Heller, L., and Lotan, G. (2015). Ecthyma gangrenosum and ecthyma-like lesions: review article. *European Journal of Clinical Microbiology & Infectious Diseases* 34 (4): 633–639.

Volkmann, E.R., Andreasson, K., and Smith, V. (2023). Systemic sclerosis. *Lancet* 401: 304–318.

Walker, S.L. and Lockwood, D.N.J. (2007). Leprosy. *Clinics in Dermatology* 25: 165–172.

Weinstien, D., Araujo, T., and Kirsner, S. (2012). Atypical wounds. In: *Wound Care Essentials Practice Principles*, 3e (ed. S. Baranoski and E. Ayello), 492–493. Philadelphia, PA: Wolters Kluwer/Lippincott Williams and Wilkins.

White, R. (1999). A new standard for the nursing assessment of leg ulcers. *British Journal of Nursing* 8 (19): 1272–1282.

Wounds International (2012). *International Case Series: Using Actisorb*. London: Wounds International.

Wounds UK (2016). *Best Practice Statement: Holistic Management of Venous Leg Ulceration*. London: Wounds UK.

Wounds UK (2018). *Best Practice Statement: Improving Holistic Assessment of Chronic Wounds*. London: Wounds UK.

Wounds UK (2019). *Best Practice Statement: Ankle Brachial Pressure Index (ABPI) in Practice*. London: Wounds UK.

Young, T. (2019). Rheumatoid arthritis and its impact on ulceration and healing. *Wounds UK* 15 (4): 40–43.

Youseff, J., Novosad, S., and Winithrop, K. (2016). Infection risk and safety of corticosteroid use. *Rheumatic Disease Clinics of North America* 42 (1): 157–176.

Zhang, D. and McMullin, G. (2022). Necrobiosis lipoidica: a review of management and the role of compression. *Wound Practice and Research* 30 (1): 11–15.

Zhou, Z., Zhang, Z.K., and Liu, T.H. (2015). Erosive pustular dermatosis of the leg mimicking lower limb cellulitis. *Clinical and Experimental Dermatology* 40 (8): 865–867.

CHAPTER 4

Musculoskeletal Factors in Leg Ulcers

Assessment and Management

RONA FRANCES CAMPBELL

There is a growing recognition that sub-optimal movement, reduced mobility and impaired biomechanical function have an impact on the development and longevity of lower limb complications that relate to chronic venous disease (CVD), venous leg ulcers (VLUs) and lymphoedema (Araujo et al. 2016; Farrelly 2018; Meulendijks et al. 2020a, 2020b).

Enhancing patient movement and addressing musculoskeletal (MSK) and biomechanical concerns is key in optimising compression therapy during an episode of ulceration. Optimal movement and mobility also helps to mitigate complications like peripheral oedema and impaired joint mobility (Wounds 2016).

Optimal physical function reflects adequate motor control, physical fitness and the ability to mobilise freely on a regular basis (Langhammer et al. 2018). Inactivity or immobility, whether because of pain, injury, systemic disease, neuropathy, non-neurological MSK disease or the ageing process, can lead to sub-optimal movement and changes in physical and biomechanical function that can increase venous hypertension (Langhammer et al. 2018).

Lower Limb and Leg Ulcer Assessment and Management, First Edition.
Edited by Aby Mitchell, Georgina Ritchie, and Alison Hopkins.
© 2024 John Wiley & Sons Ltd. Published 2024 by John Wiley & Sons Ltd.

People with CVD and VLUs are known to present with biome-chanical issues, for example impairment in ankle joint movement or gait dysfunction (Figure 4.1) (Back et al. 1995; Clarke-Moloney et al. 2007; Araujo et al. 2016). These issues can result in adverse changes in important physiological processes that ensure lower limb health and venous return, namely the veno-muscular pumps (VMPs) (Uhl and Gillot 2015; NICE 2021). The VMPs are important anatomi-cal pumps in the lower limb, and they help mediate haemodynamic homeostasis within the circulatory system and aid venous return when activated through regular MSK movement (Uhl and Gil-lot 2015). An important VMP in the lower limb is the calf muscle pump (CMP). Failure and dysfunction of this pump through a reduc-tion in ankle joint range of motion (ROM) and adverse changes in gait are major contributory factors in the development and chronicity of CVD and VLUs (Lattimer et al. 2017).

This chapter will examine the factors that influence mobility, lower limb biomechanical function and the influence of sub-optimal gait, with a focus on the lower limb VMPs and ankle joint ROM.

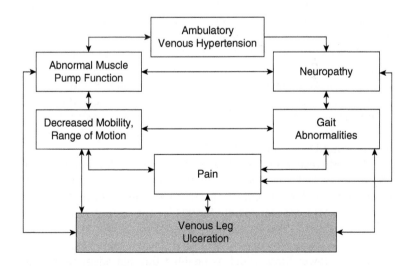

FIGURE 4.1 Biomechanical factors that influence venous leg ulceration. *Source:* Shiman et al. 2009/John Wiley & Sons. Reproduced with permission.

Understanding how these biomechanical factors affect the management of patients with CVD and VLUs is vital. These factors relating to mobility impairment are known to have a negative influence on the onset and progress of CVD, VLUs and wound healing (Padberg et al. 2004). Moreover, a loss in mobility is known to have an impact on quality of life (QoL) (Meulendijks et al. 2020b).

RISK FACTORS

There are known non-modifiable established risk factors in patients who have CVD and VLUs, such as age, sex and family history (NICE 2021). However, there is a sub-section of modifiable risk factors that relate to mobility and the biomechanical function (refer to risk factors in Chapter 5) for those who have CVD and VLUs which are poorly understood, and these relate to sub-optimal mobility and biomechanical and gait dysfunction.

During holistic lower limb assessment, screening for risk factors that relate to an individual's mobility and biomechanical function in conjunction with those relating to VLUs is important for optimal clinical outcomes, as poor mobility can have an impact on many areas within wound care management (O'Brien et al. 2014; Smith et al. 2018). However, screening for mobility risk factors for patients who have VLUs may be perceived as challenging for a nurse when evidence suggests that delivering essential care can in some cases be difficult in a busy clinical setting (Guest et al. 2018). Moreover, biomechanical and mobility factors are not always recognised as important risk factors for the development and chronicity of VLUs within wound care management (Farrelly 2018).

A poorly recognised mobility risk factor for the development and chronicity of VLUs is CMP dysfunction. The CMP is in the lower, posterior leg and is one of the important VMPs in the lower limb and foot. The VMPs are responsible for 90% of the venous return from the lower limb to the trunk (Williams et al. 2014). The CMP is responsible for approximately 65% of the net venous blood return within the lower limb, which is enabled through adequate movement at the ankle (Williams et al. 2014).

CMP dysfunction is not only a risk factor for VLUs, but also for deep vein thrombosis (DVT), and is an independent predictor of all-cause mortality (Araki et al. 1994; Back et al. 1995; Milic et al. 2009; Halkar et al. 2020). Therefore, recognition of CMP dysfunction is important not only within the context of VLU management, but in relation to the overall health of the patient.

A major biomechanical risk factor influencing CMP dysfunction is the loss of ankle joint ROM (Back et al. 1995; de Souza et al. 2022). Research suggests that when ankle joint ROM is reduced there is an increased risk of developing an ulceration (Table 4.1) (Araki et al. 1994). Once an ulcer has developed, the episode of wound healing can be prolonged compared to people with adequate ROM when using compression bandaging (Barwell et al. 2000). When movement at the ankle is impaired, there is a reduction in the functional

TABLE 4.1 Biomechanical risk factors that may contribute to developing a venous leg ulcer.

Risk factor	Explanation
Immobility	Increased risk of venous hypertension and oedema
	Reduction in joint ROM
	Sarcopenia
	Obesity
Limited ankle range of motion (ROM)	Calf muscle pump (CMP) dysfunction
	Impact on gait
	Fixed joint position
Sedentary lifestyle	Obesity
	Gait impairment
	Impact on CMP function
History of leg fracture or trauma	Impaired gait
	Damage to the venous and lymphatic anatomy
	Impaired joint ROM
Lower limb dysfunction/ structural deformities	Leg length discrepancy
	Pelvic obliquity
	Genu valgum/recuvartum
	Highly pronated or supinated foot postures
Underlying musculoskeletal disease	Diseases that cause issues with balance and proprioception
	Diseases that result in structural deformities
	Diseases that result in gait dysfunction

emptying of the venous system, which can lead to venous hypertension and VLUs (Yang et al. 1999; Houghton et al. 2021). Optimal movement of the ankle is also important for efficient ambulation. A reduction in ankle movement is known to have an impact on knee and hip function, which can lead to gait dysfunction and compromise the efficiency of the lower limb VMPs (Simonsen 2014). Pain can also cause a person to restrict movement of a joint and when this occurs at the ankle it can result in an antalgic gait pattern. An antalgic gait pattern is defined as a way of walking that offloads or reduces pain in an area of the body and can result in a limp or irregular walking pattern (Simonsen 2014).

An example of the impact in the lower limb when an antalgic gait is present is when a patient offloads a painful ulcer in the medial ankle by lifting the heel during gait. This change in the position and movement of the ankle results in a contracture of the calf muscle complex, a change in the alignment of the ankle and subtalar joint and reduced ankle joint ROM leading to an equinus foot position. Over time, this equinus foot position can become rigid which can cause malalignment at the knee, hip and pelvis. This has an impact on the CMP and will restrict its efficacy due to the malalignment of the foot and ankle.

The National Wound Care Strategy Programme (National Wound Care Strategy 2023) recognises the importance of assessing ankle joint mobility: 'joint mobility, particularly that of the ankle, is an important component of calf muscle pump function and should be carefully recorded' (National Wound Care Strategy 2023). Therefore, recognition of reduced ankle joint ROM and its impact on wound healing and gait dysfunction is important within clinical practice, as this loss can lead to complications and impaired wound healing (Wounds 2016).

LOWER LIMB VENO-MUSCULAR PUMPS

The underlying factors in the development of CVD and VLUs are multifactorial (NWCSP 2020). There are three important physiological factors that can exist in isolation or in any combination that can lead to the development and longevity of CVD and VLUs (NICE 2021).

These are valvular insufficiency, venous obstruction and CMP dysfunction (NICE 2021).

Arterial blood flow is operated by the rhythmic pumping action of the heart and through the elastic recoil of the arterial walls (Horwood 2021).The venous system is subject to lower pressures compared with, and is structurally different from, the arterial system within the systemic circulation (Kan and Delis 2001). Veins contain valves. The venous bicuspid valves in the lower limb work through antegrade pressure gradients, causing the opening and closure of the valves when there is a reversal in the pressure gradient above and below the valves moving blood flow proximally (Horwood 2019). However, in the presence of CVD these valves can fail. That coupled with the force of gravity and the fact that humans are bipedal can inhibit venous return. To overcome factors that inhibit venous return, the VMPs have evolved in the lower limb and work to activate MSK pumps through movement (Horwood 2019). These VMPs are vital in mitigating increased venous pressure by aiding venous return when standing upright and walking through a pumping action when moving, especially during walking (Padberg et al. 2004; Williams et al. 2014).

There are three VMPs located in the lower limb: one on the foot, the calf muscle complex in the posterior lower leg and the posterior thigh. These pumps, particularly the CMP, act as a peripheral heart by mechanically generating venous return from the foot pump via the CMP to the thigh pump during the cyclical, synchronised movements in the gait cycle (Ricci 2020).

Foot Pump

The foot pump is located within the venous network of the plantar and dorsal foot. There are five venous systems located in the foot: the superficial and deep veins on the plantar surface of the foot, the superficial dorsal plexus, and the marginal and dorsal arch perforating systems (Ricci 2020). The foot pump was considered historically to be insignificant in the physiological return of blood proximally in the lower limb and was theorised to work during weight-bearing only (Gardner et al. 1983). However, it is now theorised that the operation of the foot pump depends on many factors, which include compliance of the soft tissues surrounding the foot veins, the deep fascia, intrinsic muscle activity and ankle kinematics (motion) (Horwood 2019). Therefore, efficient function of the foot pump also depends on intact and fully functioning structures in the foot.

Calf Muscle Pump

The CMP can be divided into two anatomical locations (Ricci 2020). The leg pump is located in the veins of the soleus muscle and the popliteal pump ends in the popliteal vein (Ricci 2020). The medial gastrocnemius veins have a distinct plexus (network of blood vessels) of veins above the knee (Uhl and Gillot 2015; Ricci 2020). In the lower leg the lateral veins of the soleus are larger than the medial veins. These drain vertically into the peroneal veins. The medial veins of the soleus are smaller and join the posterior tibial veins horizontally (Uhl and Gillot 2015). At the popliteal level within the lower limb, the medial gastrocnemius veins are the largest veins that end uniquely as a large collector into the popliteal vein above the knee joint. When walking, with each step muscular activity exerts pressure on the venous system and there is a high-speed ejection within the venous network that propels a powerful jet of venous blood into the popliteal vein (Uhl and Gillot 2015).

Thigh Pump

The most proximal pump within the lower limb is the thigh pump. The semimembranosus muscles and the femoral vein work in tandem in this anatomical area to generate venous return during walking and movement (Uhl and Gillot 2015).

Mechanism of Action of the Veno-muscular Pumps

The VMPs are musculo-venous pumps that perform an important role in venous return in the lower limb through a chain of events that occurs through the activation of the muscles located in the lower limb during walking (Uhl and Gillot 2015). However, these are not the only mechanisms through which pressure is generated within the VMPs.

The muscle groups that make up the VMPs in the lower limb are organised into myofascial compartments of the lower limb – for example, the posterior compartment of the lower leg has a deep and superficial region, and the group of muscles is encased in a fascia (Meissner 2005; Palastanga and Soames 2018). These myofascial compartments are encased in connective fascial tissue, which further helps increase pressures within the compartments and assists antegrade blood flow.

During gait or on joint movement, muscles within these compartments in the lower limb will eccentrically (lengthen) or concentrically (shorten) contract, and this tightens the fascial compartments and associated connective tissues (Palastanga and Soames 2018). The net result is increased pressure on the venous system passing through the muscle or the compartment of the leg (Horwood 2019). This mechanism of action occurs regardless of the type of muscular contraction, whether this be eccentric or concentric contraction. These mechanisms when working optimally result in unhampered venous return (Horwood 2019).

Calf Muscle Pump Dysfunction

Research suggests that CMP dysfunction is estimated to be present in 55% of people who have CVD (Williams et al. 2014). Adequate venous return is dependent on a patent, healthy venous system, optimal gait and an operational CMP. The CMP is considered the 'second heart' and is a contributor to the cardiovascular system by enabling venous return from the lower limb to the right atrium (Halkar et al. 2020). In understanding how CMP dysfunction can develop from a mechanical aspect, it is important to understand the basic function of the ankle joint.

In terms of its structure, the appearance of the ankle joint is like that of a mortise and tenon and it is constructed at the distal ends of the tibia and fibula with the superior aspect of the talus (Palastanga and Soames 2018). The ankle joint is a synovial hinge joint. The ankle joint is classically considered to move around a single axis, within the sagittal plane, and the primary motion in this plane is dorsiflexion and plantarflexion (Brockett and Chapman 2016). The ankle joint is a complex of the talocalcaneal (subtalar), tibiotalar (talocrural) and transverse tarsal (talocalcaneonavicular) joints (Brockett and Chapman 2016). Although dorsiflexion and plantarflexion are the primary movements, there is also a smaller degree of movement in the transverse (adduction and abduction) and frontal planes (inversion and eversion) (Brockett and Chapman 2016; Palastanga and Soames 2018).

It is the movements of dorsiflexion and plantarflexion that occur at the ankle joint that influence muscle activity and tissue tension in the triceps surae (calf muscle) complex in the posterior compartment of the lower leg. These movements trigger CMP activation (Horwood 2021). Any alteration in dorsiflexion and plantarflexion clinically is of relevance and will have the greatest mechanical impact on a patient's gait and CMP function. The possible reasons behind a reduction in ankle joint ROM or biomechanical alteration are multifactorial and should be considered when taking a holistic history.

ANKLE JOINT ASSESSMENT

The ankle joint is complex and forms the link between the interface of the lower leg and the ground via the foot (Brockett and Chapman 2016). It is crucial in the operation of the VMPs in the lower limb. Its function is key not only as the simple machine that helps the CMP to function, but also as an important joint that aids sagittal plane (dorsiflexion and plantarflexion) movement in the lower limb, allowing people to walk efficiently and perform other activities of daily life (Brockett and Chapman 2016).

Given these factors and the impact of reduced ankle joint ROM, which can contribute to the development and chronicity of VLUs, it is vital that ankle joint mobility is assessed on a regular basis (NWCSP 2020). Ideally, when assessing if joint ROM is impaired, then the joint under measurement should be compared to matched controls to determine if there is an impairment (Norkin and White 2016). However, when this is not possible the contralateral limb should be used for comparison if it is not impaired (Norkin and White 2016).

Assessing ankle joint ROM can be done in several ways using quantitative and qualitative measures. There are several instruments that are available to measure joint ROM that range from tape measures to manual and digital goniometers (Figure 4.2), inclinometers and motion capture devices (Norkin and White 2016).

A goniometer is a device that measures angles and allows the rotation of an object to a defined position. It is still the most used,

(a) (b)

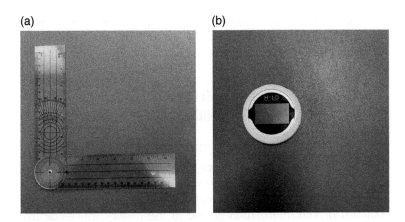

FIGURE 4.2 (a) Universal and (b) digital goniometers.

economical, portable device for the evaluation of ROM (Nussbaumer et al. 2010; Norkin and White 2016). Competency in goniometry requires that the examiner is knowledgeable in the structure and function of each joint measured and demands a specific skill set to enable accurate results (Norkin and White 2016). The use of a goniometer is not always common within nursing practice. Therefore, when in-depth assessment of ankle joint ROM using the goniometer is required, the patient should be referred to a therapist who can accurately carry out these measurements.

One method of assessing ankle ROM is by looking at, feeling and moving the joint. These skills would be within the clinical skill set of nursing:

- *Look*: Visually inspect the position of the ankle when the patient is on the couch. Look at the alignment of the ankle and check if there is any visual oedema around the ankle joint, as this can lead to a restriction in ROM.
- *Feel*: Palpate around the joint, as this enables the clinician to determine the type of oedema present, and/or if there are any unusual anatomical changes in the ankle joint or any bony pathology, like osteoarthritis or any other anatomical variation.
- *Move*: Moving the joint by way of dorsiflexing and plantarflexing the foot will enable the clinician to determine if the ankle is rigid,

semi-rigid, flexible or hypermobile. Compare to the contralateral side if this is not impaired to gain an awareness of the possible impairment on the side being assessed.

HOLISTIC HISTORY TAKING RELATING TO FACTORS THAT INFLUENCE BIOMECHANICAL LOWER LIMB FUNCTION

Taking a thorough medical history that includes social and patient-related factors like injuries is key to understanding a patient's issues and establishing information that may relate to their mobility (Day 2015). The information gained in the history will guide the practitioner in their physical examination and determine the relevant clinical tests that may be required. Thorough history taking facilitates the collection of important information that will be relevant when communicating with other practitioners involved in the care of the patient or gathering information that will be required when making a referral (Franks et al. 2016). Knowledge of the medical history that relates to lower limb function is vital, because it identifies those patients with modifiable biomechanical risk factors that can result in CMP dysfunction or gait issues that can have an impact on wound healing.

People with CVD and VLUs typically have a disproportionate number of co-morbidities and may report lower levels of activity and decreased mobility compared to the population. (Clarke-Moloney et al. 2007). Many patients with VLUs may be physically deconditioned and have compromised core strength and lower limb weakness, and may present with gait and biomechanical issues (Clarke-Moloney et al. 2007; Farrelly 2018). Therefore, identifying the patient-related factors and managing biomechanical-related issues is paramount for optimising mobility and biomechanical function.

Immobility and Impaired Mobility History

Impaired and reduced mobility is a significant issue that needs to be explored during history taking, as impaired mobility will have a deleterious impact on the lower limb in terms of the development and progression of CVD. Impaired or reduced mobility can be due to several causes and these need to be established initially so that a tailored management approach can be instigated.

Causes of immobility that are implicated in the development of VLUs can include inflammatory and non-inflammatory rheumatic diseases, peripheral arterial disease (PAD), neural disease and other acquired or congenital MSK diseases, obesity, injury or secondary to surgery or isolation (Davies et al. 2017). Mobility impairments can be the result of a dysfunction of joint ROM, especially of the ankle, which can lead to reduced CMP function and venous backflow within the lower limb (Corley et al. 2010; Ricci 2020). Impaired mobility can affect a person's QoL and this can be amplified in people with CVD (Meulendijks et al. 2020b).

Co-morbidities and Medicines

There are numerous co-morbidities that affect mobility and movement (Jordan and Osborne 2007). However, any co-morbidities that affect the musculoskeletal system must be considered when taking history as they may have a direct or indirect impact on the management of patients with CVD and VLU's. These co-morbidities can influence the course of management and be barriers to wound healing and optimal mobility (Davies et al. 2019). For example, rheumatoid arthritis (RA) can cause joint arthropathy, pain and gait dysfunction (Hennessy et al. 2012). RA may be the major underlying factor causing a reduction of ankle joint ROM. The person may be having an inflammatory disease flare and may need a medicines review to help control symptoms that can help improve joint ROM at the ankle, for example. Or a patient with VLUs and Parkinson's disease may have a festinating gait, which is characterised by a stooped posture, a narrow base of gait, a reduced stride length, shuffling steps and a propensity to freeze when approaching an object or doorway (Pirker and Katzenschlager 2017). This gait pattern will impair mobility, which will have an impact on VMP activity and balance, and can predispose a person to falling. This patient may need modification or review of their medication to help with gait impairment and physiotherapy to assist with balance and gait-related issues, or they may need a walking aid (Pirker and Katzenschlager 2017). These issues in relation to co-morbidites that relate to mobility should be identified as part of holistic assessment in order to help improve healing and mobility.

Injury History

When exploring the area of the medical history that relates to identifying any possible biomechanical risk factors, it is important to ask about any current injuries or prior injuries during the patient's life. An injury in childhood may not seem relevant to the patient in the present, but this may have great relevance within the context of the whole clinical picture. For example, an ankle sprain, previous sports injury or fracture may be the catalyst for their current lower limb issue, such as venous damage/disease and chronic oedema.

When asking about any injuries, it is important to document the date, the location and the mechanism of the injury. For example, if it was an ankle sprain gathering the information in Table 4.2 in relation to the injury is important.

Information gained in this area may also explain the reason behind a person's current level of activity, especially if it is reduced or impaired.

Falls History

It is estimated that 30% of over 65s and 50% of the over 80s will fall at least once a year (NICE 2019). Falls and the injuries that result from them can be significant issues, especially for older people (NICE 2019). VLUs are estimated to affect 1 in 500 people and become

TABLE 4.2   Important questions to ask about injury history.

Area of the injury	In what area did the injury occur?
	Were any other areas affected because of the injury?
Mechanism of injury	How did the injury occur?
	What movements occurred when the injury occurred?
Medical treatment	Did the patient seek medical help?
	Was any medical imaging undertaken?
	What was the recovery period?
Rehabilitation	What treatment was undertaken?
	Did the patient manage to complete the rehabilitation?
Outcome	Has the injury resolved itself?
	Are there any residual issues?

more ubiquitous with age (NICE 2019). People with VLUs are known to exhibit impaired muscle strength, reduced gait speed and impairments in joint ROM, and are known to be at greater risk of falling (Humphreys et al. 2016; de Souza et al. 2022). Falls can be the result of deconditioning, which is also a common biomechanical risk factor for gait dysfunction in people with VLUs (Humphreys et al. 2016). Falls account for 87% of fractures in the elderly and are estimated to cost the NHS more than £2.3 billion annually. Fractures and the immobility associated with falls can have impacts on mobility and this will have a direct negative impact on the lower limb function in terms of an increase in venous hypertension, CVD and VLUs. A history of falls can give clues to the practitioner about the possible decline of mobility or the reason for reduced mobility. Where possible, conduct a mobility screen to gather pertinent information for onward referral for specialist assessment to mitigate the risk of falls and their impact on biomechanical function, gait and complications in patients with VLUs.

Mechanisms of Falling

Understanding why people fall and the mechanism of the fall is an integral part of the inquiry. If a fall has been reported, this should lead to evidence-based interventions for the patient (Ambrose et al. 2013). Table 4.3 describes some of the common intrinsic and extrinsic reasons for falling.

Surgical History

It is important to explore whether any surgical procedure may have triggered an event for the development of CVD or VLUs. Asking about surgery should not be limited to surgery relating to the lower limb; it is important to establish all surgery that the patient has had in their lifetime. For example, coronary bypass grafting (CABG) surgery may have involved the harvesting of the great saphenous vein in the leg, and this could be the trigger for the development of CVD.

A triggering event like orthopedic surgery where post-surgical rehabilitation was not optimal may be the underlying reason for the development of CVD or VLUs. Research suggests that persistent post-surgical symptoms can result in poor-quality rehabilitation and

TABLE 4.3   Reasons for falling.

Intrinsic	Extrinsic
Sarcopenia	Footwear and clothing
Age	Home and outdoor lighting
Sex	Flooring
Gait issues and balance	Tripping hazards
Fitness	Lack of fixed grab bars
Strength and aerobic fitness	Unstable furniture
Vertigo	
Impaired vision and hearing	
Cognitive impairment	
Cardiovascular disease	
Medications	
Depression	

Source: Adapted from Ambrose et al. (2013).

decreased activity, which can have an adverse effect on a person's mobility (Hamilton et al. 2020).

Knowledge of surgical procedures will inform the clinician of any post-surgical trauma to the surrounding veins, tissues and lymphatics secondary to the surgery, which may cause the patient lower limb problems that relate to CVD in the future.

Sitting and Standing Occupations

Although there is no definitive link between the development of CVD and VLUs and certain occupations, there is evidence to suggest that people in occupations who stand or sit in a static position for long periods of time may be more at risk of developing CVD (de Lima 2019). Exploration of the patient's occupation and determining their activity at work can indicate how sedentary they are during the day and provide insight into the possible risk of CVD or developing VLUs (de Lima 2019).

Occupations that involve long periods of prolonged static standing are associated with increased MSK disorders that affect the lower back and the lower limbs (Anderson et al. 2021). Such occupations may increase the risk of developing a VLU (de Lima 2019). Standing is known to be associated with prolonged discomfort and other symptoms of venous diseases like varicose veins (Antle et al. 2018). Prolonged static standing leads to increased venous hydrostatic pressure and increased venous backflow within the peripheral venous system, which can lead to CVD and lymphoedema.

Conversely, occupations that are sedentary in nature or where prolonged sitting is involved have been reported to be associated with obesity, MSK pain and other chronic health conditions (Antle et al. 2018). Prolonged standing and sitting occupations are detrimental in terms of impaired lower limb fluid dynamics and the risk of increased venous hypertension (Uhl and Gillot 2015; Horwood 2019). Therefore, knowing a patient's occupation will allow a more tailored approach to giving advice on what can be done to improve VMP activity to help reduce venous hypertension.

For example, if the person works in retail, then encouraging them to spend less time in a static position by walking, stepping or changing position will encourage lower limb muscle pump activity and improve lower limb venous dynamics while enhancing VMP activity. In terms of sitting, encouraging people to engage in chair-based exercises and regularly getting up from the chair will again help with lower limb haemodynamics and reduce the risk of venous pooling and peripheral oedema, which can lead to CVD.

Obesity

Obesity has an impact on gait, which can impair a person's mobility and lead to a reduction in general activity; obesity is a known risk factor for the development of VLUs (Davies et al. 2017). These alterations in mobility or mobility impairment secondary to obesity can lead to reduced CMP function, which has an impact on ambulatory venous pressure (Davies et al. 2019). When abdominal obesity is present this can obstruct venous outflow and impair venous haemodynamics. Increased adipose tissue results in augmented inflammatory cytokine activity that can lead to chronic inflammation and increased endothelial permeability. This will affect microcirculatory function and can contribute to venous disease and ulceration (Meulendijks et al. 2020a). Addressing the causes and onward referral for the management (Meulendijks et al. 2020a) of the obesity are key in helping to improve physical activity and reduce the risk of chronic venous insufficiency (CVI).

Physical Activity

One of the responsibilities of healthcare practitioners is to offer lifestyle advice and discuss lifestyle modification in relation to physical activity (Department of Health and Social Care 2019). Physical activity is defined as any bodily movement produced by skeletal muscles that requires energy (Langhammer et al. 2018). It happens in many forms, in different settings and has many purposes (Department of Health and Social Care 2019). Physical activity is not limited to exercise. Many patients with CVD or VLUs may not be able to 'exercise' due to their individual physical capabilities, therefore promoting advice that is focused on being mobile and moving throughout the day is important. Reinforcing these messages during appointments may help reduce sedentary habits, which can have a positive impact on a patient's condition and quality of life.

Assessing the patient's physical activity is important to identify if they are meeting current physical activity guidelines, so that, if they are not then the clinician is aware of this and can put in place a management plan to help them achieve this or move closer to reaching activity levels within these guidelines (Knox et al. 2013; Department of Health and Social Care 2019). The guidelines can be used as a guide in terms of goals for patients to help improve mobility and activity.

They include:

- 150 minutes of moderate-intensity exercise per week.
- 75 minutes of vigorous activity.
- Strength-building activities for muscles, bones and joints at least two days a week. This could be carrying heavy bags, gym or yoga etc.
- Reducing sedentary time.
- Improving balance.

To determine a person's activity, it is important to ask:

- What types of physical activity do you do each day?
- What levels of activity occur over a week? This would include moderate or vigorous levels of activity over the week.

- What is your current physical ability? This would be a subjective report of what the person feels they may be physically capable of undertaking.
- Are there any barriers to you undertaking more physical activity?

MANAGEMENT

Walking and Mobility

Humans have evolved habitually to walk upright; this is called bipedalism (d'Août et al. 2004). Habitual bipedalism that enables walking is not only part of our physical evolution, walking is also engrained in our psyche. The ability to walk is intimately linked to our identity and emotional well-being (Hammarlund et al. 2014). Being able to walk independently is part of being autonomous in life (Pirker and Katzenschlager 2017).

Walking is an activity that people do in their everyday lives and when promoted can be a way of helping to increase a person's activity and increase their mobility. The benefit of walking is that it does not require special skill, ability or specialised equipment (Lee and Buchner 2008). Walking is accessible and is a universal form of activity that can be advocated regardless of sex, age, ethnicity, education or socioeconomic background (Lee and Buchner 2008).

Anecdotally, many patients who have VLUs state that their mobility goals are focused on being able to 'walk more'. In many cases, patients will comment on how losing the ability to walk in the way they did previously due to their lower limb condition is an issue that they find difficult to cope with and it impacts on their QoL. Patients with CVI and VLUs report leg and foot pain and this has a direct influence on their levels of activity and a deleterious impact on VMP function in the lower limb.

Active people may take thousands of steps per day. People who are not experiencing walking and mobility issues will move pain free, have adequate function and expend the least amount of energy possible to perform the task of walking, which is generally an automatic, repetitive combination of movements grouped into what is termed the gait cycle (Simonsen 2014; Gardner et al. 2016; Ricci 2020).

It is important for healthcare professionals to watch the way patients are moving and walking for the duration of their appointments to identify deficits or impairments that may require onward referral for in-depth assessment. Having a basic understanding of the concept of the gait cycle may clarify and help the clinician articulate what is being observed and aid in documentation when referring a patient to another healthcare professional.

The Gait Cycle

Complex gait analysis is beyond the scope of this book and requires skills that are outside the nursing scope of practice. However, understanding the rudiments of gait may help in recognising what is sub-optimal and this may facilitate onward referral to an allied health professional (AHP) who can undertake gait analysis and commence appropriate management.

The gait cycle is the basic terminology used to describe human locomotion. The process of walking is described in gait phases (Figure 4.3). Each gait cycle can be representative of how a person walks and the comparison of several gait cycles can be indicative of the variability of an individual's gait pattern (Baker 2013). Gait analysis assumes that cyclic motion is an important indicator of locomotor function (Baker 2013). Maintaining this optimal cyclical motion (walking) is vital in enabling the lower limb joint ROM that will enhance VMP function.

There are two main phases, the stance and swing phase, and eight sub-phases, identified as initial contact, loading response, mid stance, terminal stance, pre-swing, initial swing, mid swing and terminal swing.

The stance phase (when the foot is in contact with the ground) is typically 60% of the gait cycle and the swing phase (when the foot is off the ground) is typically 40% of the gait cycle. However, the gait cycle is variable from person to person (Ricci 2020). Typically gait-related issues occur within the stance phase of gait and this is where podiatrists or therapists will focus their treatments, for example with in-shoe foot orthoses (FO) or exercise therapy (Reina-bueno et al. 2020). However, not all gait-related issues occur in the stance phase, for example a person with foot drop will have issues in the swing phase and the stance phase due to lack of dorsiflexion of the foot and ankle, and treatments will need to be focused within the stance and swing phases.

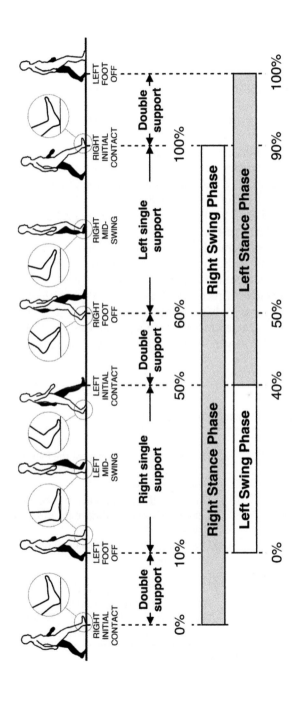

FIGURE 4.3 The gait cycle.
Source: Walha et al. (2020) / John Wiley & Sons / CC BY 4.0.

Spatial and Temporal Parameters

When considering how a person is walking, there are known spatial (space) and temporal (time) parameters that can be considered to understand how a person is moving and walking. For example, a nurse may adjust the speed at which they are walking with a patient as the patient may be walking more slowly (a temporal parameter) because they are taking shorter steps (a spatial parameter). This slower speed, shorter step length and a wider base of gait may result in a 'shuffling' gait that is detrimental to VMP function, because the sub-optimal movement of this gait pattern will result in a reduction of joint ROM and thus VMP function. Other temporal and spatial factors are listed in Table 4.4.

The causes of gait disorders include neurological, non-neurological, orthopaedic, medical and other multifactorial aetiologies; that can become more common with increasing age. Given that gait impairment is recognised as an issue for patients with VLUs, when impairment is recognised patients should be referred on for specialist gait assessment within a podiatry or physiotherapy service (Clarke-Moloney et al. 2007; Humphreys et al. 2016; Guest et al. 2018).

TABLE 4.4 Spatial and temporal parameters.

Spatial parameters	
Step length	The distance that one part of the foot travels in front of the same part of the foot during each step
Stride length	This is the distance between successive points of initial contact of the same foot with the ground
Step width	The measure of the mediolateral separation of the feet
Temporal parameters	
Stride time	The duration of one gait cycle
Cadence	The number of steps per minute
Walking speed	The distance travelled within a given time (related to cadence and stride length)

Source: Adapted from Baker (2013).

Mobility and Exercise

As previously discussed, significantly reduced ankle ROM and reductions in balance and strength are associated with the development of CMP dysfunction and can also contribute to gait dysfunction (Williams et al. 2014; de Souza et al. 2022). Considering this evidence, activities and exercises that are focused on improving these parameters would be of benefit to patients with VLUs.

The evidence base reports that progressive and aerobic exercise can be considered for those patients who have the capability of carrying out such activities (Davies et al. 2008; Araujo et al. 2016; Smith et al. 2018). If a patient is capable then dynamic, aerobic exercise would be appropriate, and encouraging walking or hobbies like tai chi and dancing would be of benefit, as these types of activities will all promote active VMP function. If the patient has balance or strength issues, then giving chair-based resistance exercises that mobilise the ankle using a TheraBand (an elastic band that adds resistance to any movement) is appropriate (Figure 4.4). If the patient is not able to use the TheraBand, then simple chair-based exercises that mobilise the ankle in the sagittal plane in dorsiflexion and plantarflexion will again help venous return and mobilise the ankle joint.

Foot Issues and Mobility

Evidence suggests that foot problems have an impact on mobility and are associated with reduced walking speeds, increased double limb support, difficulty in functional activities like rising from and sitting in a chair and impaired balance (Menz 2021). The foot is the interface between the body and the ground when weight-bearing, thus footwear can affect stability and balance in a positive or negative way, depending on the chosen footwear or how the footwear is worn (Menz 2021). Foot problems are common in older people and frequent foot pain is reported in the forefoot and toes. The most common disorders reported are:

- Hyperkeratotic lesions (callus, corns).
- Nail disorders.
- Structural foot deformities like hallux valgus (bunions) and lesser toe deformities (hammer, claw and mallet toe deformities) (Menz 2021).

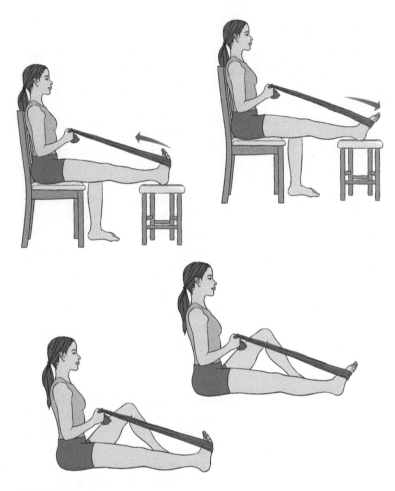

FIGURE 4.4   Seated ankle joint exercises with a TheraBand.

Identifying any foot pain or problems is important, as these issues can result in reduced mobility that negatively impacts on VMP activation.

Keeping patients walking, independently mobile and exploring the barriers behind issues related to walking and foot problems are important. Many of the issues explored and declared may be outside of the nursing scope of practice and will be within the remit of an

AHP. Therefore, it is important once these issues are identified that the patient is referred to the appropriate practitioner, such as a podiatrist or physiotherapist for further assessment and management.

Footwear

Footwear protects the feet from the environment and enables a supporting surface between the foot and the ground (Barwick et al. 2019). Footwear is also seen as part of a person's outward appearance and plays a role in identity. Some patients will choose aesthetics over comfort, fit and safety, which can often lead to sub-optimal footwear choice (Davis et al. 2013).

Similarly, shoe-wearing habits can be equally sub-optimal. Some elderly people in the United Kingdom wear slippers 80% of the day, indoors and outdoors; this can lead to a higher falls risk compared with those who wear fastened footwear (Menant et al. 2008). Walking unshod (without footwear) or when wearing socks also increases an elderly person's falls risk compared to wearing trainers (athletic shoes) or canvas-style shoes (Menant et al. 2008; Menz 2021). The heel height and design of footwear are also important factors (Menant et al. 2008). Footwear with a heel that is greater than 2.5 cm is linked to a higher falls risk compared with canvas-style shoes or trainers (Koepsell et al. 2004).

Footwear has been shown to have an influence on the haemodynamics in the lower limb in asymptomatic populations (Lerebourg et al. 2020). Unstable, rocker-soled, heelless (flat) and athletic footwear has been shown to have a positive impact on the haemodynamics in the lower limb in asymptomatic, healthy populations (Lerebourg et al. 2020). Moreover, athletic shoes have been shown to modify the spatial-temporal parameters in gait (increased step frequency and speed), which will increase muscle activity in the lower limb. This evidence suggests that unstable shoes cause instability, which increases ankle ROM during movement or gait (Lerebourg et al. 2020).

The theory of 'unstable' shoes is that certain technologies (i.e. a rocker sole) are built into the shoes that makes them unstable and this helps to train and strengthen muscles in the human locomotor system (Nigg et al. 2010). These technologies built into the shoes are reported to elicit an increase in muscle activity in approximately 80%

of the population, with the highest relative increase in the muscles that cross the ankle joint (Nigg et al. 2010). However, this is variable among subjects. This contrasts to an 'unstable' shoe that is unsafe to wear because it is ill fitting, worn-out or not appropriate for the task being undertaken, for example wearing high heels to run a marathon.

Although the evidence suggests that unstable shoes with built-in technologies can lead to a change in 'venous parameters' like blood flow in healthy populations (Lerebourg et al. 2020), it is important to note that appropriate footwear should be carefully recommended considering the patient's mobility and balance, and with safety being of paramount importance.

Fit and Condition of Footwear

The fit of footwear is important in helping a person to walk pain free and to allow optimal function during gait. Incorrectly fitting shoes have been linked to foot pain and foot disorders (Buldt and Menz 2018). There is no international sizing convention for footwear and shoe brands will use anatomical last shapes when making shoes. The last is a 3D model of a human foot that is used to construct a shoe. The last shape depends on the country the shoe is from and on the model of a typical foot from that region of the world. The style and shape of the shoe will then be determined by the footwear producer and most shoe lines are mass made. It is therefore imperative that patients check shoe fit before purchase. See Figure 4.5 for helpful suggestions when choosing footwear.

Patients may also present in footwear that they deem appropriate but are inappropriate, or may be struggling to find footwear that fits over bandaging. Due to socioeconomic factors, they may have worn-out footwear or even have had to repair shoes themselves. If this is the case and the footwear is putting the patient at risk of falling or non-healing, then referring the patient on to surgical appliances or supplying them with temporary footwear is an option.

Temporary Footwear

It is not uncommon for a patient to go into a temporary shoe, like a Darco healing sandal, during an episode of ulceration, as these better accommodate compression bandaging (Figure 4.6). However, it is

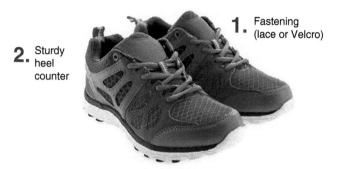

2. Sturdy heel counter

1. Fastening (lace or Velcro)

3. Rocker sole that bends where your foot bends

Top tips
- ☑ Choose a shoe with a removable insole for extra room
- ☑ Leave a thumb width gap at the end of the shoe to allow your toes to move
- ☑ Shoes with a wide opening allow for easier access for your feet

FIGURE 4.5 Tips on choosing footwear.
Source: Accelerate Footwear UK.

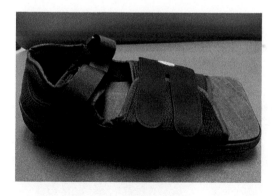

FIGURE 4.6 Darco healing sandal.

important to remember that these shoes are temporary and should be checked and replaced on a regular basis.

When transitioning a patient from bandaging into compression garments, it is important to ensure that they have a well-fitting and appropriate shoe to wear. Consider asking the patient to bring their shoes and the slippers they would normally wear so that you can assess the fit and style to see if any changes need to be made or if new footwear needs to be considered.

Bespoke or Semi-bespoke Footwear and Footwear Modifications

Some patients may have a foot shape or structure that does not fit into retail footwear, or they may require footwear modifications. Rocker-soled shoes are important for patients with CVI and VLUs, as the rocker sole enables improved ankle movement and thus enhances the action of the CMP (Figure 4.7). There are many retail shoes ranges that have rocker soles, but in some cases it may be necessary for a patient to have their shoes modified and have a specialist rocker sole added. There are other modifications that can be made to shoes to help improve gait and mobility. This requires assessment with a footwear specialist or podiatrist to ascertain what would be the most appropriate modification given the person's underlying medical issues and biomechanical function.

Advice and Education

Patient education on the important features of footwear is essential, as footwear can enhance foot function and enable improved

(a)   (b)

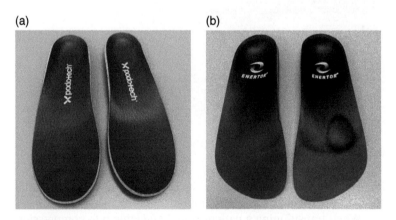

FIGURE 4.7   (a) Off-the-shelf functional foot orthoses. (b) Fully custom-made functional foot orthoses.

haemodynamics in the lower limb (Lerebourg et al. 2020). Shoes should have a fastening (this could be a lace or Velcro®) that helps to secure the shoe to the foot to enable optimal gait. A sturdy heel counter to hold the heel in place will provide stability in the rear foot during heel strike and a rocker sole will bend where the foot bends. This will enhance sagittal plane movement, aid in CMP function and offload the forefoot. Suggesting shoes with a wide opening and a removable insole will help provide extra room for oedematous feet or feet in bandaging or compression garments.

Changing footwear can be seen as a lifestyle change and must be considered among other important factors such as cost, purpose and choosing the right shoe for the right activity or occasion. Being aware of these barriers is important, as it will help identify potential issues behind why a patient is reticent to change their footwear and guide in future management. When patients do not wish to change their footwear after being given information on optimal footwear and the reasons why, then they have made an informed choice and this discussion can be revisited later when they may be more open to change.

Foot Orthoses

An orthosis is defined as 'an appliance to support, align, correct deformity or motion of parts of the body' (Mills et al. 2010). Orthotic provision in general has been reported to help people achieve optimal health and QoL, and enable them to work and live independently (Chockalingam et al. 2019).

Foot orthoses (Figure 4.7) are appliances that can be inserted into footwear to manage a number of foot and ankle pathologies (Mills et al. 2010) and can help to improve symptoms in chronic foot conditions like rheumatoid arthritis (Hennessy et al. 2012). VMPs in the lower limb rely on optimal lower limb function, so foot orthoses should be considered where lower limb function and movement are sub-optimal.

Research has reported improvements in pedobarographic examination (the study of pressure acting between the plantar surface of the foot and a supporting surface) when using orthoses (Saggini et al. 2009). Positive changes in biomechanics and the redistribution of power loads on the plantar surface of the foot were noted. This included greater activation of the external and internal plantar veins when using visco-elastic foot orthoses that corrected foot posture in patients with CVI (Saggini et al. 2009). Custom foot orthoses have been studied and, again, positive findings have been reported in terms of improved venous return in the lower limb (López-López et al. 2018). These positive findings in the biomechanical parameters, improved venous return and improved activation of the VMP of the foot and calf substantiate the use of orthoses in clinical practice.

REDUCING FALLS RISK

A fall is defined by Public Health England (Office for Health Improvement and Disparities 2022) as 'an event which causes a person to, unintentionally, rest on the ground or lower level and is not a result of a major intrinsic event'. Research has shown that 75–80% of falls where no injury was sustained are not reported (Fleming and Brayne 2008) and that there is a stigma associated with falls (Hoffman et al. 2018). This is why asking questions and screening for the risk of falls are so important, as this may help to mitigate the incidence of falls and thus the sequelae of a fall, which can have a negative impact on a patient's mobility and exacerbate CVD or VLUs in terms of prolonged healing.

Screening and Assessment of Falls

Screening will help determine if further assessment or onward referral is required. One of the simplest screening approaches is to ask if the patient has fallen in the last 12 months and then enquire about the frequency and nature of the fall(s). Observation of the patient walking is also useful to obtain objective information on how the patient is moving and if they are using walking aids, if these appear appropriate in terms of wear and height, as this may cause instability and possibly result in a fall.

It is reported in the literature that a proportion of patients with VLUs have reduced ankle ROM (Back et al. 1995; Davies et al. 2007;

Atkin et al. 2016; de Souza et al. 2022). Studies have shown that people with decreased ankle flexibility fall more often than those with adequate ankle flexibility (Menz 2021). Long-term bandaging for VLUs can alter gait by impairing the ankle ROM (Atkin et al. 2016). Therefore, patients with VLUs and a restricted ankle joint ROM are more at risk of falls. Injuries resulting from falls can lead to pain and immobility, which will have an impact on fluid dynamics in the lower limb and can result in a longer episode of ulceration.

Screening Tools for Falls

There are many validated and reliable mobility screening and assessment tools available to the practitioner and these can be used in the home or clinical setting (Table 4.5) (Tinetti et al. 1986; Podsiadlo and Richardson 1991; Bogle Thorbahn and Newton 1996).

Falls are complex, and in-depth assessment should be undertaken by a practitioner or a team to ensure the most appropriate interventions are in place to help reduce the risk of a fall. Patients who are at high risk of falls or who have a fear of falling should be referred to the appropriate service for assessment.

TABLE 4.5 Examples of screening tools for falls.

Modified falls efficacy scale	A 14-item patient-reported measure assessing confidence and activities of daily living
Timed up and go test	Assessing sitting to stand, walking two meters, turning and then sitting down. Cut-off times indicate falls risk
Thirty-second chair stand	Focused on functional ability in repeated sitting and standing from a chair
Tinetti balance tool	Assessment of balance and gait focused on chronic disabilities
Berg balance scale	An objective tool to determine a patient's ability to safely balance during pre-determined tasks

ALLIED HEALTH PROFESSIONALS AS PART
OF THE MULTIDISCIPLINARY TEAM

Populations are ageing worldwide. People are living longer and this leads to higher levels of chronic disease (Saxon et al. 2014). This will have a direct impact on the numbers within the population who have CVI and VLUs in the future.

The standards of care for long-term management of wounds have been debated within the evidence, consensus documents produced and various recommendations made (Atkin et al. 2019). The current trend within the evidence is that VLUs, especially those that are deemed long term, should be escalated to a specialist service or a multidisciplinary team (MDT) (Atkin et al. 2019). This notion is associated with the standards of best practice that are based on the UK national diabetic foot ulcer guidelines for MDT referral (Atkin et al. 2019). Recommendations for specialty skills to be integrated into best practice include podiatry, endocrinology and nutrition. While these skills within the MDT may help those who have long-term wounds, little attention is paid to addressing the area of management that enhances mobility and VMP function. This is where AHPs who have a musculoskeletal scope of practice at the core of their skill set can be used to enhance best practices within current and future guidelines.

CONCLUSION

This chapter has examined the important factors that influence mobility, biomechanical function, gait assessment and management of MSK factors within the population of people who have CVD and VLUs. The evidence elucidates the decreased levels of mobility, CMP dysfunction and physical impairments that are present within this group of patients. It is important to address these underlying MSK issues, which may be influenced by social or patient-related factors for a positive clinical outcome and may not always be within the scope of practice of wound care nursing. If this is the case, then onward referral is warranted. This ensures that the patient receives the care they need to address any underlying causes for musculoskeletal issues in order to enhance mobility, expedite wound healing and prevent the occurrence of a venous leg ulcer in the future.

REFERENCES

Ambrose, A.F., Paul, G., and Hausdorff, J.M. (2013). Risk factors for falls among older adults: a review of the literature. *Maturitas* 75 (1): 51–61.

Anderson, J., Williams, A.E., and Nester, C. (2021). Musculoskeletal disorders, foot health and footwear choice in occupations involving prolonged standing. *International Journal of Industrial Ergonomics* 81: 103079.

Antle, D.M., Cormier, L., Findlay, M. et al. (2018). Lower limb blood flow and mean arterial pressure during standing and seated work: implications for workplace posture recommendations. *Preventive Medicine Reports* 10: 117–122.

Araki, C.T., Back, T.L., Padberg, F.T. et al. (1994). The significance of calf muscle pump function in venous ulceration. *Journal of Vascular Surgery* 20 (6): 872–879.

Araujo, D.N., Ribeiro, C.D., Maciel, A.C. et al. (2016). Physical exercise for the treatment of non-ulcerated chronic venous insufficiency. *Cochrane Database of Systematic Reviews* 12 (12): CD010637.

Atkin, L., Búcko, Z., Montero, E.C. et al. (2019). Implementing TIMERS: the race against hard-to-heal wounds. *Journal of Wound Care* 28 (Sup3a): S1–S50.

Atkin, L., Stephenson, J., Parfitt, G. et al. (2016). An investigation to assess ankle mobility in healthy individuals from the application of multicomponent compression bandages and compression hosiery. *Journal of Foot and Ankle Research* 9 (1): 18.

Back, T.L., Padberg, F.T. Jr., Araki, C.T. et al. (1995). Limited range of motion is a significant factor in venous ulceration. *Journal of Vascular Surgery* 22 (5): 519–523.

Baker, R. (2013). *Measuring Walking: A Handbook of Clinical Gait Analysis*. Chichester: Wiley.

Barwell, J.R., Ghauri, A.S.K., Taylor, M. et al. (2000). Risk factors for healing and recurrence of chronic venous leg ulcers. *Phlebology* 15 (2): 49–52.

Barwick, A.L., van Netten, J.J., Hurn, S.E. et al. (2019). Factors associated with type of footwear worn inside the house: a cross-sectional study. *Journal of Foot and Ankle Research* 12: 1–9.

Bogle Thorbahn, L.D. and Newton, R.A. (1996). Use of the Berg balance test to predict falls in elderly persons. *Physical Therapy* 76 (6): 576–583.

Brockett, C.L. and Chapman, G.J. (2016). Biomechanics of the ankle. *Orthopaedics and Traumatology* 30 (3): 232–238.

Buldt, A.K. and Menz, H.B. (2018). Incorrectly fitted footwear, foot pain and foot disorders: a systematic search and narrative review of the literature. *Journal of Foot and Ankle Research* 11 (1): 1–11.

Chockalingam, N., Eddison, N., and Healy, A. (2019). Cross-sectional survey of orthotic service provision in the UK: does where you live affect the service you receive? *BMJ Open* 9 (10): e028186.

Clarke-Moloney, M., Godfrey, A., O'Connor, V. et al. (2007). Mobility in patients with venous leg ulceration. *European Journal of Vascular and Endovascular Surgery* 33 (4): 488–493.

Corley, G.J., Broderick, B.J., Nestor, S.M. et al. (2010). The anatomy and physiology of the venous foot pump. *Anatomical Record: Advances in Integrative Anatomy and Evolutionary Biology* 293 (3): 370–378.

D'Août, K., Vereecke, E., Schoonaert, K. et al. (2004). Locomotion in bonobos (Pan paniscus): differences and similarities between bipedal and quadrupedal terrestrial walking, and a comparison with other locomotor modes. *Journal of Anatomy* 204 (5): 353–361.

Davies, J.A., Bull, R.H., Farrelly, I.J., and Wakelin, M.J. (2007). A home-based exercise programme improves ankle range of motion in long-term venous ulcer patients. *Phlebology* 22 (2): 86–89.

Davies, J., Bull, R., Farrelly, I., and Wakelin, M. (2008). Improving the calf pump using home-based exercises for patients with chronic venous disease. *Wounds UK* 4 (3): 48–57.

Davies, H.O., Popplewell, M., Bate, G. et al. (2019). Publication of UK NICE Clinical Guidelines 168 has not significantly changed the management of leg ulcers in primary care: an analysis of the health improvement network database. *Phlebology* 34 (5): 311–316.

Davies, H.O.B., Popplewell, M., Singhal, R. et al. (2017). Obesity and lower limb venous disease–the epidemic of phlebesity. *Phlebology* 32 (4): 227–233.

Davis, A., Murphy, A., and Haines, T.P. (2013). 'Good for older ladies, not me': how elderly women choose their shoes. *Journal of the American Podiatric Medical Association* 103 (6): 465–470.

Day, J. (2015). Diagnosing and managing venous leg ulcers in patients in the community. *British Journal of Community Nursing* 20 (Sup12): S22–S30.

de Lima, D.C. (2019). Varicose veins and occupational health: symptoms, treatment and prevention. *Revista Brasileira De Medicina do Trabalho* 17 (4): 589.

Department of Health and Social Care (2019). Physical activity guidelines: adults and older adults. https://www.gov.uk/government/publications/physical-activity-guidelines-adults-and-older-adults

de Souza, I.N., de Oliveira, L.F.F., de Almeida, I.L.G.I. et al. (2022). Impairments in ankle range of motion, dorsi and plantar flexors muscle strength and gait speed in patients with chronic venous disorders: a systematic review and meta-analysis. *Phlebology* 37 (7): 496–506.

Farrelly, I. (2018). The adversarial relationship between wounds and biomechanics in the lower limb. *Wounds UK* 14 (5): 70–76.

Fleming, J. and Brayne, C. (2008). Inability to get up after falling, subsequent time on floor, and summoning help: prospective cohort study in people over 90. *BMJ* 337: a2227.

Franks, P.J., Barker, J., Collier, M. et al. (2016). Management of patients with venous leg ulcers: challenges and current best practice. *Journal of Wound Care* 25 (Sup6): S1–S67.

Gardner, A.M.N., Ch, M., and Fox, R.H. (1983). Pump of the preliminary report. *Bristol Medico-Chirurgical Journal* 98 (July): 109–112.

Gardner, A.W., Montgomery, P.S., Casanegra, A.I. et al. (2016). Association between gait characteristics and endothelial oxidative stress and inflammation in patients with symptomatic peripheral artery disease. *Age* 38 (3): 64.

Guest, J.F., Fuller, G.W., and Vowden, P. (2018). Venous leg ulcer management in clinical practice in the UK: costs and outcomes. *International Wound Journal* 15 (1): 29–37.

Halkar, M., Inojosa, J.M., Liedl, D. et al. (2020). Calf muscle pump function as a predictor of all-cause mortality. *Vascular Medicine* 25 (6): 519–526.

Hamilton, D.F., Beard, D.J., Barker, K.L. et al. (2020). Targeting rehabilitation to improve outcomes after total knee arthroplasty in patients at risk of poor outcomes: randomised controlled trial. *BMJ* 371: m3576.

Hennessy, K., Woodburn, J., and Steultjens, M.P.M. (2012). Custom foot orthoses for rheumatoid arthritis: a systematic review. *Arthritis Care & Research* 64 (3): 311–320.

Hoffman, G.J., Ha, J., Alexander, N.B. et al. (2018). Underreporting of fall injuries of older adults: implications for wellness visit fall risk screening. *Journal of the American Geriatrics Society* 66 (6): 1195–1200.

Horwood, A. (2019). The biomechanical function of the foot pump in venous return from the lower extremity during the human gait cycle: an expansion of the gait model of the foot pump. *Medical Hypotheses* 129 (March): 109220.

Horwood, A. (2021). The venous foot pump: modelling its function in gait. *Podiatry Review* 78 (3): 19–24.

Houghton, D.E., Ashrani, A., Liedl, D. et al. (2021). Reduced calf muscle pump function is a risk factor for venous thromboembolism: a population-based cohort study. *Blood* 137 (23): 3284–3290.

Humphreys, C., Moffatt, C., and Hood, V. (2016). Risk of falling for people with venous leg ulcers: a literature review. *British Journal of Community Nursing* 21 (Sup3): S34–S38.

Jordan, J.E. and Osborne, R.H. (2007). Chronic disease self-management education programs: challenges ahead. *Medical Journal of Australia* 186 (2): 84–87.

Kan, Y.M. and Delis, K.T. (2001). Hemodynamic effects of supervised calf muscle exercise in patients with venous leg ulceration: a prospective controlled study. *Archives of Surgery* 136 (12): 1364–1369.

Kim, S.J., Shin, Y.-K., Yoo, G.E. et al. (2016). Changes in gait patterns induced by rhythmic auditory stimulation for adolescents with acquired brain injury. *Annals of the New York Academy of Sciences* 1385 (1): 53–62.

Knox, E.C.L., Esliger, D.W., Biddle, S.J.H., and Sherar, L.B. (2013). Lack of knowledge of physical activity guidelines: can physical activity promotion campaigns do better? *BMJ Open* 3 (12): e003633.

Koepsell, T.D., Wolf, M.E., Buchner, D.M. et al. (2004). Footwear style and risk of falls in older adults. *Journal of the American Geriatrics Society* 52 (9): 1495–1501.

Langhammer, B., Bergland, A., and Rydwik, E. (2018). The importance of physical activity exercise among older people. *BioMed Research International* 7856823.

Lattimer, C.R., Franceschi, C., and Kalodiki, E. (2017). Optimizing calf muscle pump function. *Phlebology* 33 (5): 353–360.

Lee, I.-M. and Buchner, D.M. (2008). The importance of walking to public health. *Medicine & Science in Sports & Exercise* 40 (7): S512–S518.

Lerebourg, L., L'Hermette, M., Menez, C., and Coquart, J. (2020). The effects of shoe type on lower limb venous status during gait or exercise: a systematic review. *PLoS One* 15 (11): e0239787.

López-López, D., Araújo, R., Losa-Iglesias, E. et al. (2018). Influence of custom foot orthoses on venous status: a quasi-experimental study. *Journal of the Mechanical Behavior of Biomedical Materials* 79: 235–238.

Meissner, M.H. (2005). Lower extremity venous anatomy. *Seminars in Interventional Radiology* 22 (3): 147–156.

Menant, J.C., Steele, J.R., Menz, H.B. et al. (2008). Optimizing footwear for older people at risk of falls. *Journal of Rehabilitation Research and Development* 45 (8): 1167–1181.

Menz, H.B. (2021). Foot problems, footwear, and falls. In: *Falls in Older People: Risk Factors, Strategies for Prevention and Implications for Practice* (ed. S. Lord, C. Sherrington, and V. Naganathan), 119–129. Cambridge: Cambridge University Press.

Menz, H.B., Auhl, M., Tan, J.M. et al. (2016). Biomechanical effects of prefabricated foot orthoses and rocker-sole footwear in individuals with first metatarsophalangeal joint osteoarthritis. *Arthritis Care & Research* 68 (5): 603–611.

Meulendijks, A.M., Franssen, W.M.A., Schoonhoven, L., and Neumann, H.A.M. (2020a). A scoping review on chronic venous disease and the development of a venous leg ulcer: the role of obesity and mobility. *Journal of Tissue Viability* 29 (3): 190–196.

Meulendijks, A.M., Welbie, M., Tjin, E.P.M. et al. (2020b). A qualitative study on the patient's narrative in the progression of chronic venous disease into a first venous leg ulcer: a series of events. *British Journal of Dermatology* 183 (2): 332–339.

Milic, D.J., Zivic, S.S., Bogdanovic, D.C. et al. (2009). Risk factors related to the failure of venous leg ulcers to heal with compression treatment. *Journal of Vascular Surgery* 49 (5): 1242–1247.

Mills, K., Blanch, P., Chapman, A.R. et al. (2010). Foot orthoses and gait: a systematic review and meta-analysis of literature pertaining to potential mechanisms. *British Journal of Sports Medicine* 44 (14): 1035–1046.

National Institute for Health and Care Excellence (NICE) (2021). Leg ulcer - venous. https://cks.nice.org.uk/topics/leg-ulcer-venous

Norkin, C.C. and White, D.J. (2016). *Measurement of Joint Motion: A Guide to Goniometry*. Philadelphia, PA: FA Davis.

Nussbaumer, S., Leunig, M., Glatthorn, J.F. et al. (2010). Validity and test-retest reliability of manual goniometers for measuring passive hip range of motion in femoroacetabular impingement patients. *BMC Musculoskeletal Disorders* 11: 1–11.

National Wound Care Strategy Programme (NWCSP) (2020). Lower limb assessment essential criteria. https://www.nationalwoundcarestrategy.net/wp-content/uploads/2021/04/CQUIN-20-21-Lower-Limb-Assessment-Essential-Criteria-Final.pdf

O'Brien, J., Finlayson, K., Kerr, G., and Edwards, H. (2014). The perspectives of adults with venous leg ulcers on exercise: an exploratory study. *Journal of Wound Care* 23 (10): 496–509.

Padberg, F.T. Jr., Johnston, M.V., and Sisto, S.A. (2004). Structured exercise improves calf muscle pump function in chronic venous insufficiency: a randomized trial. *Journal of Vascular Surgery* 39 (1): 79–87.

Palastanga, N. and Soames, R. (2018). *Anatomy and Human Movement: Structure and Function*, 7e. Edinburgh: Churchill Livingstone.

Pirker, W. and Katzenschlager, R. (2017). Gait disorders in adults and the elderly: a clinical guide. *Wiener Klinische Wochenschrift* 129 (3–4): 81–95.

Podsiadlo, D. and Richardson, S. (1991). The timed 'Up & Go': a test of basic functional mobility for frail elderly persons. *Journal of the American Geriatrics Society* 39 (2): 142–148.

Reina-Bueno, M., Vázquez-Bautista, C., Palomo-Toucedo, I.C. et al. (2020). Custom-made foot orthoses reduce pain and fatigue in patients with

Ehlers-Danlos syndrome. A pilot study. *International Journal of Environmental Research and Public Health* 17 (4): 1359.

Ricci, S. (2020). Anatomy and venous hemodynamics of gait phases. *Journal of Theoretical and Applied Vascular Research* 5 (3): 0831.

Saggini, R., Bellomo, R.G., Iodice, P., and Lessiani, G. (2009). Venous insufficiency and foot dysmorphism: effectiveness of visco-elastic rehabilitation systems on veno-muscle system of the foot and of the calf. *International Journal of Immunopathology and Pharmacology* 22 (3_suppl): 1–8.

Saxon, R.L., Gray, M.A., and Oprescu, F.I. (2014). Extended roles for allied health professionals: an updated systematic review of the evidence. *Journal of Multidisciplinary Healthcare* 7: 479–488.

Shiman, M.I., Pieper, B., Templin, T.N. et al. (2009). Venous ulcers: a reappraisal analyzing the effects of neuropathy, muscle involvement, and range of motion upon gait and calf muscle function. *Wound Repair and Regeneration* 17 (2): 147–152.

Simonsen, E.B. (2014). Contributions to the understanding of gait control. *Danish Medical Journal* 61 (4): 1–23.

Smith, D., Lane, R., McGinnes, R. et al. (2018). What is the effect of exercise on wound healing in patients with venous leg ulcers? A systematic review. *International Wound Journal* 15 (3): 441–453.

Tinetti, M.E., Williams, T.F., and Mayewski, R. (1986). Fall risk index for elderly patients based on number of chronic disabilities. *American Journal of Medicine* 80 (3): 429–434.

Uhl, J.-F. and Gillot, C. (2015). Anatomy of the veno-muscular pumps of the lower limb. *Phlebology* 30 (3): 180–193.

Williams, K.J., Ayekoloye, O., Moore, H.M., and Davies, A.H. (2014). The calf muscle pump revisited. *Journal of Vascular Surgery: Venous and Lymphatic Disorders* 2 (3): 329–334.

Wounds UK (2016). Best practice statement: Holistic management of venous leg ulceration. https://wounds-uk.com/best-practice-statements/holistic-management-of-venous-leg-ulceration

Yang, D., Vandongen, Y.K., and Stacey, M.C. (1999). Effect of exercise on calf muscle pump function in patients with chronic venous disease. *British Journal of Surgery* 86 (3): 338–341.

Hammarlund, C.S., Andersson, K., Andersson, M. et al. (2014). The significance of walking from the perspective of people with Parkinson's disease. *Journal of Parkinson's Disease* 4 (4): 657–663.

National Institute for Health and Care Excellence (NICE) (2019). Falls risk assessment. https://cks.nice.org.uk/topics/falls-risk-assessment

National Wound Care Strategy (2023). Data collection form for CQUIN Audit CCG13. Assessment, diagnosis, and treatment of lower leg wounds (v4.1). https://www.nationalwoundcarestrategy.net/cquin

Nigg, B.M., Federolf, P., and Landry, S.C. (2010). Gender differences in lower extremity gait biomechanics during walking using an unstable shoe. *Clinical Biomechanics* 25 (10): 1047–1052.

Office for Health Improvement and Disparities (2022). Falls; applying All Our Health. https://www.gov.uk/government/publications/falls-applying-all-our-health/falls-applying-all-our-health

CHAPTER 5

Assessment of Leg Ulceration

KAREN STAINES AND ABY MITCHELL

A leg ulcer is a break in the skin below the knee that has not healed within a two-week period (NICE 2021). A lower limb assessment is essential to identify the risk factors for developing leg ulceration and delayed healing. There is currently no pathway for preventing primary leg ulcers and management in clinical practice tends to be reactive rather than proactive. According to the Commissioning for Quality and Innovation system (CQUIN; CCG11), all patients should receive a full lower limb assessment following referral to a service within 28 days of a non-healing wound. A holistic lower limb assessment includes patient assessment, leg assessment and wound and skin assessment (Wounds UK 2022) and it is essential to identify contributory and causative factors to aid in diagnosis (Mitchell 2020). Accurate and timely wound assessment underpins effective clinical practice, decision-making, improving patient-centred goals and reducing morbidity and costs associated with long-term wound care. Furthermore, early assessment, diagnosis and intervention are essential to reduce the burden of venous disease and improve quality of life (Mitchell and Elbourne 2020). Fundamentally this is where understanding and patient partnership start.

Lower Limb and Leg Ulcer Assessment and Management, First Edition.
Edited by Aby Mitchell, Georgina Ritchie, and Alison Hopkins.
© 2024 John Wiley & Sons Ltd. Published 2024 by John Wiley & Sons Ltd.

ASSESSMENT

It is essential to establish the underlying cause of leg ulceration to avoid misdiagnosis and unnecessary delays in healing (Wounds UK 2016). All patients with a wound on the lower limb should be assessed to determine the vascular status of the limb prior to commencing treatment with strong compression therapy. In the absence of red flags, mild compression therapy can be commenced immediately to prevent deterioration while the person awaits full assessment, including assessment of the ankle brachial pressure index (ABPI). This is referred to as 'early intervention' and is advocated by the National Wound Care Strategy; it is explained in more detail in Chapter 9. Wound care should be considered a specialist segment of healthcare that requires additional training to assess, diagnose and manage (Guest et al. 2015). Leg ulcer assessment is a complex skill and should only be undertaken by healthcare professionals who have the appropriate level of skills and proficiency (Mitchell 2017). A structured assessment is key to gathering and interpreting data about the patient, confirming the patient's specific requirements and reasons for assessment.

Good history taking is pivotal to decision-making and will form the basis for multifaceted diagnoses including medical, psychosocial and psychological. (See Chapter 7 for a focus on developing personalised assessment.) A full medical history should also include any co-morbidities or surgical procedures, which may be causative factors in the development of a leg ulcer.

HISTORY TAKING

Age

Increasing age leads to degenerative changes and atrophy of the smooth muscle layer in the vein, which increases susceptibility to dilation (Robertson 2013) and thus the presence of venous disease. The presence of peripheral arterial disease (PAD) also increases with age.

Family History

A family history of venous disease is commonly associated with valve dysfunction leading to venous hypertension (Ortega et al. 2021). Ask the patient if any first-degree relative has a history of telangiectasis, varicose veins, blood clots in the lower limbs, a current or previous leg ulcer, phlebitis, pulmonary embolism or any other venous problems (Cirqui et al. 2007). If both parents have varicose veins, the offspring have a 90% chance of developing them (Collares and Faintuch 2017).

Medical History

Check the patient's medical status and whether ongoing medical support is required for any pre-existing conditions.

Medications

Medications and their side effects may cause a delay in wound healing, make the person increase the risk of wound infection or be a contributory factor in ulceration. There are certain medications that can exacerbate and further increase the risk of leg ulceration, as discussed (see Chapter 8). It is important to discuss medications with the person and the prescriber.

Previous Surgery

Limb, abdominal, bypass or amputation surgery may cause disruption and damage to the circulatory system. A venous thrombus episode (VTE) can occur in between 10% and 14% of patients after major abdominal surgery (Theochari et al. 2022).

Deep Vein Thrombosis

People who have a history of deep vein thrombosis (DVT) have an increased risk of ulceration due to damage to the deep veins.

Previous Trauma

There is an increased risk of DVT following a fracture of the lower limb (Mioc et al. 2018). Any break in skin integrity from trauma can also influence the disruption to the lymphatic system (Minasian et al. 2022). The superficial lymphatics can be found in the dermis layer of the skin, resulting in an increase in localised oedema if these become damaged.

Haemorrhoids and Constipation

Ask the patient if they are suffering from haemorrhoids and/or constipation. The results of the CHORUS study found that over 50% of patients who had a history of haemorrhoids and constipation also had venous disease with a CEAP classification (see Table 5.2) up to C2 (Godeberge et al. 2019).

Diabetes/Associated Peripheral Neuropathy

People diagnosed with diabetes are at greater risk of having small vessel disease and nerve damage, with one in four patients having peripheral neuropathy (NHS 2022). This can result in pressure damage occurring due to a lack of sensation without the patient feeling pain. Furthermore, uncontrolled blood glucose levels can mean that the person with diabetes has an increased risk of infection and delayed wound healing. See Box 5.1 on monofilament testing.

Box 5.1 Monofilament Testing for Neuropathy

Monofilament testing is used in the presence of diabetes or when there is concern about peripheral neuropathy being present. Using a monofilament is an inexpensive portable test for assessing the loss of protective sensations in the foot. Monofilaments are single-fibre nylon threads that generate a buckling stress; the higher the value or weight of the thread, the harder it is to bend.

In normal practice a 10 g monofilament is used at various points on the plantar aspect of the foot. The patient is assessed with their eyes closed or head turned so that they cannot see where the monofilament is being placed. They are to tell the clinician when they feel their foot being touched. A lack of response needs to be checked, but will denote a lack of sensation and the protective function.

This patient will then have a reduced pain response, which has clinical implications for management and use of compression therapy. Use local guidelines and referral mechanisms.

Cancer Diagnosis or Treatment

Cancer itself can cause occlusion, depending on tumour location. Cancer treatment can affect the lymphatic system, leading to an increased risk of oedema. Radiotherapy and chemotherapy can adversely impact the immune system and destroy cells, which delays wound healing (Deptuła et al. 2019).

Inflammatory and Auto-immune Conditions

People who have underlying auto-immune conditions can have an increased risk of developing ulceration. Conditions such as pyoderma gangrenosum and vasculitis may need medical management to guide medication as well as wound management and compression therapy; read more about this in Chapter 3.

Haematological Disorders

Disorders of the blood may have contributed to the presenting ulceration or reduced healing potential, depending on the type of haematological disorder, such as sickle cell disease (SCD), anaemia or haemophilia. People diagnosed with SCD are 10 times more at risk of developing a leg ulcer than the general population (Young 2020). See Chapter 3.

Respiratory Disorders

Chronic obstructive pulmonary disease (COPD) or similar respiratory disorders may have increased oedema due to breathlessness. Caution may be needed to ensure that compression therapy will not exacerbate breathlessness. A quarter of patients with COPD have cor pulmonale (right-sided heart failure), which can lead to increased oedema and shortness of breath (Robinson and Scullion 2021).

Cardiac Vascular History

Previous myocardial infarction or angina may indicate a reduction of oxygenated blood that increases the chance of developing leg ulcers and causes a delay in healing. People with a diagnosis of heart failure need to be carefully monitored and discussed with the wider multidisciplinary team to ensure that any treatment will not cause an increase in cardiac oedema. For most people, unless they are in unstable heart failure, compression is a safe and necessary intervention. See Chapter 8.

Phlebitis

Inflammation of the veins can again cause long-term damage and be a causative factor for ulceration.

Hypertension

Patients may have hypertension from an underlying condition of high cholesterol, previous myocardial Infarction (MI), transient ischaemic attack (TIA), stroke or kidney disease and are at a greater risk of cardiovascular disease. If not well controlled, this may also result in an abnormal ABPI.

Infection

A local or systemic infection will delay wound healing.

Pregnancy

Ask if the patient is pregnant. Cyclical changes in females' progesterone levels affect the vein wall and valves. The risk increases during pregnancy whereby blood volume is increased, and the enlarging uterus can restrict venous return (Nicholls 2005). Females who have a history of pregnancy have an 82% higher risk of varicose veins compared to those who have never been pregnant (Ismail et al. 2016).

Allergies or Known Sensitivities

Patients with venous leg ulcers are prone to increased sensitivity. This may occur after prolonged use of certain dressings or emollients. The most frequent allergen groups are fragrances (30.5%), antimicrobials (19.5%), topical excipients (19.5%), rubber accelerators (13.5%) and topical corticosteroids (8%) (Tavadia et al. 2003). It is important to check any known allergies and consider food allergies, as some dressings have food products within them such as shellfish and ovine products. Allergies such as latex and lanolin may also have an influence on the choice of treatment.

Diet and Nutritional Status

Individuals who are overweight are just as likely to be malnourished as those who are slight in build. Highly exuding wounds result in a loss of protein that is essential for cell regeneration. Having a well-balanced diet is a key factor to consider in wound healing (Hess 2020). The prevalence of venous leg ulcers (VLUs) is significantly higher in patients who have obesity compared to patients who do not (Daniels-son et al. 2002; Van Rij et al. 2008). A high body mass index (BMI) will add extra pressure on the venous system and increase the risk of valvular incompetence (Atkin 2019). Additional intra-abdominal pressure in patients with a BMI >40 or >35 (with obesity-related complications) can hinder venous and lymphatic drainage and a high BMI can increase the risk of varicose veins (Iannuzzi et al. 2002). Obesity can result in a reduction of mobility, increased aggravation of limited joint and ankle mobility (Belczak et al. 2021) and a sedentary lifestyle. People who are suffering from active ulceration are more likely to be obese (Carruthers et al. 2014). Discuss diet and signpost to a dietician where appropriate.

Sleep Pattern and Behaviour

The importance of discussing sleep behaviour and asking the direct question 'Where do you sleep at night?' is fundamental to the success of the treatment and an important discussion point within the assessment. If the individual does not sleep in a bed at night, this results in an increase in dependent oedema. Riser recliner chairs do have some benefits and are useful during the day to raise the feet intermittently. However, most of these chairs, unless they lay flat, do not elevate the legs sufficiently for effective venous return and some dependent oedema is likely to remain. It is recommended that patients should aim to raise their legs approximately 15 cm (6 in.) from the bed to reduce oedema (Vascular Society for Great Britain and Ireland 2023).

Smoking

Smokers have an increased risk of cardiovascular disease. Smoking damages the lining of the arteries, including the coronary arteries. The damage encourages the build-up of fatty materials in arteries, which can lead to MI and stroke. Smoking causes vasoconstriction, which leads to hypoxia. Neutrophils and monocytes (cells that help prevent infection) are reduced, as is collagen, which means that there is less tensile wound strength and a delay in wound healing due to the reduction of oxygenated blood essential for tissue repair (Wang et al. 2021).

Pain

Ask the person about the pain they feel. Pain associated with venous insufficiency occurs after standing or sitting for long periods of time. Does the pain improve when the legs are elevated? If there is pain or discomfort lying down at night, consider restless leg syndrome or intermittent claudication (Collares and Faintuch 2017). See Chapter 6 for a more detailed exploration of pain and its impact.

Stress

Stress in both family and work environments may worsen prognosis and accelerate the progression of coronary heart disease and atherosclerosis in women (Wang et al. 2006).

Alcoholism

Alcohol can increase the risk of arterial disease by narrowing the arteries and reducing blood flow. Alcohol works as a vasoconstrictor, causing veins to tighten and constrict (Kawano 2010).

Mobility

Studies show that regular exercise protects against the development of VLUs (Wittens et al. 2015; Smith et al. 2018). The calf muscle pump function is reduced in patients with VLUs and non-functioning of the calf muscle pump in permanent immobility leads to an outflow disorder, which may result in oedema and skin changes (Suehiro et al. 2014). Co-morbidities resulting in reduced mobility that are found to be associated with VLUs include rheumatic diseases, PAD and neuropathy (Seitz et al. 2010; Matic et al. 2016). Note that any limb deformity including of the foot is especially important in patients who have rheumatoid arthritis or diabetes, for instance Charcot's foot. Assess ankle mobility and action of the calf muscle pump to aid in venous return (Chapter 4 explores the biomechanical fundamentals).

Quality of Life

Consider whether the person has any symptoms that affect their quality of life (NICE 2023). Concerns could include malodour, exudate, finding appropriate footwear and social isolation.

Loneliness and Isolation

Leg ulceration can be lonely and isolating. Malodour or poor exudate management can add to this significantly, as can difficulty finding appropriate footwear. Signpost patients to support services such as Lindsay Leg Clubs (www.legclub.org). Leg Clubs were initially set up in 1995 to offer community-focused support to patients in a social non-medical environment. Healthcare professionals work in collaboration with volunteers to support health promotion. The social aspect of meeting others with the same condition can prevent social isolation and support integration into their local community. However, it is worthy of note that not all areas of the UK have Leg Clubs. Legs Matters (https://legsmatter.org) is an organisation that provides advice on leg care and foot health that is accessible for patients and healthcare professionals.

Family/Carer Support

Discuss long-term support with the patient. This could be a relative, carer, friend or neighbour who may be willing to support with the application and removal of compression hosiery or wraps. Attendance allowance is not means tested and patients should be signposted to apply for this if help with personal care is required.

Employment

Ask the patient what they do for work. People who have occupations that require prolonged standing are more are risk of developing venous disease (Atkin 2019). The sustained pressure of standing for long periods of time is thought to lead to venous distention and secondary valvular incompetence (Nicholls 2005).

Psychological Status

Assess the patient's psychological status. There is increasing recognition of the role that psychological status plays in the development and outcomes of chronic disease (Moffatt et al. 2009). The nature of leg ulceration can affect the most important spheres of human life: physical, psychosocial and emotional. Leg ulcers are accompanied by numerous symptoms, including pain, pruritus, joint deformation, swelling, discharge and unpleasant odour. These symptoms can diminish quality of life (QoL) by restricting physical activities, influencing mobility, causing sleeplessness, depressing mood, limiting professional, social and familial relationships and leading to financial difficulties (Platsidaki et al. 2017). Family members can experience a significant impact on their lives too. This impact depends on the duration and the severity of the disease, the treatment that is followed and, above all, the relationship with the patient. Patients with leg ulcers demonstrate higher anxiety levels in comparison with healthy people (Platsidaki et al. 2017). This could be explained by the associated stressors of living with leg ulcers, which lead to negative emotions and anxiety. Understanding the person's emotional state of mind can determine their ability to engage with the assessment and management process, which is particularly important for long-term conditions (Table 5.1). See Chapter 7 for a greater exploration of the impact on QoL and further discussion of self-care, personalisation and psychosocial support.

Good history taking in leg ulcer management can provide health-care practitioners with the essential information required to ensure that care is effective and patient centred based on individual values, beliefs and expectations.

TABLE 5.1   Psychological assessment.

Mental health history	Has the patient been detained under the Mental Health Act?
	Do they have capacity and ability to answer questions during the assessment?
	Is there a risk of self-harm?
	A patient's ability to engage may be affected by their understanding and capacity, which are fundamental to gaining a therapeutic relationship with the healthcare provider (Wounds UK 2019b).
	It is also important to remember that just because someone is making a decision that the professional feels is clinically unwise, this does not mean they do not have capacity, and it is their right to do so if they have capacity.
Current mental health	Is the patient at risk?
	Do they require an advocate or an assessment to review their mental capacity?
Clinical depression	Is the patient currently or have they in the past been diagnosed with depression?
	Is this exacerbated by the patient's current mental state?
	Research suggests that there is a direct association between having a leg ulcer and depression (Upton et al. 2014). This may be influenced by changes in their daily activities of living (Platsidaki et al. 2017).
Anxiety	Does the patient appear anxious?
	Are there any areas of particular concern?
	Anxiety can be raised, with consequent inability to work and feelings of inadequacy to care for and provide for the family (Platsidaki et al. 2017).
Belief systems	What are the patient's belief systems around medical management and self-management?
	What is their understanding of how the wound will heal?
	A study by Walburn et al. (2017) found that there was an association between slower healing leg ulcers and patients who had negative beliefs and perceptions about the ability to heal the ulcer.

TABLE 5.1 (Continued)

Understanding own health needs	Does the patient understand the nature of leg ulceration and what they can do to help themselves? Supported self-management (NHS 2020) should be encouraged following a mental capacity assessment. How is the patient currently managing anxiety around their health or current problem? Additional mental health support may be appropriate.
Expectations	What is the patient's expectation (hopes and fears) of this assessment? It is important to identify small goals that are achievable. It is important to work collaboratively with the patient and build trust. Patients tend to have fewer symptoms of their condition and have higher satisfaction with the treatment they receive if they have trust in the healthcare professional delivering their care (Birkhäuer et al. 2017).
Motivation	How motivated is the patient towards treatment and lifestyle change? Motivation is an inherent part of the healing process.
Perception of and living with an ulcer – body image challenges	How is having a leg ulcer affecting the patient's self-image, hobbies and social life? Salomé et al. (2016) found that patients with leg ulcers had negative feelings about their bodies with low self-esteem.
Loss of status, self-esteem and independence	Is the patient dependent on others to support them with daily activities? Have they lost their independence, which can lead to a loss of self-esteem? The symptoms associated with leg ulcers, e.g. pain, malodour and exudate, can reduce functionality and culminate in a feeling of low self-esteem (Salomé 2020).
Psychological assessment – dependence on nursing services	Assess the patient's level of dependence on nursing services. Patients may suffer from social isolation, malodour or wound exudate leakage (Platsidaki et al. 2017).

(Continued)

TABLE 5.1 (Continued)

Quality of life	Assess the patient's quality of life with the use of a validated tool, e.g. the Quality of Life Wound Checklist (Green et al. 2018).
Concordance, adherence and ability to tolerate treatment	A patient may choose not to adhere to a plan of care for a variety of reasons, especially if incorrect compression is applied and is not effective, or feels uncomfortable.
	Ensure that treatment planning is patient centred and that patients are empowered to become active participants in their own care.
	The care plan should respond to the patient's individual needs, values and preferences.

EXAMINATION

Practitioners who manage people with leg ulceration need to be competent in recognising clinical signs and symptoms of PAD and chronic venous insufficiency (CVI). CEAP is a standardised classification system based on the current understanding of venous pathology, signs, symptoms and manifestations of the disease process (Lurie et al. 2020). The issues of concern are categorised as follows:

- **C**linical presentation
- **E**tiology
- **A**bnormalities found
- **P**athophysiology of the problem encountered

The clinical presentation classification is divided into six categories and further subdivisions (Table 5.2). Determination of CEAP classification requires an interprofessional team of health professionals, specialists and assessors (Zegarra and Tadi 2022).

A comprehensive assessment of the limb is vital to identify early indications of venous disease, assess for the presence of arterial disease, and strategies to maintain the patient's QoL and reduce the prevalence of ulceration or adverse limb events (Tummala and Scherbel 2018).

TABLE 5.2 The CEAP standard for identifying venous disease.

Category	Description
C0	No visible or palpable signs of venous disease. This category is often overlooked – however, early intervention at this stage can have excellent results. Patients report tired, heavy legs.	This section has been subdivided into two categories: ■ Patients with venous symptoms and no signs of venous disease, with reflux or obstruction identified during routine investigations. ■ Patients with venous symptoms, no venous signs and no pathological findings. 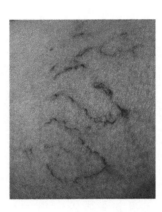 **FIGURE 5.1** Signs of telangiectasis.
C1	Telangiectasis or spider veins are dilated venules or arterioles measuring less than 1.0 mm in diameter (Figure 5.1).	Telangiectasis can appear anywhere on the lower extremities (Thomson 2016), but quite often in the thigh region caused by dilation of the capillaries just under the surface of the skin. Reticular veins have a diameter of less than 3 mm. These are often tortuous and located in the subdermal or subcutaneous tissue (Eklof et al. 2004) and are the first visible signs of venous problems.

(Continued)

TABLE 5.2 (Continued)

Category	Description
C2	Varicose veins. Swollen or enlarged veins.

Varicose veins are a significant indicator of chronic venous insufficiency (CVI) affecting an estimated 30% of the population (this is considered to be underreported) (Onida and Davies 2016). For this category, these are subcutaneous, dilated and tortuous veins measuring more than 3 mm in diameter when the patient is in a standing position (Collares and Faintuch 2017). Varicose veins are caused by damage to the valves that prevent the backflow of blood from the deep to the superficial venous system. Venous valve damage is serious enough that backflow and blood pooling cause vein walls to stretch beyond repair. This makes it increasingly difficult for the venous system to pump blood back to the heart. Varicose veins can change in severity from mild to moderate and may be bumpy in appearance, ranging from reddish to purple or blue in colour (Figure 5.2).

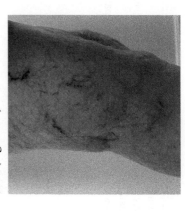

FIGURE 5.2 Signs of enlarged veins.

C2r	Recurrent varicose veins.	The incidence of recurrent varicose veins after surgery is reported to be between 20% and 80% (Winterborn et al. 2004; Blomgren et al. 2004).
C3	Oedema. Swelling for more than 3 months in duration, which mostly involves the toes and feet and can extend up into the thigh. Less likely to resolve on limb elevation and skin changes indicative of lymphoedema are likely to follow (see Chapter 2).	In CVI this tends to be pitting oedema (excess fluid in the body, causing swelling when under pressure and the skin remains indented), which gets worse during the day and is resolved partially when the patient goes to bed at night. This should not be confused with cardiac or renal oedema, which is non-pitting. Other symptoms of cardiac and renal oedema include shortness of breath, bilateral oedema, fatigue, urine retention and oedema extending to other parts of the body.
C4	Changes in skin and subcutaneous tissue secondary to venous disease.	Often associated with changes that cause discomfort, pain, sleep disturbances, absenteeism in the workplace, disability and deteriorated quality of life (Ruggiero et al. 2016).

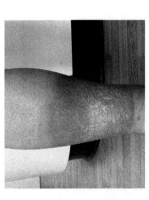

FIGURE 5.3 Signs of hyperpigmentation, staining and hyperkeratosis. Courtesy of Accelerate / Andrew Joyce.

(Continued)

TABLE 5.2 (Continued)

Category	Description
C4a	Hyperpigmentation. A red/brown discoloration of the skin (this is a deep brown in darker skin) caused by leakage and breakdown of red blood cells from the capillary network into the skin. Presentation can be small, localised patches or extend over the gaiter region.	This can be quite a distressing symptom to the patient as it can look like dirty marks on the skin (Figure 5.3). A note of caution is that although this is a sign of venous disease, it does not disappear when the ulcer is healed and as the patient ages may still be present with arterial disease (Lymphoedema Framework 2006).
C4a	Varicose eczema, an inflammatory condition caused by the irritation of blood products that have leaked into the skin and present as red, itchy, scaly or flaky skin that may have blisters and crusts (NICE 2022).	Varicose eczema (Figure 5.4) can present as wet or dry and can be localised or may involve the whole gaiter region. Occasionally, if the patient scratches the eczema this can lead to a much more widespread manifestation. It can often be confused with contact dermatitis and irritant eczema. Both of these are also commonly found in combination with varicose eczema and leg ulceration.

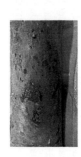

FIGURE 5.4 Varicose eczema.

| C4b | Atrophie blanche (AB; white atrophy), angular scars on the lower leg or foot. | AB is mainly located on the lower leg. This is a condition whereby white, 'lacy' areas of vascular tissue are interspersed with visibly engorged capillaries, which are seen as tiny red dots below the surface of the skin and are often surrounded by regions of skin hyperpigmentation (Figure 5.5) (McVittie and Holloway 2015). AB is caused by low blood flow as a result of fibrin plugs causing occlusion to the vessels, increasing the propensity to ulcerate (McVittie and Holloway 2015). These patches can be small or extensive, arising on areas of the skin that have never ulcerated or areas where there was a previous ulceration. AB results in localised hypoxic areas that can lead to ulceration. It can be classified as idiopathic (the absence of related diseases) or secondary (as a consequence of other systemic conditions, most commonly CVI). Patients describe excruciating neuropathic stabbing or shooting pain. This is likely to be caused by a combination of localised ischaemia and inflammation of the capillary walls and can make the introduction of compression intolerable. (For pain associated with AB, see Chapter 6.) The patient can experience painful, purpuric lesions that progress to punched-out ulcers. These will heal with porcelain-white, stellate scars (Harper and Crane 2022). |

(Continued)

TABLE 5.2 (Continued)

Category | **Description**

Lidodermatosclerosis (LDS), chronic inflammation and hardening (fibrosis) of the dermis and subcutaneous tissue of the lower limb (NICE 2022).

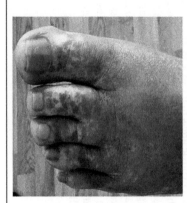

FIGURE 5.5 Atrophie blanche.

LDS is often present in venous disease and is thought to be caused by leakage and laying down of the fibrin from the capillary network, fat necrosis, inflammation and scarring. Progressive fibrosis leads to increased skin fragility and atrophic skin surface, with loss of sweat glands and hair follicles. The presentation is a hard, woody layer just below the surface of the skin, often beginning around the ankle region and gradually extending up to the mid-calf region over the years. This process can give rise to an 'inverted champagne bottle'–shaped leg whereby soft swelling accumulates in the calf, distorting the leg shape as a result of fibrinous tissue replacing the fatty layer and oedema being trapped above, usually in the knee and thigh (Figure 5.6).

The skin around the ankle becomes too tight to stretch. Acute stages of LDS are often misdiagnosed as cellulitis and phlebitis (Miteva et al. 2010). Unlike cellulitis, its borders do not change quickly, and the patient will not be pyrexic. LDS can be acute or chronic. In the acute phase it can be very painful. Chronic pain with LDS tends to be more of a dull ache (Miteva et al. 2010). Unless treated with compression, the leg will continue to become increasingly inflamed and break down. Compression may need to be introduced gradually with analgesia if AB is present. Generally, acute LDS progresses to a chronic state. It is important to note that chronic LDS does not always begin with an acute episode. This presents as areas of pale to dark brown leathery skin that is too tight to pinch up (it may be harder to spot in dark skin tones).

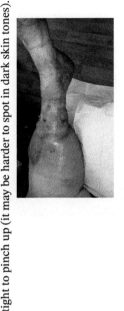

FIGURE 5.6 Lipodermatosclerosis and venous staining. Courtesy of Accelerate.

(*Continued*)

TABLE 5.2 (Continued)

Category	Description
C4c	Corona phlebectatica (ankle flare) is a distended myriad of tiny varicose veins caused by perforator vein incompetence, which causes the blood to pool and stretch the blood vessels.

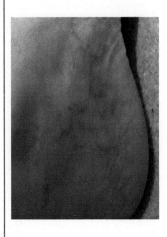

FIGURE 5.7 Signs of ankle flare.

Look for a fan-shaped pattern of several small intradermal veins commonly located around the medial or lateral aspects of the ankle and foot (Figure 5.7) (Collares and Faintuch 2017).

Category	Description
C5	A person's leg will always be at risk of reoccurrence of ulceration and so they must be transitioned into the correct dose and type of compression hosiery stockings once healed to prevent reoccurrence. This is discussed further in Chapter 9. If venous leg ulcers have not healed within 12 weeks of treatment, the patient should be referred to appropriate specialist services (Wounds UK 2022).
	Healed.

C6	Venous leg ulcer. A leg ulcer is defined as a break in the skin that has failed to heal in two weeks (NICE 2021).	These typically occur in the medial or gaiter region. They are the most common type of leg ulcer and in the United Kingdom 420000 leg ulcer patients are managed by the NHS (Guest et al. 2018).
C6r	Recurrent active venous ulcer.	When a venous leg ulcer has healed, prevention of recurrence is vital. Regular review and reassessment are essential, together with educating the patient to keep vigilant for any signs of changes to the lower limb (Wounds UK 2022).

Source: Adapted from Lurie et al. (2020).

ARTERIAL DISEASE

While venous leg ulceration is reportedly the most commonly occurring type of ulceration, healthcare practitioners need to develop competence in recognising clinical symptoms of PAD, ischaemic changes and arterial pain (Figure 5.8). These are discussed further in Table 5.3 and the 6 Ps of PAD are listed in Table 5.4.

A simple way for healthcare practitioners to be cognisant of this variety of clinical presentations related to PAD is the 6 Ps of PAD, described in Table 5.4. See Chapter 8 for a discussion of clinical management in the presence of PAD.

Effective wound treatment and preventative care depend on accurate and thorough assessment, leading to a diagnosis that triggers action and is tailored to the individual patient, their skin and their wound. Assessment should involve a thorough inspection of the skin, and this should include finding out about the patient's baseline skin tone. This is vital so that any changes to patients' skin, for example signs of inflammation and haemosiderin, are observed and monitored in the same way. Skin inspection and awareness of skin tone should be carried out as part of a holistic assessment. The use of a validated skin tone classification tool is a simple way of assessing skin tone across healthcare settings (Figure 5.9).

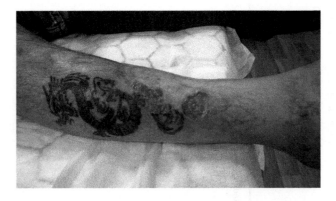

FIGURE 5.8 Arterial ulceration. Courtesy of Accelerate.

TABLE 5.3 Identifying arterial disease in the lower limb.

Ischaemic limb changes – acute limb ischaemia is a sudden decrease in limb perfusion threatening the viability of the limb due to artery occlusion, vascular bypass graft or stent (Cai and Forsyth 2022).	Cold limbs – note if the limbs are cold in a warm environment and feel the difference between the two limbs.	In the presence of arterial disease, the limb may range from very pale to mottled blue due to the lack of oxygenated blood. Limbs may have a deep red/purple hue in pale skin tones. Dependent rubor (when the limb is in a dependent position) is caused by the dilation of dermal arterioles and capillaries in the presence of increased hydrostatic pressure (Mintz et al. 2013) in the foot, as an attempt to adequately oxygenate the limb. This results in the pooling of arterial blood. N.B. It can often be mistaken for cellulitis or a well-perfused limb. In darker skin tones these colour changes are important to note and to compare with another limb; dependent rubor will present as darker than other areas and paler if the person is hypoxic.
		Buerger's test (Buerger 1924) identifies the position of the rubor (in a healthy limb this should stay the same whether elevated or dependent). To assess dependent rubor ask the patient to lie flat on their back and gently elevate their limb to above the heart at a 90° angle (hold this for approx. 30 seconds). Lower the limb noting any changes in colour. If dependent rubor is the cause for colour change, the limb will become pale on elevation; redness or a darkening of the skin in darker skin tones will gradually return once the limb is lowered (Eder et al. 2019).
		Although this remains a very beneficial test when vascular assessment equipment may not be available, it has been replaced in part by the pole test (1994), whereby a handheld Doppler is used when the limb is elevated to a height of 77 cm. If Doppler sounds can still be heard, this is a good indication that there is adequate arterial flow to the foot (Eder et al. 2019).

(Continued)

TABLE 5.3 (Continued)

Loss of sensation, hair loss, atrophic skin changes with white skin tones turning paler, trophic changes to nails and muscle wastage resulting in weakness in the legs. Non-healing foot or leg ulcer.	Assess for any lower limb changes.	These are all symptoms of peripheral arterial disease (PAD). The arteries become hardened when plaque attaches to the artery walls and blood flow to the lower limb is restricted.
Lower limb oedema.	Dependent oedema – check the limb for dependent oedema.	Patients with arterial disease may still have significant limb oedema (Nickles et al. 2023). This can result in the patient being unable to sleep at night with their legs elevated because of ischaemic night pain. For most patients relief is found by spending the night in a chair with their legs down, although this may then cause an increase in oedema from limb dependency and further reduce the arterial blood flow (Woelk 2012). There is some evidence to suggest that patients with lower limb oedema and peripheral arterial disease may benefit from some compression therapy (Nickles et al. 2023), but caution should be exercised and this should only be instigated through specialist experts within tissue viability or under vascular guidance.
Absent pedal pulses.	Feel for pedal pulses and note any absence.	Refer to the section on ankle brachial pressure index assessment. The palpation of pedal pulses on its own is insufficient to detect the presence or absence of arterial disease.

Ischaemic pain.	Pain is associated with the lack of oxygen to the lower limb. Assess the patient's experiences of pain.	This can present in several ways depending on severity.

There can be intermittent claudication. The muscles of the lower limb require increased blood flow when walking and exercising. Patients with PAD have a decreased blood supply to the lower limb when this is maximised, and no further perfusion can be supplied to the lower extremity muscles. The supply and demand mismatch causes temporary ischaemia of the muscles that presents as pain, cramping and fatigue (Zemaitis et al. 2022). The pain disappears at rest when the oxygen demand is reduced. Record how far the patient can walk before the onset of pain.

Night pain occurs when legs are elevated at night. Blood pressure drops during sleep. In patients with PAD this reduced blood pressure is not sufficient to maintain perfusion in the lower limb. Relief can be gained by hanging the legs over the edge of the bed.

Rest pain occurs even when sitting. It often involves the foot and indicates a severe reduction in arterial blood flow required for normal tissue metabolism (see Chapter 6 for pain assessment and management).

TABLE 5.4 The 6 Ps of peripheral arterial disease (PAD).

Pain
Pallor
Poikilothermia
Pulselessness
Paraesthesia
Paralysis or power loss

FIGURE 5.9 Skin tone tool.
Source: Wounds UK (2021). Reproduced with permission.

WOUND ASSESSMENT

The holistic assessment of a wound is essential to identify causative and contributory factors, support diagnosis and determine factors that may contribute to delayed wound healing. Wound assessment should include assessment of the wound bed, care and intervention planning, evaluation of treatment and interventions and continual reassessment. Accurate and timely wound assessment underpins effective clinical decision-making, appropriate patient-centred goals, and reduced morbidity and costs associated with the burden of wound care (Posnett and Franks 2008).

It is important that clinicians understand the factors that influence wound healing as part of the holistic assessment (Table 5.5).

On the first presentation build up a picture of the origin of the ulcer. This presentation will help to identify the patient's specific

TABLE 5.5   Intrinsic and extrinsic factors that affect wound healing.

Intrinsic

Oxygenation: oxygen is essential for cell metabolism and energy production. Hypoxic wounds are at increased risk of infection, reduced angiogenesis (the development of new blood vessels), reduced epithelialisation, fibroblast (connective tissue cell) proliferation, collagen synthesis and wound contraction (Guo and DiPietro 2010).

Infection: once the skin is injured, micro-organisms that are normally on the skin surface access underlying tissue. Infected wounds become 'stuck' in the inflammatory phase. The pathogenic microbes compete with the fibroblasts for nutrients and other resources (Guo and DiPietro 2010).

Venous insufficiency: increased venous pressure over time leads to a chronic inflammatory response, which can cause the breakdown of tissue resulting in venous leg ulceration (Wounds UK 2016).

Diabetes: prolonged wound hypoxia, dysfunction in fibroblasts and epidermal cells, impaired angiogenesis and neovascularisation (natural formation of new blood vessels) decrease host immune resistance and neuropathy (Guo and DiPietro 2010).

Peripheral arterial disease: decreased blood flow to the lower extremities and wound, reducing the amount of oxygen and nutrients to the wound bed.

Temperature: the cooler the wound, the longer it will take to heal. Higher temperatures promote vascular dilation.

Necrotic tissue or foreign bodies: both prolong the inflammatory response and increase the risk of infection.

Oedema: affects the permeability of vascular membranes, inflammation or tissue trauma. Also, fluid can leak into the surrounding tissue.

Dehydration: fluids are required for oxygen profusion, hydration of the wound bed, transportation of nutrients, as a solvent for vitamins, minerals, glucose, amino acids and to transport waste away from cells.

Extrinsic

Age: skin loses its elasticity with ageing. Collagen is reduced and blood flow can be restricted due to other chronic conditions. Other factors that delay wound healing in older people are altered inflammatory response, delayed T-cell infiltration and alterations in chemokine production, and reduced macrophage phagocytic capacity.

Sex: oestrogen helps to regulate a variety of genes associated with regeneration. Older males and post-menopausal women are at a higher risk of chronic wounds (Oh and Phillips 2006).

Co-morbidities: conditions such as diabetes, chronic venous insufficiency, peripheral arterial disease and immune deficiency disorders are known to delay the wound healing process. Additional screening for these co-morbidities in patients with wounds is recommended.

(Continued)

TABLE 5.5 (Continued)

In diabetes narrowed blood vessels lead to decreased blood flow and oxygen to a wound. Elevated blood sugars decrease red blood cells, which carry nutrients to the tissue, and lower the efficacy of white blood cells (neutrophils and monocytes) in fighting infection.

Obesity: reduces the availability of oxygen to the wound. Skin folds can harbour bacteria and damage can be caused by skin-to-skin friction and increase the risk of pressure ulcer development (Mitchell 2018). Obesity can also be connected to stress, anxiety and depression.

Medications: steroids, non-steroidal anti-inflammatory drugs, chemotherapy – many medicines interfere with clot formation or platelet function, inflammatory responses and cell proliferation.

Nutrition: nutrition is required to provide adequate support for the increased energy demands during the healing process. Inadequate protein leads to skin fragility, decreased immune function and poor wound healing. The body requires 30–35 Kcal daily to heal a wound and 40 Kcal if the patient is underweight.

Lifestyle factors: smoking causes vasoconstriction, which leads to hypoxia. Neutrophil and monocyte (cells that help prevent infection) activity is reduced and fibroblast proliferation and migration are reduced. Collagen is reduced in smokers, which means less tensile wound strength. Alcoholism diminishes host resistance, making the body more at risk of infection. Alcohol decreases phagocytic function (phagocytosis is a three-stage process in which neutrophils, monocytes and macrophages engulf and destroy micro-organisms, other foreign antigens and cell debris). Release of cytokines (small secreted proteins released by cells that have a specific effect on the interactions and communications between cells) is suppressed and angiogenesis is reduced.

Immunocompromised conditions: cancer, radiotherapy, AIDS. Chemotherapy and radiation can slow wound healing. Processes such as cellular replication, inflammatory reactions and tissue repair are compromised. Radiation therapy can cause permanent tissue damage.

Stress and anxiety: stress delays wound healing by altering the multiple physiological pathways required in the repair processes (Gouin and Kiecolt-Glaser 2011). Stressors can lead to negative emotional states, for example anxiety and depression, which have an impact on physiological processes and behavioural patterns that influence health outcomes (Guo and DiPietro 2010).

Pain: ineffective wound pain management can delay wound healing and contribute to lack of concordance with treatment (Frescos 2011).

Source: Adapted from Mitchell (2020), with permission of the British Journal of Nursing.

treatment pathway. Many wounds start as the result of a trauma and some wounds appear spontaneously or for no obvious reason. Ask the patient some specific questions:

- When and how did the wound occur?
- Where is the wound located?
- Is this the first episode of a wound?
- Have you been diagnosed with a leg ulcer before?
- What was the time taken to heal the previous ulcer?
- How long have you not had an ulcer for?
- What were the past treatments (successful and unsuccessful)?

TIMES (Tissue viability, Inflammation or Infection, Moisture balance, Edge of wound, Surrounding skin or peri-wound area) is a framework used to focus on specific wound bed parameters to aid management and guide treatment. It should be used as part of a holistic assessment (Atkin 2019) (Table 5.6).

During the initial assessment, clues with respect to the location of the ulcer and basic clinical descriptors may point to the likely cause and diagnosis (Chapter 1). Leg ulcers do not always fit into two distinct categories. Observations in clinical practice indicate that there is a belief that three types of ulceration exist: venous, arterial and mixed aetiology. In reality there are many other, perhaps less commonly observed types of ulceration, which are examined in Chapter 3. Basic clinical descriptors of unusual aetiologies may include the following:

- Atypical site for the suspected aetiology. Be wary if the ulcer is in an unusual location and develops spontaneously.
- Atypical tissue type. Observe for wounds that bleed easily: appear to scab over quickly and or break down recurrently; look healthy but fail to show normal signs of healing.
- Atypical history. Did it occur very quickly or spontaneously? Is it not progressing as expected? Observe for clusters of small ulcers, blistering and ulcers that rapidly increase in size.
- Atypical shape or depth.
- Atypical edges. Observe for any raised or rolled edges or discoloured wound margins.

TABLE 5.6 TIMES wound assessment.

T – Tissue viability (Figure 5.10). Repair and regeneration or non-viable tissue?	Is the wound showing signs of regeneration and repair, such as granulation tissue or epithelial cells, or is the wound bed displaying non-viable tissue, for example slough, necrosis or eschar? Consider if the amount of devitalised or non-viable tissue is influencing wound healing or facilitating infection (Atkin 2019).
	Identify the site of the wound, which may give an indication of whether an ulcer is venous, arterial or mixed aetiology. Classically venous ulcers present in the gaiter area of the leg, but be mindful that there are always exceptions to these rules.
	Measure the wound size. This should be documented in the patient's notes and updated on dressing changes. If taking photographs, adhere to any local guidelines and seek permission from the patient (Ousey and Cook 2012).
	Identify the wound depth, if necessary take a measurement using a sterile probe. This procedure should only be carried out by qualified practitioners who are familiar with anatomical structures in close proximity to the wound. Also look for tracking, cavities or fistulae from the wound bed.
	Consider debridement. The type of debridement needs to be determined by the clinical presentation, the patient's preferences and circumstances, and variations in clinical skills (Atkin 2019).
	Assess the extent of tissue involvement. Does the wound involve the epidermis, dermis, fat, fascia? Review if there is exposed muscle and/or bone.
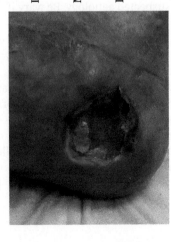 **FIGURE 5.10** Repair and regeneration.	Document any wound odour. A slight odour may be associated with an occlusive dressing type. Fungating and necrotic wounds are often malodorous. If a wound is heavily colonised this can cause malodour (Edward-Jones 2018).

Consider using an odour assessment tool when documenting odour:

- Strong odour – evident when entering the room, dressing is intact.
- Moderate odour – evident when entering the room, dressing removed.
- Slight odour – evident during dressing change.
- No odour – no odour during dressing change (Haughton and Young 1995).

Hypergranulation, also known as overgranulation, can exercise clinicians; healthy granulation is often misdiagnosed as hypergranulation in lower leg wounds.

Granulation develops in the proliferation stage and is a critical stage in wound healing. Hypergranulation is when the granulation tissue 'over grows beyond the wound surface' (Mitchell and Llumigusin 2021) and can inhibit healing, often due to adverse conditions at the wound bed.

Healthy granulation tissue: very vascular, pink and moist. Usually at the level of the surrounding skin except when oedematous or simply very active tissue, responding well to the treatment regime.

Unhealthy granulation tissue: darker tissue bed, can be very flat or raised and is friable, bleeding easily when touched. Raised or hypergranulating wound beds also are protruding, not just a raised mound, and these protrusions are jelly-like when pushed and bleed readily. The wound healing gets stuck and the energy appears to go to growing upwards rather than into the maturation phase. This may be exacerbated by infection or biofilm. The clinician will be seeing a wound that is *not* reducing in width.

When is a raised granulating wound bed healthy and not a concern? The raised granulation tissue remains pink and healthy, even globular in nature, but on weekly review the clinician will find that the width of the wound continues to contract and exudate is controlled.

Despite the raised tissue, the edges are still flattening and contracting. Healing is continuing. This is therefore not true adverse hypergranulation tissue that needs clinical attention; carry on with standard wound management. Adopt a wait-and-see approach (Vuolo 2010).

It is important to note that true hypergranulation is more common in surgical wounds and uncommon in leg ulceration. Non-healing hypergranulation may also be suspicious; see Chapter 4 on unusual aetiologies.

(Continued)

TABLE 5.6 (Continued)

I – Infection or Inflammation (Figure 5.11).

Inflammation (or the inflammatory response) is a normal stage of wound healing. If the wound is red, hot, swollen or painful within the first 1–7 days of injury occurring, then this is a normal inflammatory response and unless the wound is physically dirty it is not likely to be infected.

Chronic inflammation, however, is problematic and is often caused through a high bacterial burden in the wound bed. This is frequently related to the presence of biofilm.

Biofilms are made up of micro-organisms that gather in islands across the wound bed and attach themselves to the wound surface. They are protected within a polysaccharide matrix that is impervious to antimicrobials; this can delay wound healing and cause chronic inflammation (Steven et al. 2012) as the normal inflammatory response of phagocytosis, often referred to as the 'clearing-up phase', is unable to occur as the micro-organisms are protected by the matrix, and so the wound bed itself is attacked. This causes a state of ongoing inflammation that impedes wound healing.

Biofilms are almost impossible to see with the naked eye. However, if a wound is static with no signs of overt infection, it is highly likely that a biofilm will have been formed (Stoodley et al. 2002).

The clinical indications of a biofilm may present as:

- No response to antimicrobial treatment.
- Delayed healing beyond expectations.
- Friable granulation tissue that bleeds easily on contact.
- Low-level inflammation and erythema.
- Increase in wound exudate.
- Wound breakdown following completion of antibiotics.
- Signs of secondary infection (IWII 2016).

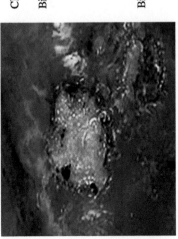

FIGURE 5.11 Infection and inflammation of the tissue.

The opposite of a biofilm infection is a spreading infection. This is when the microbial burden in the wound increases and the person is at risk of becoming unwell as infection spreads and there is a risk of systemic infection.

Assess for signs of infection, which may be indicated by swelling, localised heat or pain, erythema, purulent discharge (white, yellow or brown and might be slightly thick in texture), increased exudate, malodour and pyrexia (Wilson 2012).

Measure the patient's core temperature. Laboratory investigations for inflammation markers such as C-reactive protein (CRP) may be indicated.

Assess the wound for any foreign bodies present in the wound bed, which may be a source of infection.

The wound infection continuum guides the clinician to the signs and symptoms of wound infection to support accurate diagnosis and to enable the appropriate use of antimicrobial wound dressings and antibiotics for systemic infection.

The diagnosis of wound infection should be made using a combination of clinical presentation and clinical judgement. Routine swabbing is not indicated in leg ulcer management. However, if it is decided that a swab is rationalised, then use the Levine technique to collect cultures.

Do not delay the commencement of antibiotics for spreading infection while waiting for a swab result, but keep in mind that antibiotics do not promote wound healing in a leg ulcer that is not clinically infected (NICE 2020).

(*Continued*)

TABLE 5.6 (Continued)

M – Moisture balance. Is there too much or too little exudate?	A moist wound bed has been shown to improve healing and reduce pain, discomfort and infection (Winter 1962). Whereas contact with wound fluid is beneficial to the healing process in acute wounds, it contains substances detrimental to cell proliferation and can inhibit healing of hard-to-heal wounds (Cutting and White 2002). Large amounts of exudate can be indicative of infection or unmanaged oedema.
	Exudate usually occurs as a result of vasodilation in the inflammatory phase. Exudate is mainly water, but also contains electrolytes, nutrients, proteins, inflammatory mediators, protein-digesting enzymes such as matrix metalloproteinases (MMPs), growth factors, neutrophils, macrophages, platelets and waste cells (Cutting 2004).
	Assessment of exudate is an essential part of wound management and should include type, colour, amount, odour (if any) and viscosity at each dressing change. Table 5.7 describes the exudate and its significance.
	If the wound is too dry, this will inhibit the epithelial cell's ability to migrate across the wound bed, thus an overly dry wound bed is also detrimental to wound healing.

E – wound Edge (Figure 5.12).Epithelial edges or non-viable edges?

Wound margins tend to change in appearance as the wound heals or deteriorates (Wilson 2012).

Classically the edges of an arterial ulcer will be 'punched out' in shape and the wound will be deep from the edges. This is sometimes termed 'cliff edges'.

Typically in venous ulceration a less conforming edge that slopes gradually is noted.

It is unlikely that epithelial advancement will occur if high levels of exudate, underlying pathology, biofilm or infection have not been addressed (Atkin 2019).

The edge of the wound should be flattened and advancing across the granulation tissue. If rolled edges are present (hyperbole), this is a sign of a long-standing wound where epithelial advancement has been hindered due to an overly dry or high bacterial burden in the wound bed over a continued period of time.

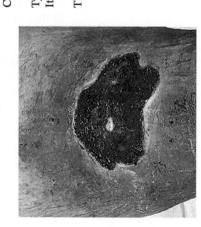

FIGURE 5.12 Epithelial wound edges.

S – Surrounding skin

Assess the peri-wound skin for moisture damage or compromise. Peri-wound moisture-associated dermatitis may indicate that more absorbent dressings or frequent dressing changes are required or that the dose of compression therapy is sub-optimal.

Regular washing, cleansing and moisturising of the surrounding skin are an integral part of lower limb management. See Chapter 8 for more.

Source: Adapted from Mitchell (2020) with permission of the British Journal of Nursing.

TABLE 5.7 Descriptions of exudates and their significance.

Type	Consistency	Colour	Significance
Serous	Thin, watery	Clear, straw-coloured	Often considered normal, but increased volume may indicate infection (e.g. *Staphylococcus aureus*). May also be due to fluid from urinary or lymphatic fistula.
Fibrinous	Thin, watery	Cloudy	May indicate the presence of fibrin strands, which would indicate a response to inflammation.
Sero-sanguineous	Thin, slightly thicker than water	Clear, pink	Presence of red blood cells indicates capillary damage (e.g. after surgery or a traumatic dressing removal).
Sanguineous	Thin, watery	Reddish	Low protein content due to venous or congestive cardiac disease, malnutrition or enteric or urinary fistula.
Purulent	Viscous, sticky	Opaque, milky, yellow or brown, sometimes green	White blood cells, bacteria, slough or from enteric or urinary fistula. Bacterial infection (e.g. *Pseudomonas aeruginosa*).

TABLE 5.7 (Continued)

Type	Consistency	Colour	Significance
Haemopurulent	Viscous	Reddish, milky	Established infection. May contain neutrophils, dying bacteria, inflammatory cells, blood leakage due to dermal capillaries, some bacteria.
Haemorrhagic	Viscous	Dark red	Capillaries break down easily and bleed due to infection or trauma.

Source: Adapted from World Union of Wound Healing Societies (2007), Wounds UK (2013) and Nichols (2016).

SKIN ASSESSMENT

The skin surrounding wounds often has compromised integrity caused by tissue inflammation. Surrounding skin is more susceptible to irritation, maceration and loss of epithelium as a result of moisture damage and wound exudate (Dini et al. 2020). Observation of the peri-wound via fluorescent imagery (MolecuLight) indicates for most wounds an elevated level of bacteria that can transfer into the wound bed (Sharpe et al. 2022). Early recognition of the risk of skin breakdown is an essential part of prevention. The skin should be assessed holistically as part of the patient's regular assessment and reassessment (Table 5.8):

- Ask the patient about their normal skin well-being, including skin hygiene, integrity and management (Mitchell 2022).
- Note any changes in the skin colour or discoloration (refer to Table 5.2).

TABLE 5.8   Skin assessment.

Dry, flaky skin and varicose eczema. Also known as gravitational eczema or venous stasis (Atkins et al. 2020).	A good skincare regime is required with washing and thorough drying of skin. Using soap substitutes alongside emollients can support skin integrity (Wounds UK 2020). Varicose eczema may be treated with a course of topical steroids (NHS Inform 2022).
Hyperkeratosis – thick, scaly skin – is caused by increased production of keratin, a protein in the skin, causing thickness in the stratum corneum. The extent to which this can build up varies and increases the risk of infection as the thick moist scales are a breeding ground for bacteria (Wounds UK 2016).	Remove thick plaques by gently debriding with a gloved hand, forceps or debridement pad or cloth (Wounds UK 2016).
Excoriation – red, inflamed skin caused by wound exudate or lymphorrhoea.	Consider wound dressing and apply barrier film to protect the surrounding skin.
Maceration – white, soggy skin saturated by poor fluid management.	Increase the frequency of dressing changes and consider the type of super-absorbent dressing and its placement. Dressings should be placed distally to the leg ulcer to prevent exudate from running down the limb. Check and encourage limb elevation to aid venous return (Brown 2017). Evaluate the efficacy of compression therapy and whether it is at a therapeutic dose.

- Note any changes in firmness or moisture.
- Assess the peri-wound (Table 5.6).
- Assess the peri-wound for localised maceration caused by the removal of skin dressings and dressing adherence that has affected the skin barrier by stripping away parts of the epidermis (Mitchell and Hill 2020).

DIAGNOSTIC ASSESSMENT

Ankle brachial pressure index (ABPI) testing is a non-invasive way to assess an individual's vascular status and identify the presence, absence or degree of PAD. It forms a significant part of the overall holistic assessment (Wounds UK 2019a). A Doppler ultrasound measures the amount of blood flow in a patient's arteries in the lower limb using high-frequency sound waves. Vascular flow studies detect abnormal blood flow in the arteries and veins. The purpose of ABPI testing is to assess the degree of arterial perfusion at the ankle (Wounds UK 2019a) and as such it does not diagnose the cause of the ulcer.

Modalities for assessing vascular status are as follows (Wounds UK 2019a):

- Ankle brachial pressure index (ABPI) – an automated or hand-held device is used to exclude the significance of arterial disease and record the arterial blood flow at the ankle compared with pressure at the arm (brachial).
- Toe brachial pressure index (TBPI) – an automated or handheld device is used to record the arterial blood flow at the toe compared with blood flow at the arm (brachial). The cuff is placed on the hallux to obtain toe pressure. This method is often used in practice if a cuff cannot go around the ankle due to pain, ulceration, lymphoedema or obesity, or if it has not been possible to occlude the vessels in the lower leg, so instead using the smaller vessels in the toe, which tend to become damaged only in more advanced disease, is recommended.
- Pulse oximetry – a secondary investigation by using a pulse oximeter to measure blood oxygen levels. The flow of oxygenated blood can be assessed on a limb after the application of compression therapy to see if it decreases as the compression therapy has been applied. This may be useful to add confirmation that a limb is suitable for compression and is sometimes used within GP practices. It is important to note that this method is not reliable at excluding PAD.

Modalities for assessing arterial disease (medical) include the following:

- Arterial duplex scan – an ultrasound scan of the arteries, which is usually first line within vascular services. It can show the structure and formation of the vessels as well as detecting the rate of blood flow.

- Computer tomography angiogram (CTA) – used for looking at the arterial system from the aorta and below. Using a contrast radioactive highlights any narrowing in the arteries.
- Magnetic resonance angiogram (MRA) – like CTA but uses lower levels of radioactive dye with magnetic fields, which may be a safer option for patients who also have renal disease.

The following should undergo ABPI testing (Wounds UK 2019a):

- Patients presenting with a lower limb wound irrespective of suspected aetiology to assess for PAD.
- Patients who are considered high risk, e.g. those with diabetes or who are immobile.
- Patients presenting with lower limb changes.
- Patients with stigmata of disease but no ulceration, to halt the progression and initiate early intervention.
- Patients with any symptoms of PAD, to confirm or exclude disease.
- Patients with early or established lower limb swelling, as early intervention can halt the progression and identify treatment choices.
- Patients who are currently receiving treatment with compression therapy, as part of reassessment and before the issue of any new garments. This is to ensure that their arterial status has not altered.
- All these patients at regular reassessment intervals of 3, 6 or 12 months. Frequency depends on ongoing assessment outcomes, cardiovascular risk status, patient needs and local guidelines.

Many people may not understand the vascular assessment process. It is important to inform the patient about how it works, why it is being conducted and how the results will be interpreted, using plain language and terms the person can easily understand. Some people may find the procedure difficult to tolerate, particularly if they are unable to lie flat due to pain or mobility issues, breathing problems or weight issues. The misconception that ABPI testing in the incorrect position is 'better than not doing it' should be challenged, as it can cause incorrect readings and discrepancies in results and is therefore not advocated (Wounds UK 2019a).

Factors that may affect the patient's ability to undergo ABPI testing in the usual way include (Staines 2018; Wounds UK 2019a):

- Unmanaged pain.
- Surgery to arm or leg.
- Lymph node clearance.
- Cancer-related treatment.
- Circumferential ulceration (consider TBPI).
- Cellulitis (not a contraindication, but dependent on level of pain as to whether a cuff can be applied to the limb).
- Amputation.
- Friable skin.
- Mental health–related issues.
- Cognitive impairment, e.g. dementia.
- DVT (not a total contraindication, but dependent on pain and if active treatment has been started for a period of 48 hours).
- Critical limb ischaemia.
- Neurological disease.

There are some conditions that may lead to inaccurate results of the vascular assessment and may warrant onward referral (Table 5.9).

In recent years, advances in technology have resulted in new developments for ABPI testing. Automated devices can simplify and speed up an accurate assessment compared to traditional Doppler testing, although not all clinical environments have access to these devices. The latest guidance from the National Institute for Health and Care Excellence (NICE 2023) is that there is not enough evidence to support their use as a direct alternative to the handheld Doppler and they may need to be reserved for use in research or in conjunction with the handheld Doppler by a healthcare professional already experienced in the assessment of peripheral vascular disease. At the time of writing it is noted that a national response to the NICE guidance is being prepared by a senior consortium of lower limb professionals.

TABLE 5.9 Presenting conditions that may lead to inaccurate Doppler results.

Peripheral oedema	Inaccurate results could elevate ankle brachial pressure index (ABPI) through inability to occlude the artery due to oedema.
Diabetes	Small vessel disease – calcification of arteries will lead to false high readings as arteries cannot be occluded.
Atherosclerosis	Hardening the arteries due to disease – may lead to high ABPI.
Uncontrolled pain	May lead to raised blood pressure and inability to keep the limb still to perform the procedure.
Renal disease	Blood pressure fluctuations may lead to inaccuracy.
Cardiac arrhythmias	Including atrial fibrillation – when the pulse is irregular may miss the incoming return of the pulse.

Source: Adapted from Staines (2018).

HOW TO PERFORM A HANDHELD DOPPLER

Equipment needed:

- Handheld Doppler 5–8 MHz (5 MHz probe for a larger limb, 8 MHz probe for a normal limb).
- Ultrasound gel (alternative gels such as lubricants should not be used).
- Sphygmomanometer cuff 23–33 or 31–40 cm in accordance with the leg/arm circumference.
- Paper towels.
- Cling film.
- Disinfectant wipes to clean and decontaminate the equipment.

Before undertaking the procedure, explain to the patient what is going to happen. Ensure that the patient understands and knows what is involved (Beldon 2011).

Measure the Brachial Systolic Blood Pressure

Step 1

The patient should lie as flat as possible for 10–15 minutes with no external pressure on the proximal vessels (Vowden and Vowden 2018). They should avoid smoking or caffeine, as this can affect the results of the test. Lying flat for 10–15 minutes removes the effect of gravity on the blood flow and minimises hydrostatic pressure variance. If a patient is unable to lie flat due to breathing difficulties, ask them to lie as low as is tolerable. The position for the procedure should be recorded (Young 2015). Examination without resting may lead to lower ankle systolic pressure and reduced ABPI (Vowden and Vowden 2018). Patients should be informed that they may experience some discomfort during the procedure when the blood pressure cuff tightens and that they may ask to stop if the procedure becomes too painful.

Step 2

Apply the sphygmomanometer cuff firmly to the arm above the elbow (see Figure 5.13). It is important to measure the circumference of the arm first and select the appropriately sized cuff (the bladder of the cuff should fit around at least 80% of the limb but not more than 100%). If the cuff does not fit properly, it is likely that the reading will be inaccurate. If the cuff is too small, a considerable overestimation can occur (Vowden and Vowden 2018). Locate the brachial artery (with fingers) and apply contact gel on the skin to aid conduction. The Doppler probe must be kept at 45–70° to the skin towards the patient's face until the arterial sign is audible and clear (Beldon 2011). Do not press the probe into the patient's skin as it may occlude the vessel.

Step 3

Keep the probe still and start to inflate the cuff until the audible sound disappears. Inflate a further 20 mmHg and be careful not to move the probe from the line of the artery during deflation (Vowden and Vowden 2018). A rapid deflation of the cuff may miss the highest pressure and underestimate the ABPI (Vowden and Vowden 2018). Record the reading: this is the brachial systolic pressure. N.B. If the

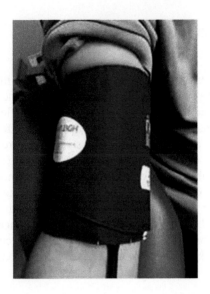

FIGURE 5.13   Applying the sphygmomanometer cuff.

patient has cardiac rhythm alterations, such as atrial fibrillation, consider releasing the cuff more slowly. Repeat the same procedure on the opposite arm. Record each reading immediately so as not to confuse readings later. Use the highest of the two values to calculate the ABPI. Note that if a difference of more than 15 mmHg is detected between the two values, then a referral for vascular review is indicated as this may be indicative of undetected PAD. It is worth noting that before a referral it is prudent to consider rechecking.

Measure the Ankle Systolic Pressure

Step 1

Cover any wounds with cling film or film dressing.

Step 2

Locate the pedal foot pulses to assess the arteries. There are four pedal pulses that can be used: posterior tibial artery (PTA), anterior tibial artery (ATA), peroneal tibial artery and dorsalis pedis artery (see Figure 5.14). Palpate pedal pulses and document which ones if

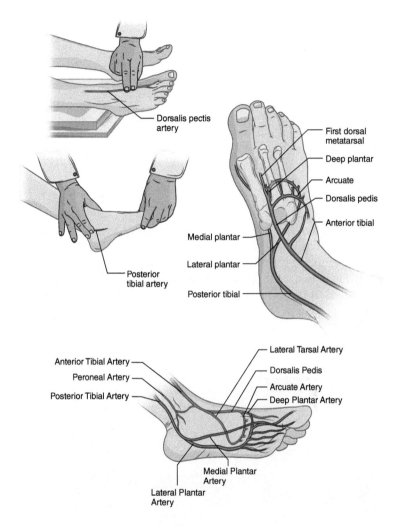

FIGURE 5.14 Arterial pulses of the foot.

any are palpable. The two most common arteries used in this procedure are the dorsalis pedis and the posterior tibial arteries, but studies have demonstrated that the peroneal should be included in this test: as a smaller vessel this may be the first one to be occluded (Taylor and Holland 1990). The dorsal pedis and anterior tibial pulses are from the same artery, so choose one or the other. These are easier to access when the blood pressure cuff is applied to the leg.

Step 2

Apply the cuff firmly at the ankle just above the malleolus. Placing the cuff above the ankle will elevate the pressure and the ABPI (Vowden and Vowden 2018) (see Figure 5.15). Ensure that the cuff is the right size for the ankle circumference.

Step 3

Examine the foot and apply contact gel. Continue as for the brachial pressure and record in the same way. Remember that the foot arteries are not parallel with the skin and sometimes the probe must be adjusted to have a clear signal. Repeat this step for at least two of the pedal pulses. If the pulse is irregular, a slow deflation of the cuff will help with accuracy.

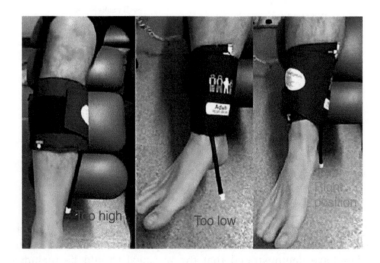

FIGURE 5.15   Lower limb cuff position. Courtesy of Accelerate.

Step 4

Note the mmHg at the point of the sound returning (when the pulse becomes audible again). This is the absolute pressure and inclusion of this in the documentation is important, as it is an indicator of overall perfusion to the limb.

Step 5

Note down the sounds – these are as valuable as the ABPI measurement.

- Triphasic signal – this is represented by three sounds together very quickly and indicates that the arteries are working well and the artery has good elasticity. There are three parts to the waveform that can be seen visually if the Doppler device has a display window or heard if the transmission is clear (Figure 5.16).
- Biphasic signal – this can be recognised as two sounds heard together and indicates that the arteries are losing some of their elasticity, which may be due to the ageing process. There are only two parts to this waveform visually.
- Monophasic signal – A single almost 'banging' sound indicates the presence of advanced arterial disease and the artery will have little or no elasticity in the vessel.

Calculation and Interpretation of the Ankle Brachial Pressure Index

The ABPI for each leg is calculated separately by taking the highest reading of the foot pulse readings and dividing by the highest of the brachial readings:

$$\frac{\text{ankle systolic BP}}{\text{brachial systolic BP}} = \text{ABPI}$$

The ABPI values are reported numerically, for example 0.82 or 1.30, which indicates to the assessing clinician that the patient had an arterial flow of oxygenated blood of approximately 82% or 130%. Compression therapy may be safely used in venous leg ulcer patients with an ABPI >0.8 (Table 5.10).

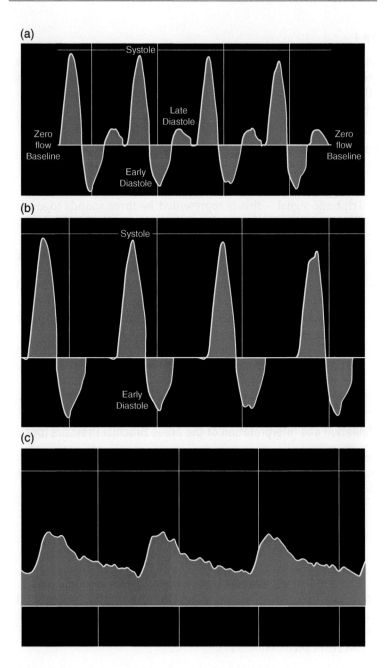

FIGURE 5.16 Waveforms. (a) Triphasic; (b) biphasic; (c) monophasic.

TABLE 5.10 Ankle brachial pressure index (ABPI) indicators for compression therapy.

ABPI = 1.01–1.3	No indicators of peripheral vascular disease	Apply high levels of compression therapy
ABPI = 0.81–1.0	Mild peripheral disease	May have high levels of compression therapy – monitor ABPI
ABPI = 0.51–0.8	Significant arterial disease	May have reduced compression – refer to specialist nurse/ vascular
ABPI <0.5	Severe arterial disease	No compression – urgent referral to vascular
ABPI >1.3[a]	Measure toe pressures or refer to specialist	May have compression therapy – liaise with specialist nurse/ vascular

[a] A high ABPI may not always be indicative of peripheral vascular disease, but could be a false high from poor technique. A toe Doppler will be able to confirm the presence of arterial disease if calcification in the arteries has rendered them difficult to compress. Calcification does not usually affect the smaller vessels in the toes (Whayman 2014). It is also useful to consider the absolute pressures as an indicator of perfusion.
Source: Adapted from Harding et al. (2015).

ABPI is a useful test to determine arterial sufficiency. It is important that healthcare professionals understand normal values so that abnormal values can be recognised.

Medical factors that may affect the patient's ability to undergo ABPI assessment include:

- DVT or suspected DVT.
- Cellulitis.
- Lymph node clearance.
- Amputation (the automated ABPI device has an amputation function).
- Surgery to arm/leg.
- Friable skin.
- Mental health–related issues.
- Dementia.

- Neurological disease (this may affect the patient's ability to stay still).
- Cancer-related treatment.

Remember that when undertaking ABPI assessment, practitioners should always refer to their own local protocol, as there are local variances between clinical services.

RED FLAGS FOR THE URGENT TREATMENT OF PATIENTS WITH VENOUS LEG ULCERS

- Infection of the leg or foot, identified by symptoms of increasing pain, redness, oedema and local heat with purulent discharge.
- Critical limb-threatening ischaemia.
- Suspected untreated DVT.
- Suspected skin malignancy.

REASSESSMENT AND RECURRENCE

Leg ulcer assessment should be an ongoing process until the wound is healed. When the wound is healed, maintenance and prevention of recurrence are vital (Wounds UK 2016). The recurrence rate in venous leg ulcers is estimated to be as high as 50.4% within the first 12 months (Finlayson et al. 2018). Doppler ABPI reassessment is essential every three months, or more frequently if changes in the lower limb are observed.

CONCLUSION

Good assessment and history taking are pivotal to decision-making, diagnosis, treatment and partnership working with patients with leg ulcers. Communication between healthcare professionals and patients is essential to gain trust, partnership and understanding. Consideration must be given to patients with any additional vision, hearing or literacy needs. It is essential for practitioners to have cultural competence and awareness to ensure that patients' cultural needs and beliefs are met. Assessment is not just something that happens at the beginning of treatment, it should be ongoing throughout. Identifying leg ulcer aetiology, causes and risk factors is essential to ensure that treatment options and strategies are appropriate and effective. Having an in-depth understanding of the patient you are working with will help you find the most successful treatments.

REFERENCES

Atkin, L. (2019). Venous leg ulcer prevention 1: identifying patients who are at risk. *Nursing Times* 115 (6): 24–28. https://www.nursingtimes.net/clinical-archive/tissue-viability/venous-leg-ulcer-prevention-1-identifying-patients-who-are-at-risk-28-05-2019/

Atkins, E., Mughal, N.A., Place, F., and Coughlin, P.A. (2020). Varicose veins in primary care. *BMJ* 370, m2509. https://doi.org/10.1136/bmj.m2509.

Belczak, S., Ramos, R., and Pereira de Godoy, J. (2021). Association between obesity and the aggravation of limited range of ankle mobility in chronic venous disease. *Phlebology* 37 (3): 196–199.

Beldon, P. (2011). How to . . . Ten top tips for doppler ABPI. *Wounds international* 2 (4): https://woundsinternational.com/journal-articles/how-toten-top-tips-for-doppler-abpi.

Birkhäuer, J., Gaab, J., Kossowsky, J. et al. (2017). Trust in the health care professional and health outcome: a meta-analysis. *PLoS One* 12 (2): e0170988. https://doi.org/10.1371/journal.pone.0170988.

Blomgren, L., Johansson, G., Dahlberg-Åkerman, A. et al. (2004). Recurrent varicose veins: incidence, risk factors and groin anatomy. *European Journal of Vascular and Endovascular Surgery* 27 (3): 269–274.

Brown, A. (2017). Managing exudate and maceration in venous leg ulceration within the acute health setting. *British Journal of Nursing* 26 (Sup20): S18–S24. https://doi.org/10.12968/bjon.2017.26.sup20.s18.

Buerger, L. (1924). *The Circulatory Disturbances of the Extremities: Including Gangrene, Vasomotor and Trophic Disorders.* Philadelphia, PA: W.B. Saunders.

Cai, P. and Forsyth, J. (2022). Acute limb ischaemia. Vascular surgery – II. *Surgery* 40 (7): 450–459.

Carruthers, T.N., Farber, A., Rybin, D. et al. (2014). Interventions on the superficial venous system for chronic venous insufficiency by surgeons in the modern era: an analysis of ACS-NSQIP. *Vascular and Endovascular Surgery* 48: 482–490.

Cirqui, M., Denenberg, J., Bergan, J. et al. (2007). Risk factors for chronic venous disease: the San Diego Population Study. *Journal of Vascular Surgery* 46 (2): 331–337.

Collares, F. and Faintuch, C. (2017). *Varicose Veins: Practical Guides in Interventional Radiology*. New York: Thieme Medical Publishers.

Cutting, K.F. (2004). Exudate: composition and functions. In: *Trends in Wound Care: Volume III* (ed. R. White), 41–49. London: Quay Books.

Cutting, K.F. and White, R.J. (2002). Avoidance and management of periwound maceration of the skin. *Professional Nurse* 18 (1): 33–36.

Danielsson, G., Eklof, B., Grandinetti, A., and Kistner, R.L. (2002). The influence of obesity on chronic venous disease. *Vascular and Endovascular Surgery* 36 (4): 271–276. https://doi.org/10.1177/153857440203600404.

Deptuła, M., Zieliński, J., Wardowska, A., and Pikuła, M. (2019). Wound healing complications in oncological patients: perspectives for cellular therapy. *Advances in Dermatology and Allergology* 36 (2): 139–146. https://doi.org/10.5114/ada.2018.72585.

Dini, V., Janowska, A., Oranges, T. et al. (2020). Surrounding skin management in venous leg ulcers: a systematic review. *Journal of Tissue Viability* 29: 169–175.

Eder, S., Dissemond, J., Vanscheidt, W. et al. (2019). Buergers test/pole test: simple clinical tests to screen the arterial perfusion before compression therapy. *Phlébologie* 49 (02): 108–110. https://doi.org/10.1055/a-0865-7947.

Edward-Jones, V. (2018). Microbiology and malodourous wounds. *Wounds UK* 14 (4): 72–75.

Eklof, B., Rutherford, R.B., Bergan, J.J. et al. (2004). Revision of the CEAP classification for chronic venous disorders: consensus statement. *Journal of Vascular Surgery* 40 (6): 1248–1252.

Finlayson, K.J., Parker, C.N., Miller, C. et al. (2018). Predicting the likelihood of venous leg ulcer recurrence: the diagnostic accuracy of a newly developed risk assessment tool. *International Wound Journal* 15 (5): 686–694.

Frescos, N. (2011). What causes wound pain? *Journal of Foot Ankle Research* 4 (Suppl 1): P22. https://doi.org/10.1186/1757-1146-4-S1-P22.

Godeberge, P., Sheikh, P., Zagriadskiï, E. et al. (2019). Hemorrhoidal disease and chronic venous insufficiency: concomitance or coincidence; results of the chorus study (chronic venous and Hemorrhoidal Diseases Evaluation and Scientific Research). *Journal of Gastroenterology and Hepatology* 35 (4): 577–585. https://doi.org/10.1111/jgh.14857.

Gouin, J.P. and Kiecolt-Glaser, J.K. (2011). The impact of psychological stress on wound healing: methods and mechanisms. *Immunology and Allergy Clinics of North America* 31 (1): 81–93. https://doi.org/10.1016/j.iac.2010.09.010.

Green, J., Corcoran, P., Green, L., and Read, S. (2018). A new quality of life wound checklist: the patient voice in wound care. *Wounds UK* 14 (4): 40–45.

Guest, J.F., Gerrish, A., Ayoub, N. et al. (2015). Clinical outcomes and cost-effectiveness of three alternative compression systems used in the management of venous leg ulcers. *Journal of Wound Care* 24 (7): 300–310.

Guest, J., Fuller, G., and Vowden, P. (2018). Venous leg ulcer management in clinical practice in the UK: cost and outcomes. *International Wound Journal* 15 (1): 29–37.

Guo, S. and DiPietro, L.A. (2010). Factors affecting wound healing. *Journal of Dental Research* 89 (3): 219–229. https://doi.org/10.1177/002203 450935912.

Harding, K., Dowsett, C., Fias, L. et al. (2015). Simplifying venous ulcer management: consensus recommendations. Wounds International London. https://woundsinternational.com/consensus-documents/simplifying-venous-leg-ulcer-management-consensus-recommendations

Harper, C. and Crane, J. (2022). Atrophie blanche. In: *StatPearls*. Treasure Island, FL: StatPearls Publishing https://www.ncbi.nlm.nih.gov/books/NBK544285.

Haughton, W. and Young, T. (1995). Common problems in wound care: malodorous wounds. *British Journal of Nursing* 4 (16): 959–963. https://doi.org/10.12968/bjon.1995.4.16.959.

Hess, C.T. (2020). Checklist for successful wound healing outcomes. *Advances in Skin & Wound Care* 33 (1): 54–55. https://doi.org/10.1097/01.asw.0000617008.87552.bc.

Iannuzzi, A., Panico, S., Ciardullo, A.V. et al. (2002). Varicose veins of the lower limbs and venous capacitance in postmenopausal women: relationship with obesity. *Journal of Vascular Surgery* 36: 965–968.

International Wound Infection Institute (IWII) (2016). Wound infection in clinical practice. Wounds International. https://woundsinternational.com/consensus-documents/wound-infection-in-clinical-practice-principles-of-best-practice

Ismail, L., Normahani, P., Standfield, N., and Jaffer, U. (2016). A systematic review and meta-analysis of the risk for development of varicose veins in women with a history of pregnancy. *Journal of Vascular Surgery: Venous Lymphatic Disorders* 4 (4): 518–524.

Kawano, Y. (2010). Physio-pathological effects of alcohol on the cardiovascular system: its role in hypertension and cardiovascular disease. *Hypertension Research* 33 (3): 181–191. https://doi.org/10.1038/hr.2009.226.

Lurie, F., Passman, M., Meisner, M. et al. (2020). The 2020 update of the CEAP classification system and reporting standards. *Journal of Vascular Surgery and Venous Lymphatic Disorders* 8 (3): 342–352. https://doi.org/10.1016/j.jvsv.2019.12.075.

Lymphoedema Framework (2006). International consensus: Best practice for the management of lymphoedema. https://www.lympho.org/uploads/files/files/Best_practice.pdf

Matic, M., Matic, A., Djuran, V. et al. (2016). Frequency of peripheral arterial disease in patients with chronic venous insufficiency. *Iranian Red Crescent Medical Journal* 18 (1): e20781. https://doi.org/10.5812/ircmj.20781.

McVittie, E. and Holloway, S. (2015). Aetiology and management of atrophie blanche in chronic venous insufficiency. *British Journal of Community Nursing* 20 (Supp 12): S8–S13.

Minasian, R.A., Samaha, Y., and Brazio, P.S. (2022). Post-traumatic lymphedema: review of the literature and surgical treatment options. *Plastic and Aesthetic Research* 9: 18. https://doi.org/10.20517/2347-9264.2021.128.

Mintz, B., Jaff, M., and Mintz, J. (2013). *Atlas of Clinical Vascular Medicine.* Chichester: Wiley.

Mioc, M.-L., Prejbeanu, R., Vermesan, D. et al. (2018). Deep vein thrombosis following the treatment of lower limb pathologic bone fractures – a comparative study. *BMC Musculoskeletal Disorders* 16: 213.

Mitchell, A. (2017). Assessing the value of practice-based leg ulcer education to inform recommendations for change in practice. *British Journal of Community Nursing* 22 (Supp 12): S28–S34.

Mitchell, A. (2018). Adult pressure area care: preventing pressure ulcers. *British Journal of Nursing* 27 (18): 1050–1052. https://doi.org/10.12968/bjon.2018.27.18.1050.

Mitchell, A. (2020). Assessment of wounds in adults. *British Journal of Nursing* 29 (20): S18–S24.

Mitchell, A. (2022). Skin assessment in adults. *British Journal of Nursing* 31 (5): 274–278. https://doi.org/10.12968/bjon.2022.31.5.274.

Mitchell, A. and Elbourne, S. (2020). Lower limb assessment. *British Journal of Nursing* 29 (1): 18–21.

Mitchell, A. and Hill, B. (2020). Moisture-associated skin damage: an overview of its diagnosis and management. *British Journal of Community Nursing* 25 (3): S12–S18. https://doi.org/10.12968/bjcn.2020.25.Sup3.S12.

Mitchell, A. and Llumigusin, D. (2021). The assessment and management of hypergranulation. *British Journal of Nursing* 30 (5): S6–S10. https://doi.org/10.12968/bjon.2021.30.5.S6.

Miteva, M., Romanelli, P., and Kirsner, R. (2010). Lipodermatosclerosis. *Dermatologic Therapy* 23 (4): 375–388.

Moffatt, C., Franks, P.J., Doherthy, D.C. et al. (2009). Psychological factors in leg ulceration: a case-control study. *British Journal of Dermatology* 161 (4): 750–756. https://doi.org/10.1111/j.1365-2133.2009.09211.x.

National Institute for Health and Care Excellence (NICE) (2020). Leg ulcer infection: antimicrobial prescribing. NICE guideline [NG152]. https://www.nice.org.uk/guidance/ng152/chapter/Recommendations#treatment

National Institute for Health and Care Excellence (NICE) (2021). Leg ulcer – venous. https://cks.nice.org.uk/topics/leg-ulcer-venous

National Institute for Health and Care Excellence (NICE) (2022). Venous eczema and lipodermatosclerosis: how should I assess the person?

https://cks.nice.org.uk/topics/venous-eczema-lipodermatosclerosis/diagnosis/assessment

National Institute for Health and Care Excellence (NICE) (2023). Leg ulcer – venous. https://cks.nice.org.uk/topics/leg-ulcer-venous

NHS (2020). Universal personalised care: implementing the comprehensive model. https://www.england.nhs.uk/wp-content/uploads/2019/01/universal-personalised-care.pdf

NHS (2022). Causes: Peripheral neuropathy. https://www.nhs.uk/conditions/peripheral-neuropathy/causes

NHS Inform (2022). Varicose eczema. https://www.nhsinform.scot/illnesses-and-conditions/skin-hair-and-nails/varicose-eczema

Nicholls, S.C. (2005). Sequelae of untreated venous insufficiency. *Seminars in Interventional Radiology* 22 (3): 162–168.

Nichols, E. (2016). Wound assessment part 2: exudate. *Wound Essentials* 11 (1): 36–44.

Nickles, M.A., Ennis, W.J., O'Donnell, T.F. Jr., and Altman, I.A. (2023). Compression therapy in peripheral artery disease: a literature review. *Journal of Wound Care* 32 (Supp 5): S25–S30. https://doi.org/10.12968/jowc.2023.32.sup5.s25.

Oh, D.M. and Phillips, T.J. (2006). Sex hormones and wound healing. *Wounds* 18 (1): 8–18.

Onida, S. and Davies, A. (2016). Predicted burden of venous disease. *Phlebology* 31 (1): 74–79.

Ortega, M.A., Fraile-Martínez, O., García-Montero, C. et al. (2021). Understanding chronic venous disease: a critical overview of its pathophysiology and medical management. *Journal of Clinical Medicine* 10 (15): 3239. https://doi.org/10.3390/jcm10153239.

Ousey, K. and Cook, L. (2012). Wound assessment made easy. Wounds UK. https://wounds-uk.com/made-easy/wound-assessment-made-easy

Platsidaki, E., Kouris, A., and Christodoulou, C. (2017). Psychosocial aspects in patients with chronic leg ulcers. *Wounds: A Compendium of Clinical Research and Practice* 29 (10): 306–310. https://doi.org/10.25270/wnds/2017.10.306310.

Robertson, L.A. (2013). Incidence of varicose veins, chronic venous insufficiency and venous reflux in the general population and associated risk factors: the Edinburgh Vein Study follow up. PhD thesis, Edinburgh Research Archive. https://era.ed.ac.uk/handle/1842/8149.

Robinson, T. and Scullion, J.E. (2021). *Oxford Handbook of Respiratory Nursing*. Oxford: Oxford University Press.

Ruggiero, M., Grande, R., Naso, A. et al. (2016). Symptoms in patients with skin changes due to chronic venous insufficiency often lead to emergency care service: an Italian observational study. *International Wound Journal* 13 (5): 967–971.

Salomé, G. (2020). Body image of people with venous ulcers. *Journal of Contemporary Nursing* 9 (2): 225–230. https://doi.org/10.17267/2317-3378rec.v9i2.2930.

Salomé, G.M., de Almeida, S.A., de Jesus Pereira, M.T. et al. (2016). The impact of venous leg ulcers on body image and self-esteem. *Advances in Skin & Wound Care* 29 (7): 316–321. https://doi.org/10.1097/01.asw.0000484243.32091.0c.

Seitz, C.S., Berens, N., Brocker, E.B., and Trautmann, A. (2010). Leg ulceration in rheumatoid arthritis–an underreported multicausal complication with considerable morbidity: analysis of thirty-six patients and review of the literature. *Dermatology* 220 (3): 268–273. https://doi.org/10.1159/000284583.

Sharpe, A., Dowsett, C., Welch, D. et al., (2022). Wound preparation by cleansing and debridement using Alprep® Pad. Wounds UK. https://wounds-uk.com/best-practice-statements/wound-preparation-by-cleansing-and-debridement-using-alprep-pad

Smith, D., Team, V., Barber, G. et al. (2018). Factors associated with physical activity levels in people with venous leg ulcers: a multicentre, prospective, cohort study. *International Wound Journal* 15 (2): 291–296. https://doi.org/10.1111/iwj.12868.

Staines, K. (2018). Safe compression and accurate ABPI – overcoming barriers. *Wounds UK* 14 (1): 64–67.

Steven, L., Hill, K., Williams, D. et al. (2012). A review of the scientific evidence for biofilms in wounds. Wound repair and regeneration. *Wound Repair and Regeneration* 20: 647–657.

Stoodley, P., Sauer, K., Davies, D.G., and Costerton, J.W. (2002). Biofilms as complex differentiated communities. *Annual Review of Microbiology* 56: 187–209. https://doi.org/10.1146/annurev.micro.56.012302.160705.

Suehiro, K., Morikage, N., Murakami, M. et al. (2014). A study of leg edema in immobile patients. *Circulation Journal* 78 (7): 1733–1739. https://doi.org/10.1253/circj.cj-13-1599.

Tavadia, S., Bianchi, J., Dawe, R.S. et al. (2003). Allergic contact dermatitis in venous leg ulcer patients. *Contact Dermatitis* 48 (5): 261–265.

Taylor, K.J. and Holland, S. (1990). Doppler US. Part I. Basic principles, instrumentation, and pitfalls. *Radiology* 174 (2): 297–307. https://doi.org/10.1148/radiology.174.2.2404309.

Theochari, C.A., Theochari, N.A., Mylonas, K.S. et al. (2022). Venous thromboembolism following major abdominal surgery for cancer: a guide for the surgical intern. *Current Pharmaceutical Design* 28 (10): 787–797. https://doi.org/10.2174/1381612828666220217140639.

Thomson, L. (2016). Sclerotherapy of telangiectasias or spider veins in the lower limb: a review. *Journal of Vascular Nursing* 34 (2): 61–62.

Tummala, S. and Scherbel, D. (2018). Clinical assessment of peripheral arterial disease in the office: what do the guidelines say? *Seminars in Interventional Radiology* 35 (5): 365–377.

Upton, D., Andrews, A., and Upton, P. (2014). Venous leg ulcers: what about well-being? *Journal of Wound Care* 23 (1): 14–17. https://doi.org/ 10.12968/jowc.2014.23.1.14.

Van Rij, A.M., De Alwis, C.S., Jiang, P. et al. (2008). Obesity and impaired venous function. *European Journal of Vascular and Endovascular Surgery* 35 (6): 739–744. https://doi.org/10.1016/j.ejvs.2008.01.006.

Vascular Society for Great Britain and Ireland (2023) Lymphoedema and limb swelling. https://www.vascularsociety.org.uk/patients/conditions/ 1/lymphoedema_and_limb_swelling

Vowden, P. and Vowden, K. (2018). The importance of accurate methodology in ABPI calculation when assessing lower limb wounds. *British Journal of Community Nursing* 23 (Sup3): S16–S21. https://doi.org/10.12968/ bjcn.2018.23.Sup3.S16.

Vuolo, J. (2010). Hypergranulation: exploring possible management options. *British Journal of Nursing Tissue Viability* 19 (Suppl. 2): S4–S8.

Walburn, J., Weinman, J., Norton, S. et al. (2017). Stress, illness perceptions, behaviors, and healing in venous leg ulcers: findings from a prospective observational study. *Psychosomatic Medicine* 79 (5): 585–592. https:// doi.org/10.1097/psy.0000000000000436.

Wang, X.-H., Leineweber, C., Kirkeeide, R. et al. (2006). Psychosocial stress and atherosclerosis: family and work stress accelerate the progression of coronary disease in women. The Stockholm Female Coronary Angiography study. *Journal of Internal Medicine* 261 (3): 245–254.

Wang, W., Zhao, T., Geng, K. et al. (2021). Smoking and the pathophysiology of peripheral artery disease. *Frontiers in Cardiovascular Medicine* 8: 704106. https://doi.org/10.3389/fcvm.2021.704106.

Whayman, N. (2014) 'Doppler assessment: getting it right', Wounds UK. https://wounds-uk.com/wound-essentials/doppler-assessmentgett ing-it-right

Wilson, M. (2012). Understanding the basics of wound assessment. *Wound Essentials* 7 (2): 8–12.

Winter, G.D. (1962). Formation of the scab and the rate of epithelialisation of superficial wounds in the skin of domestic pig. *Nature* 193: 293–294.

Winterborn, R.J., Foy, C., and Earnshaw, J.J. (2004). Causes of varicose vein recurrence: late results of a randomized controlled trial of stripping the long saphenous vein. *Journal of Vascular Surgery* 40 (4): 634–639.

Wittens, C., Davies, A.H., Baekgaard, N. et al. (2015). Editor's choice – management of chronic venous disease: clinical practice guidelines of the European Society for Vascular Surgery (ESVS). *European Journal of Vascular and Endovascular Surgery* 49 (6): 678–737. https://doi. org/10.1016/j.ejvs.2015.02.007.

Woelk, C.J. (2012). Management of critical limb ischemia. *Canadian Family Physician/Le médecin de famille canadien* 58 (9): 960–963.

World Union of Wound Healing Societies (2007). *Wound Exudate and the Role of Dressings: A Consensus Document*. London: MEP.

Wounds UK (2013). Best practice statement: effective exudate management. https://wounds-uk.com/best-practice-statements/best-practice-statement-effective-exudate-management.

Wounds UK (2016). Quick guide: Management of hyperkeratosis of the lower limb. https://www.wounds-uk.com/resources/details/quick-guide-management-of-hyperkeratosis-of-the-lower-limb

Wounds UK (2019a). Best practice statement: Ankle brachial pressure index (ABPI) in practice. https://wounds-uk.com/best-practice-statements/ankle-brachial-pressure-index-abpi-practice

Wounds UK (2019b). Best practice statement: Addressing complexities in the management of venous legs ulcers. https://wounds-uk.com/best-practice-statements/addressing-complexities-management-venous-leg-ulcers

Wounds UK (2020). Best practice statement: Management of lower limb skin tears in adults. https://wounds-uk.com/best-practice-statements/management-lower-limb-skin-tears-adults.

Wounds UK (2021). Best practice statement: Addressing skin tone bias in wound care: assessing signs and symptoms in people with dark skin tones.https://wounds-uk.com/best-practice-statements/addressing-skin-tone-bias-wound-care-assessing-signs-and-symptoms-people-dark-skin-tones.

Wounds UK (2022). Best practice statement: Holistic management of venous leg ulceration. https://www.wounds-uk.com/resources/details/holistic-management-venous-leg-ulceration-second-edition

Young, T. (2015). Unit 5. How to undertake a doppler ultrasound. *Practice Nursing* 22 (11): 1–4.

Young, T. (2020). Leg ulceration in sickleell disease. *Wounds UK* 16 (1): 72–77.

Zegarra, T. and Tadi, P. (2022). CEAP classification of venous disorders. In: *StatPearls*. Treasure Island, FL: StatPearls Publishing https://www.ncbi.nlm.nih.gov/books/NBK557410/.

Zemaitis, M., Boll, J., and Dreyer, M. (2022). *Peripheral Arterial Disease*. Bethesda, MD: National Library of Medicine.

CHAPTER 6

Holistic Management of Pain

FRAN WORBOYS AND ALISON HOPKINS

Pain is a common feature of all types of leg ulceration and lower limb swelling. It is essential that pain as a symptom is understood and that the complexities of managing this common side effect are recognised. Pain is more than a physical response to a stimulus and the clinician needs to understand and manage the associated psychological features that may exacerbate or diminish the pain sensations. It is critical that a plan to address these aspects includes more than analgesia: that the clinician prioritises understanding of the patient's lived experience of their pain so that the underlying features of the pain cycle are included in the treatment plan. The clinician needs to understand the various theories relating to pain, the different types of pain and factors that have an impact on the pain experience, which will inform their understanding of the phenomenon of pain. Myths associated with the pain experience will be addressed in this chapter.

THE PAIN EXPERIENCE

Pain is a significant common experience as well as the most devastating aspect related to living with non-healing wounds (Woo et al. 2008; Price et al. 2008) and, reportedly, the worst aspect of having a leg ulcer (Briggs et al. 2012).

Lower Limb and Leg Ulcer Assessment and Management, First Edition.
Edited by Aby Mitchell, Georgina Ritchie, and Alison Hopkins.
© 2024 John Wiley & Sons Ltd. Published 2024 by John Wiley & Sons Ltd.

The International Association for the Study of Pain (IASP) defines pain as 'an unpleasant sensory and emotional experience associated with, or resembling that associated with, actual or potential tissue damage' (Raja et al. 2020). This is useful in framing the nature of pain beyond the physical domain, while raising further questions about how pain is perceived and in what way it relates to tissue injury. However, it does not entirely do justice to the complexity of the pain experience and what it means to live with pain.

There have been numerous qualitative studies that have sought to find a deeper understanding of what pain is and how it affects lives. A number of these have focused on patients living with leg ulcers and the personal narratives have been able to enhance understanding of the character of non-healing and the complexity of lives caught up in an endless pain narrative (Walshe 1995; Krasner 1998; Rosenburg et al. 2022).

Pain has been found to dominate the lives of people with leg ulcers (Green et al. 2017), with participants describing the pain as 'unceasing [in] nature, severity and timing, especially through the night'. In a study looking at a specific wound dressing on chronic venous leg ulcer patients, pain was termed as unrelenting with persistent wound pain fluctuating over a 24-hour period, alongside intermittent bursts of spontaneous pain (Flanagan et al. 2006). Key themes included unpredictability and the challenge of living with fatigue and activity restrictions.

Leren et al. (2020) in their review conclude that pain is a 'serious problem for patients' and that the issues that subsequently flow from unresolved pain are significant and disrupt the lives of the patient and their families. People with leg ulcers have a significant risk of their pain becoming long-standing and persistent, with 'chronic pain, insomnia, depression and suicidal ideation being inextricably linked' (Taverner et al. 2014). Clinicians need to be vigilant from the first assessment, as much suffering can be reduced if patients' stories are listened to and effective management is put into place from the outset.

Clinicians need to be aware of the impact that pain has on their patients, but there has been concern that practitioners have either not understood its impact or have placed a low importance on pain management (EWMA 2002; Price et al. 2007; Taverner et al. 2011). A recent Australian study (Frescos 2018) assessing pain in chronic wounds found that although almost all wound care practitioners participating in the study (n = 1298) asked patients about their wound pain experience, this reduced to 38% when considering how many assessed wound pain at every consultation/dressing change. Pain is a common feature experienced by leg ulcer patients and so its presence and impact need to be the concern of practitioners.

Pain has been described as being 'whatever the experiencing person says it is, existing whenever the experiencing person says it does' (McCaffery 1968), yet if practitioners do not assess, review and ask the questions, this cannot be ascertained. Pain is also as much about what the patient does not say (WUWHS 2004) as what they do, and this requires patience, observation, perception and understanding to facilitate awareness. The recognition of pain and how it is to be managed form part of the therapeutic partnership and the overall healing outcomes that practitioners need to have with patients.

THEORIES OF PAIN

Pain Theory Evolution

Numerous theories have sought to explain the physiological processes behind the pain experience, with the ancient Greeks being the first to discover the nervous system. Pain theory in its simplest form postulated that if there was a linear progression between the point of trauma or injury and the sensation experienced, it would associate cause with effect, which could be related to expectation. Skuse (2021) describes how, in the seventeenth century, Descartes proposed a theory of pain that articulated the idea that pain was located in the brain, with nerves being responsible for stimulating a response. The rationale arose out of Descartes' study of phantom limb pain and the observation that pain was being experienced from a site that was no longer part of the body. In his bell-cord theory he identified a link between an injury and the pain experienced, such that a signal is sent to the brain and it reacts like the ringing of a bell. This simple model was suggestive of a pain pathway, but it did little to explain the complexities and nuances of the pain experience, where the injury might be the same but the pain narratives between different people in similar situations or the same person in another setting could be poles apart.

In the nineteenth century the physiology of the nerves was revealed, with differentiation between the cell body, the dendrite and the axon. The work of individuals such as Charles Bell, Otto Deiters who saw the nervous system as a railroad (Ehrlich 2022), Emil du Bois-Reymond and his identification of nerve impulses, C.S. Sherrington and Jean-Martin Charcot brought a new dimension of understanding about nerves, the nervous system and the way impulses travel to the brain. Sherrington discovered that nerves do not touch one another but communicate by 'synapse' across a small space to the next one, due to chemical and electrical exchanges. This forms the neural circuitry within the body. Sherrington also identified the specialised receptors at the end of nerves that detect motor and sensory activity while linking nerves to muscle activity. These receptors, known as nociceptors, detect damage and danger by reacting to noxious stimuli (mechanical, thermal and chemical). They send electro-chemical impulses along the peripheral sensory nerve towards the spinal cord and from there to the brain (Molnár and Brown 2010).

In the twentieth century, the study of the nervous system continued with what is termed modern brain science. The work of Santiago Ramón y Cajal identified individual cells that are now known as neurons (Ehrlich 2022). The continued discoveries within the fields of neurology and neuroscience are the backdrop for theories of pain that have since developed. These models have evolved alongside our understanding of psychology, including emotions and belief systems, the body, and people's relationships to one another, their environment and the world.

Gate Theory

One of the most influential pain theories has been work by Melzack and Walls (1965; Katz and Rosenbloom 2015), which introduced the concept of a gate mechanism within the nervous system that had the ability to select the pain impulses travelling to the brain. They proposed that nociceptive pain signals are transmitted from the peripheral nervous system to the brain, where a pain response is elicited. A specialised group of cells within the spinal cord functions as a gate, enabling these impulses to be either allowed or blocked from travelling to the brain. Where the gate is open pain is experienced,

TABLE 6.1 Gate theory and influences.

	Emotional	Cognitive and behavioural	Physical
Opens the gate	Anxiety Worry Tension Depression	Focusing on the pain Boredom Other reactions	Extent and type of injury Low-level activity
Closes the gate	Happiness Optimism Relaxation	More involvement and interest in life's activities Distractions or focus on other activities Other reactions	Medication Counter-stimulation, e.g. rubbing

Source: Adapted from Upton and Upton (2015).

but where the gate is closed there is less pain. Pain signals are thereby modulated, with specific influences for deciding whether this gate should be open or shut being multivariant, and having as much to do with emotional, psychological and environmental factors as with the injury or disease process itself. See Table 6.1.

The theory has helped with understanding the function of the different nerve fibres (Melzack 1996). The small peripheral nerve fibres directly communicate damage, with noxious stimuli opening the gate, whereas activation of the large peripheral fibres can mediate to close the gate. Non-painful sensations such as massaging, rubbing around an area or the application of heat may have a soothing effect, because in these instances the large peripheral fibres are being activated, inhibiting other pain signals (Upton and Upton 2015).

This theory has enabled insights into nursing the patient in pain. It has assisted with understanding some of the influences that determine pain from a physiological perspective, but also in considering the challenges and variables relating to pain management. Despite this, the theory continued to emphasise the presence of a pathway to define the nature and experience of pain, which meant that persistent pain was not so easily addressed within this model.

Biopsychosocial Model

With the development of successive theories and associated research, it has become increasingly recognised that pain does not equate with injury. Theories around pain and what contributes to the pain narrative have increasingly sought to understand the complexity of the experience. This has led to the recognition of the biopsychosocial model as the most comprehensive and accepted model to date, with pain now accepted as a biopsychosocial phenomenon and essential in understanding the pain experience (Upton and Solowiej 2010; Dueñas et al. 2016).

This model emphasises the dynamic relationship between the biological, social and psychological domains of a person's life. As there is no single pain centre in the brain, different parts are activated according to the stimuli. These stimuli are always individually perceived and experienced, being influenced by the biopsychosocial variables. This is termed the neurosignature (Lyman 2021) and is unique to each person. Within this model the phenomenon of pain will include:

- Sensory aspects, as the brain seeks to determine where the danger is coming from. This will include pathophysiological causes such as wound aetiology, prolonged inflammation, hypersensitivities, venous insufficiencies, local infection and pressure from neo-plasms (Hollinworth 2005) as well as ischaemia and dermatitis (Briggs et al. 2012), odour and exudate (Phillips et al. 2018). The release of inflammatory molecules as part of the immune response will contribute to inflammatory processes and the further sensitisation of nerves (Zhang and An 2007).
- Psychological, where the brain decides that the stimuli is a threat.
- Emotional responses, such as moods, anxiety, depression, fear and stress. See Table 6.2.
- Cognitive components, involving our memories, thoughts and beliefs, which will include cultural backgrounds and religious thinking, although these must not be used to infer stereotypes. Beliefs also relate to self-efficacy and the extent to which people believe that they can cope with pain, as well as to expectations. These are important determinants within the therapeutic relationship and in being able to tolerate pain.

TABLE 6.2 Impact of pain on the person.

	Effect of excessive pain

Stress
Woo (2010)
Upton and
  Solowiej (2010)
Wynn and
  Holloway (2019)
	Pain is a major source of stress leading to:
	■ Delayed healing.
	■ Increased activity on the body's immune and hormonal systems, which raises the peripheral immune response, increasing sensitivity to pain and amplifying chronic stress.
	■ Driving of inflammation, prolonging the inflammatory phase of wound healing, which increases pain and contributes to non-healing.

Anxiety Colloca and Beneddetti (2007) Woo (2015)	Pain is a major source of anxiety leading to: ■ More anxiety being experienced. ■ Nocebo effect: heightened anxiety in the anticipation of pain giving higher ratings to the pain experience and self-reported pain intensity. ■ Increased sensitivity to pain: lower pain threshold and tolerance. ■ Predictor of procedural pain: increased wound-related pain at dressings and between changes. ■ Delayed healing: impact of inflammatory mediators. Drives inflammation that increases pain. ■ Cycle of pain, stress, worsened pain and delayed wound healing.
Fear Dueñas et al. (2016)	■ Increases the peripheral immune response, increasing sensitivity to pain. ■ Can become a self-fulfilling prophesy as the brain's alarm system is elevated. ■ Combined with anxiety amplifies to the brain that all is not well.
Lack of sleep Upton and Andrews (2013) Green et al. (2017)	■ Causes inflammation, which increases pain. ■ Debilitates and adds to the pain cycle. ■ Lack of sleep can contribute to increased pain.
Negative emotions and moods, feeling threatened, lack of control, helplessness Bair et al. (2003) Woo et al. (2008) Ballantyne and Sullivan (2015) Dueñas et al. (2016)	■ Can worsen short-term pain, which may transition into long-term pain. ■ Pain is rated as more intense.

The importance of this model relates to the interconnectedness of the component parts that produce the neurosignature. Practitioners need to interpret this alongside patients, because it is individual and helps to account for why people have different pain experiences. It is also of value because it can be used to decipher and explain persistent pain, which can be a major component of living with a leg ulcer. As this model has developed it can be described as not just biopsychosocial but also as having an existential component: the meaning that is given to the pain experience (Dezutter et al. 2015).

Today's scientific research is taking a step further to determine pain. Lyman (2021) writes that 'pain is not detected by the brain, it is created by it' and that it is 'a conscious translation of our unconscious brain's decision that the body is in danger' (Lyman 2021). In understanding what this means for our leg ulcer patients it is helpful to look at what some of these influences are in more detail. As Lyman (2021) also writes, 'Pain is a decision made by the brain – the vast majority of which is outside our conscious control – to tell our conscious mind that we are in danger.'

CAUSES OF PAIN

The World Union of Wound Healing Societies (2004) provides useful descriptions that help establish the broad term of wound-related pain to be broken down into a number of causes that should assist a clinician in their joint exploration of pain with the patient. These are described as follows:

- Background pain from the underlying aetiology of the leg ulceration and the wound itself, such as local inflammation or oedema.
- Pain incidents such as daily activity and walking.
- Procedural or operative pain from the wound treatment itself or the dressing change.

Patients are unlikely to be experiencing just one kind of pain and so it is important that different types are distinguished.

TYPES OF PAIN

Nociceptive pain is caused by the stimulation of peripheral nerve fibres, which sense and respond to affected or damaged areas of the body. The sodium channels within the nerves can act as a volume to the pain intensity (Lyman 2021). Nociceptive pain may be defined as 'an appropriate physiological response to a painful stimulus. It may involve acute or chronic inflammation' (WUWHS 2004). Typically this is short-lived (acute) when due to infrequent trauma or procedure, or it can be cyclic in nature if it becomes a regular occurrence (Acton 2007). The sensations experienced are typically localised, with constant aching and throbbing (Table 6.2). Where the innervation becomes persistent there is an overstimulation of nociceptors; the prolonged inflammatory response may cause heightened sensitivity in both the wound (primary hyperalgesia) and the surrounding skin (secondary hyperalgesia) (WUWHS 2004).

Neuropathic pain develops due to damage to the somatosensory system (NICE 2022), thereby occurring when there has been either peripheral or central nervous system dysfunction or damage. The effect is to elicit altered sensations, which are often unpleasant. Descriptors of neuropathic pain include burning, tingling, pins and needles and electrical shocks located in and through the affected area. Related sensitivity to often non-painful stimuli such as light touch, pressure or changes in temperature can provoke intense pain, which can become persistent. This enhanced sensitivity is known as hyperalgesia or allodynia and is dependent on which nerve fibres are affected (Wulf and Baron 2002; WUWHS 2004; Sandkühler 2009). Neuropathic pain can be difficult to treat, so requires recognition and management that includes specific pharmacological preparations.

Nociceptive and neuropathic pain may manifest in distinct ways with patients using different words or descriptors to describe their experience (Box 6.1). Finding words that resonate with the individual will aid in the communication and evaluation of any strategy.

However, on occasions nociceptive and neuropathic pain may also be difficult to distinguish from one another as symptoms overlap and become similar (Jenkins 2020b). This, alongside their joint presentation in the same person, makes for a complex pain profile. When nociceptive pain is inadequately managed, persistent pain may develop with both nociceptive and neuropathic properties

---

Box 6.1   Pain Descriptors That May Help Communicate the Lived Experience

Nociceptive	Neuropathic
Throbbing	Shooting
Sharp	Burning
Dull	Stabbing
Sore	Tingling
Aching	Numb
	Prickling
	Itchy

Source: Adapted from NICE (2022) and EWMA (2002).

(Taverner et al. 2014), although non-healing wounds seem to be associated with neuropathic pain. Hypersensitivity is poorly understood by clinicians and leads to a 'lack of belief in the extent of the patient's pain' (Hopkins and Worboys 2005). Understanding the patient's lived experience of pain, influenced by variables such as wound care procedures, is critical if we are to determine an effective treatment plan. This influences the clinician's approach to compression therapy and the management plan being suggested (see Chapter 8).

Pain has been described as acute and short-lived or chronic and persistent if of over seven weeks' duration (EWMA 2002). However, there has been more recent debate as to the use of the term 'chronic' and how to define where acute pain ends and long-term pain begins. It has been suggested that another name for chronic pain is persistent pain, with certain characteristics being presented that can be helpful for the practitioner in understanding their patient's journey. The debate continues (Nicholas et al. 2019). Definitions of persistent pain are debated (Upton and Upton 2015; Nicholas et al. 2019), but the characteristics relate to the following:

■ Pain persisting over seven weeks (Wulf and Baron 2002) and over longer periods. This will be the experience of many leg ulcer patients.

- The specified duration of 'long period' is classified as being over three months (Treede et al. 2015). A high percentage of leg ulcer patients do not have their wounds healed in under 12 weeks, so that the potential for long-term pain complexities is great.
- Pain that exists beyond the period of expected healing (Treede et al. 2015). For venous leg ulcer management this will be 12 weeks, but it is harder to determine for other aetiologies.
- Pain that may continue post healing. This is an important reminder for clinicians as patients may be left with residual sensations or even pain after healing; healing the wound is only one of the desirable outcomes for managing patients with lower limb wounds and conditions.
- 'Pain that stopped being a symptom and has become the disease' (Lyman 2021; Wulf and Baron 2002).

PAIN CYCLES: NEVER-ENDING PAIN

Pain can be disruptive, life altering and self-perpetuating. Cycles of pain relate to the never-ending narrative of living with pain. Energy, sleep, mood and activity are all interrelated and if a patient is struggling in one area it will have an impact on the others. Upton and Andrews (2013) found a significant correlation between wound pain and sleep disruption. If a patient is anxious, fearful or depressed, this will affect their sleep. Lack of sleep and the necessity of having to cope with pain decrease energy and make it difficult to be active. Pain together with lack of exercise and movement increases pain, particularly where ankle range of motion is affected (Davies et al. 2007). This in turn affects mood (Upton 2014).

Pain cycles are self-perpetuating and in wound care include those that relate to wound care procedures and specifically dressing changes. Upton and Upton (2015) talk about pain at dressing change, which can easily become a perpetual cycle of pain leading to more dressing. The cycle goes like this. There is pain at dressing change, which leads to stress and related anticipatory pain when dressing time approaches. The patient may then adopt avoidance behaviour, which can cause delayed wound healing, exacerbating pain and initiating the need for more dressings, which are now perceived as being painful. As patients become more anxious or stressed in anticipation of pain, they will also rate their pain higher (Colloca and Beneddetti 2007). Within this cycle it is easy to see how a patient may be labelled non-concordant as they seek to alleviate the cycle they are in. Perhaps less obvious is the role that nurses can play to alleviate or even negate the discomfort experienced.

IMPACT OF PAIN ON PEOPLE'S LIVES

The experience of pain is individual, but numerous studies have highlighted commonly encountered factors that can potentiate pain. It is important to understand and identify what is likely to increase pain so that there can be mediation and appropriate care can be given and planned for. Table 6.2 identifies some of these considerations.

Stress, anxiety and fear are closely linked and well documented as being influencers and predictors of increased pain that delays healing. The impact on sleep is a common feature of quality-of-life studies (Green et al. 2017; Hellström et al. 2016; Taverner et al. 2014; Upton and Andrews 2013). Green et al. (2017) found that 'the lack of sleep seemed to accentuate the debilitating nature of the condition and made day-to-day functioning more challenging'.

CAUSES OF PAIN

The literature is inconclusive about whether the severity of the pain is predicted by the wound aetiology. Experience can tell us it can be, but clinicians need to be mindful not to be affected by the experiences of others. It remains critical that clinicians come to the assessment with an open mind and ready to listen to the patient's experience. The myth that pervaded for many years was that arterial ulcers are more painful than venous and so clinicians were already making a value judgement on how much pain a patient was likely to be in. It is now recognised that this is erroneous.

Briggs et al. (2007) found that severity of the pain cannot be predicted by the wound type, size or duration of the leg ulcer. Hellström et al. (2016), in their study of elderly patients, found that pain intensity varied with wound type, those with multiple ulceration of different diagnoses scoring the highest (Table 6.3). Of note is that

TABLE 6.3   Leg ulcer types.

Leg ulcer type	Findings	Implications
Venous leg ulceration	50% no pain 31% scored 5–10	A significant proportion experienced severe pain. When 50% can experience no or resolved pain, the patient in pain can be ignored or disbelieved.
Arterial leg ulceration	27% no pain 54% scored 5–10	There remain some patients who experience nil or resolved pain. However, a significant number experience severe pain.
Mixed venous/ arterial leg ulceration	39% no pain 47% scored 5–10	It is of note that despite arterial disease, a significant number of patients experience nil or resolved pain. However, nearly 50% experience severe pain.

Source: Adapted from Hellström et al. (2016).

over 70% of patients with bilateral ulceration were identified as having significant pain. 'Higher pain intensity was associated with increasing odds of having sleep disturbances' and increased rapidly, with a score of over 4 on a numerical rating scale. Hellström et al. (2016) also found a number of patients who reported no pain and still had significant sleep disturbances, thus this remains a critical question in assessment. While a number of patients said they had no pain associated with their ulceration, it remains significant that a high proportion had scores of 5–10 in severity; this may be related to a wound, infection, erosions or unmanaged swelling. This group needs to feel heard and have their experiences explored if pain is to be successfully managed.

Certain conditions may predispose to articulations of particularly painful experiences. This includes inflammatory processes manifesting as part of the underlying pathology. Thus, sickle cell disease, vasculitis including pyoderma gangrenosum, and atrophie blanche may all experientially be found as extremely painful. See Chapter 3 on unusual aetiologies and Chapter 8 on compression therapy and its role in reducing inflammation.

PAIN MANAGEMENT SOLUTIONS: ASSESSMENT

Managing pain can be a significant challenge for those with leg ulceration and the clinicians caring for that person. Management is rooted in intelligent assessments to understand the patient's story in relation to their current circumstances and presenting symptoms. WUWHS (2004) suggests a layered approach in assessing pain at wound-related procedures consisting of initial, ongoing and review assessments.

This guidance is a helpful way of approaching the whole impact of pain in a more fundamental way. Wound care procedures are just one aspect of living with a leg ulcer and if pain management is to be meaningful, the assessment needs to encompass all stages of the experience for that patient. WUWHS (2004) talks about assessments needing to be carried out by experienced practitioners with good listening skills. Factors such as feelings, perceptions and beliefs, along with the meaning and impact of pain for that person and the surrounding family, require exploration. The need for establishing a conversation with the patient is paramount to acknowledging the patient's experience (Jenkins 2020b; Ballantyne and Sullivan 2015). Patients need to be able to tell their story, some of which will be about presenting issues, and to feel that they are being listened to in a non-judgmental but informed way. See Box 6.2.

Box 6.2   Asking Questions to Understand Patients' Pain

Remember: Assess and document regularly!
Be prepared to listen.
Do not form preconceived ideas.

✓ The pain history
✓ Pain trends
✓ Where is the pain?
✓ What is it like?
✓ What makes it worse?
✓ What makes it better?

Comprehension and the ability to communicate thoughts and beliefs underpin the use of any assessment tool. Where there are language barriers it is important that translation solutions are sought. In situations where cognitive differences exist or other forms of communication are required, an acknowledgement of this need alongside appropriate and alternative ways of communicating will be required. Equally practitioners need to be aware that patients may be reticent in disclosing information. Green et al. (2017) found that patients did not always disclose their issues with clinicians during consultation, even when these had been identified as important; this underlines the need for clinicians to create a safe space where the disclosure of sensitive or personal information can be heard and holistic care can be provided.

There are numerous assessment tools available to the practitioner (Feldt 2000; Hockenberry et al. 2005; Woo et al. 2008), although Leren et al. (2020) found that they were used inconsistently. Some of these tools are more age specific or helpful where cognitive ability needs to be addressed. Others are very comprehensive, but can be lengthy and time consuming to complete in the clinical field. Organisations may also have their own guidance about which tools should be used for a cohort of patients. What is important is that the practitioner becomes cognisant with the tool they are using and that there is consistency with other clinicians to monitor and evaluate progress, including any interventions within ongoing care. Where tools are used it is helpful to have them embedded within a narrative that explores the wider context of the lived experience.

Validated quality-of-life assessment frameworks such as the Quality-of-Life Scale or the Sickness Impact Profile provide much more detailed information. They may be less easy to use in clinical settings where transient staff are not familiar with the tool, or where time has not been allowed for a more detailed exploration of the patient narrative. Green et al. (2017) have developed an assessment template that goes beyond physical considerations to consider quality-of-life factors and concerns.

Validated assessment scales are of value at all stages of leg ulcer management, whether as part of an initial assessment or for ongoing monitoring (Table 6.4), and are recommended for review at dressing changes. They are not mutually exclusive and when used with other quality-of-life frameworks can be the source of rich information to inform and evaluate care in an intelligent and comprehensive way.

TABLE 6.4 Assessment scales.

Type of assessment tool	Description	Comments
Visual scales	Visual analogue scale (VAS). This includes the Wong-Baker Faces scale, which presents as a range of faces from happy with 'no hurt' through to upset with 'hurts worse'. Numerical values are attached to the faces with the higher scores indicating the worse pain.	Can be useful for children, but less so for those with cognitive impairment such as those with dementia. Simple, replicable and communicable.
Numerical	Numerical rating scale (NRS). A numerical value is placed against the pain rating (0–10 or 0–100), so no pain may be rated as 0 and the worst possible pain as 10.	Some people find it difficult to engage with numbers and find words or pictures easier. Some find the variation in pain during the day difficult to score, especially if it is episodic neuropathic pain. Simple, replicable and communicable.
Verbal	Visual rating scale (VRS). Uses a scale of descriptor words, such as 'none', 'mild', 'moderate' or 'severe'.	Can be used on a standalone basis or with other scales. Simple, replicable and communicable.

Source: Adapted from WUWHS (2004).

Pain diaries written by the patient are of value to explore the pattern and nature of 'why I have pain' (EWMA 2002; Mudge and Orsted 2010; Upton 2014). These may be helpful where patients are interested in and able to write a narrative, albeit they do not suit everyone.

Where patients have multiple causes and experiences of pain, these scales offer limited information. Leg ulcer patients may present with any number of variables that are contributing to their pain status, but without a narrative or surrounding detail they can offer only a snapshot of a trend towards either having pain or being without pain. Recognising this and ensuring the patient's experience is heard and solutions offered are vital. Enabling the patient to describe their pain, 'giving them descriptive words to choose' (Acton 2007), can help in conversation and understanding.

The clinical team needs to provide a consistent approach to the exploration so that the outcome of the clinical or pharmacological interventions can be observed. Box 6.3 gives some guidance on what areas can be explored with the patient. The practitioner also needs to be aware of what will be the preferred or best way of gaining insight and this will depend on the choice of tool for that patient as well as how the conversation is framed.

Those who have learning disabilities or are cognitively impaired, such as those with a form of dementia, will need to have their pain described or interpreted in different ways. The Wong-Baker Faces scale may not be helpful for those with cognitive impairment (Upton and Upton 2015). Alternative tools may enable a clinician to explore pain through the person's own descriptors or the use of non-verbal cues (Box 6.4). These scenarios can be better explored with carers who know the patient well and can provide new evidence or comparators. Body language is always an important indicator of

---

Box 6.3   Understanding the Pain Experience

When and for how long.
Type of pain descriptors: nociceptive or neuropathic or a mix.
Severity using a visual or numeric tool.
Impact and consequences on sleep and daily life.
Factors that exacerbate or reduce the pain, coping strategies.
Relief rating with analgesia or other interventions.
Adverse effects of current or future treatment.

Source: Adapted from Acton (2007).

Box 6.4   Alternative Tools for Exploring Pain

When your patient has learning difficulties or is cognitively impaired, use an established pain tool to document the pain assessment. This will include the following:

- The perception of pain from a main carer
- Impact on breathing
- Vocalisation or changes
- Facial expression
- Body language
- Consolability

Source: Adapted from International Association for the Study of Pain (2019).

---

whether someone is in pain and so non-verbal cues must not be ignored (Feldt 2000).

Exploring the pain experience within children is another area that requires special mention. Carter and Simons (2014), in their comprehensive book focusing on the stories of children's pain, thoughtfully and comprehensively look at neonatal pain in through to adolescence. In their introduction they write that 'through attending to stories ... we have a chance to start to understand what is important to the children, young people, and families for whom we care. If we ignore their stories, we are ignoring who they are as well as what we can do for and with them.' Stories are an important part of our assessment, but also our ongoing review and management. Children will have different experiences and diverse ways of articulating and viewing the world. Understanding, cognition and stage of development will all play a part. What is important is that clinicians who care for young people with leg wounds are aware that articulation of pain and suffering may be different and that management modalities will need to take account of the childhood experience, level of understanding and expression.

Interpretation of patient narratives must also be done with understanding and without prejudice. Cultural characteristics are often thought to influence the reporting of pain, but clinicians need to be greatly aware of biases, including unconscious ones, that are present in how people are managed, especially when the patient belongs to a different racial or ethnic group. There is an increasing awareness of health inequalities and disparity in treatments due to race and socioeconomic group, with an adverse association between non-white patients and the treatment of chronic pain (Morales and Yong 2021). Equality of access may also be affected by age. Leren et al. (2020) found that increasing age did report a reduction in pain intensity score, but no difference between genders or ulcer durations; however, Taverner et al. (2014) found that older adults are less likely to report pain due to stoicism and less likely to receive a pain assessment and adequate analgesia.

MANAGING PAIN

For management to be effective, it needs to be linked to what is triggering or exacerbating the pain being experienced and is a particular concern at dressing change. However, this exploration of pain and its impact demonstrates that pain management in lower limb wounds is far more than careful removal of a dressing. This may be underlying disease pathology, local wound factors such as infection (Mudge and Orsted 2010) or excess exudate, wound care procedures or psychological and social factors. Existing co-morbidities may have a negative impact contributing to either background or principal pain, further complicating the pain profile. At times the complexity of pain management can seem immense for both patient and practitioner, particularly where persistent pain exists. Despite this, it is important to acknowledge the power that practitioners have to make a positive difference in the lives of their patients. See Table 6.5 for a summary of the key actions to consider. Do we understand and acknowledge the potency we hold as clinicians to make a positive difference to our patients?

In determining the management of pain, WUWHS (2004) writes that treatment of the underlying cause and associated pathologies is the most important consideration in the management of wound pain: 'Treat, where possible, the underlying aetiology of the wound or associated pathologies.' Certainly, the correct management for the

TABLE 6.5 Key messages that will make a difference to patients.

Domain	Practice
Competent and skilled practitioners	Develop the necessary knowledge and skills related to lower limb management to become competent practitioners.
	Use your skills and knowledge in an informed way to manage expectations, bring confidence to the patient and deliver therapeutic care.
	Early intervention to commence therapeutic management.
	Use language that is positive, thoughtful and encouraging.
Assessment	Make sure that your patient feels heard and validated.
	Ensure that their pain is not dismissed.
	Be certain that you acknowledge and understand their pain experience.
	Recognise and respond to non-verbal as well as verbal indicators of pain.
	Make sure that assessment is without prejudice or bias.
	Use validated tools.
Management	Offer explanation to inform and discuss.
	Treat the cause.
	Refer on for unusual aetiologies and vascular implications.
	Medication management. Liaise with the medical prescriber and consider:
	■ Is the medication effective?
	■ Is it being taken appropriately?
	■ Are there medication side effects such as hyperalgesia that are negating the therapeutic intervention?
	Wet wounds, frequent infection and unmanaged oedema all add to the pain experience, so:
	■ Manage exudate. Ensure effective limb oedema management. Skin care protects surrounding skin and promotes skin integrity. Apply appropriate absorbent dressings.
	■ Manage infection episodes. Know the infection continuum and when antibiotics are required. Early detection will avoid pain amplification.
	■ Manage oedema. Oedema can cause 'heavy' legs with dull, aching and persistent pain. Apply effective and therapeutic regimens that are comfortable and well tolerated.
	Refer on in a timely manner for complexities that require specialist intervention. This will help to avoid further complexities occurring and will include:
	■ Pain team.
	■ Tissue viability team.
	■ Foot care team.
	■ Psychological support.

TABLE 6.5 (Continued)

Domain	Practice
Dressing change	Listen to the patient's fears or experience related to previous dressing changes.
	Is analgesia required at the outset? Are there any triggers?
	Engaging the patient in conversation will help to distract them away from focusing on pain. Focus them on breathing during the procedure.
	Give control to the patient, allowing self-removal of dressing and adjusting treatment to reduce pain. Offer 'time out' as required.
	Consider cleaning and debriding techniques and what makes the experience painful. Does exposure to air or washing the leg cause more pain. Could other methods/preparations be used?
	Skin care: ensure that skin conditions like eczema and fungal infections, which cause irritation and pain, are being effectively managed.
	Consider the dressing: does this increase pain? If so, consider other dressings that minimise trauma such as those that are non-adherent, have an optimum wear time to manage exudate thereby avoiding frequent dressings, or have a gentler action on the wound.
	Consider the compression:
	▪ Is the compression effective?
	▪ Know the art as well as the science of compression bandaging.
	▪ Have compression garments been correctly fitted to the patient? Are they comfortable?
Managing expectations	The person giving the treatment influences the pain experience for the patient. Aim for therapeutic relationships that are based on trust.
	Use constructive words and phrases that are positive and encouraging.
	Expectation influences perception, so:
	▪ Be aware of and talk about the patient's expectations of care.
	▪ Be mindful that professional expectations may not be the same as the patient's.
	Offer transparency in care and be prepared to identify and reconcile any differences in expectations.

(Continued)

TABLE 6.5   (Continued)

Domain	Practice
Empowerment	Empower through listening and acting on patient experience.
	Enhance patient skills by linking their experience to clinical knowledge.
	Encourage self-belief and efficacy.
	Offer peer support including Leg Club frameworks.
	Support the patient to develop their own strategies.
Coping strategies	Promote positive conversations.
	Signpost and/or refer for specialist support where needed:
	■ Clinical psychologists.
	■ Psychotherapies: counselling such as talking therapies and mindfulness techniques.
	■ Patient activation schemes.
	■ Life coaching.
	Refer to occupational therapy for functional aids and adaptations.
Staying active	Discuss and encourage mobility and activity.
	Enhance ankle range of motion – teach TheraBand exercises.
	Encourage occasions for social interaction. This could be related to a craft-making activity.
	Consider social prescribing opportunities.
	Signpost to activity classes: swimming, gym, dance, walking.

presenting aetiology is an essential part of pain management. Patients with chronic venous insufficiency will require therapeutic strong compression therapy. If ischaemia is present, vascular intervention will be necessary to restore the blood supply. Where presentation of the ulcer(s) is unusual to the clinician, referral to a specialism such as dermatology will be required to diagnose and commence systemic therapy or some other form of intervention (see Chapter 4).

Analgesia

Analgesia forms a vital and foundational part of managing pain. The practitioner needs to understand the analgesic options and be able to work with the patient and the medical prescribing team to facilitate the best possible regimen for the patient. Decisions on what will be beneficial are not always straightforward and considerations need to include contraindications, allergies, previous reactions as well as drug interactions, existing medication, and drug dependency history. The World Health Organization analgesic ladder, developed in 1986, is often used to help rationalise decision-making. It is important to note that this often-referenced model has been critiqued and suggestions for modifications made (Anekar et al. 2023). Co-analgesics that work alongside these medications include anticonvulsants and antidepressants that target neuropathic pain. Knowledge of the type of pain, and where possible what is either causing or exacerbating it, will assist in this decision-making process. Where people are already on strong analgesics for other pathologies or lifestyle choices, medication will need to be carefully considered, as pain tolerance and thresholds will already be affected. If pain is mostly related to specific events, such as wound care procedures, analgesic options should specifically target those occasions, but both background and incident pain must be well controlled if pain intensity is to be minimised during dressing changes (WUWHS 2004).

The use of opioids within leg ulcer management requires thoughtful application. Opioids work well in acute pain scenarios, but they can be addictive (Jenkins 2020a). Where persistent pain exists the use of opioids is likely to be problematic with little benefit (Ballantyne and Sullivan 2015; Jenkins 2020a). Long-term use can contribute to the inflammatory effect, with the potential of adding to the pain experienced. The tendency to increase the dose of the opioid is likely to lead to a state of hyperalgesia that, rather than controlling the pain, instead increases perception and sensitivity to pain (Lyman 2021). Dependency on the opioid may also lead to bouts of drowsiness and inactivity, which are opposite to the management need to get people moving and active. Dependency may also be problematic as patients encounter withdrawal symptoms when they step down from taking the opioid.

Patients have a choice in taking analgesia. This can be a source of frustration to clinicians if advice has been given to take medication to alleviate discomfort around a specific regimen, such as wound care procedures, and this is ignored. Patients may be labelled as non-concordant in these instances (see Chapter 7 for exploration of this topic). However, it is important to remember that choice resides with the patient, who may have valid reasons for or beliefs about not taking the medication. Perhaps this is also a timely place to remember that 'in the case of persistent pain, the most effective treatments we often have are non-pharmacological' (Lyman 2021). Alleviating and managing pain do not solely reside in the pharmacological, with other solutions increasingly being recognised and resourced. The clinician plays an important front-line role in these options and solutions.

Compression Therapy

Compression therapy is the treatment for venous insufficiency and management of lower limb oedema, where there are no vascular contraindications (see Chapter 8). Tolerance of compression therapy is multifactorial, but discomfort or increase in pain may be experienced. The participants in Taverner et al.'s (2014) study describe how compression therapy or exercise worsened their pain. The patients developed coping strategies to manage this. Unfortunately, the reason for the increased pain from compression therapy was not explored, but it tells us that exploration and identifying why and where it is painful are paramount. People expect to have pain with an injury and that this pain will diminish with effective treatment. When the wound is not healing but treatment carries on, the presence of continual pain at this stage is described as 'pain without purpose' because a benefit, in this case the healing, was not being seen; one can surmise that the compression therapy was not provided at a therapeutic level and thus was ineffective, creating a non-healing wound. This allowed the participants to enter a 'chronic pain state' that was associated with insomnia, depression, pain at night, loss of mobility and suicidal ideation. Compression therapy may be a difficult treatment to tolerate and thus it is incumbent on the practitioner to increase their own knowledge and skills to enable the patient to have this successful treatment (Hopkins and Worboys 2005).

Unfortunately, the skill of the practitioner is rarely mentioned in the literature when discussing the issue of pain and discomfort with compression therapy. Compression therapy applied at an inappropriately high level is noted and identified as a risk for pain and non-concordance (Boxall et al. 2019), but delivering an inadequate dosage of compression will also lead to increased pain and exudate because the venous disease and inflammation are not being treated; this leads to a lack of trust in treatment efficacy and thus a lack of adherence to a regime that is not beneficial to the patient. Nevertheless, correctly fitting and skilled compression therapy, including appropriate compression garments, leads to a reduction in pain and improvement in quality of life (Berszakiewicz et al. 2021).

Psychosocial Management

Distraction

Distraction is a potent reliever of pain as it can refocus the person's attention away from the pain experience. Preoccupation with pain accompanied by low moods and anxiety can draw the patient into a world dominated by pain. A cohort of patients with lower limb wounds and oedema will be housebound and/or have sedentary life-styles. Social interaction may be limited, with emotional moods being negatively impacted. Bringing attention to pain even by introducing words may increase the pain experienced (Hall and Stride 1954).

Distraction offers a way of focusing attention away from potentially harmful stimuli elsewhere. Opioids are naturally produced in the body to decrease pain and in distraction opioids are produced to enable the blocking of nociceptive signals. Increasingly there is evidence of virtual reality being used as a distraction device in a variety of clinical settings for the purpose of managing pain (Indovina et al. 2018). Hoffman et al. (2011) found reductions in pain when used with burns patients.

Expectation

Pain can be manipulated through beliefs and expectations. Expectation influences perception and this has a physiological dimension; if pain relief is expected the body will produce opioids including endorphins to manage the pain. Studies looking at the placebo effect have clearly demonstrated the power of perception (Wager et al. 2007). The 'nocebo' effect occurs when negative expectations are transferred to the patient, causing this negativity to become the patient's perception. Alternatively, positive and constructive words and ideas will have a positive effect. See Box 6.5 for examples. Setting realistic patient-centred goals will also be beneficial and can link into a sense of progress.

Box 6.5 The Nocebo Effect

The nocebo effect can be triggered by phrases such as:

- 'You're a high-risk patient.'
- 'You have a chronic condition.'
- 'You have chronic pain.'
- 'This will hurt.'
- 'You are non-compliant.'

These place emphasis on the side effects or negative impact of treatment as opposed to the positive.

In contrast, positive words and concepts, including use of metaphors, help to rewire the brain.

They encourage feelings of safety, offer positive reinforcement, reduce a sense of danger and provide hope. This is particularly of relevance where therapies may be new to the patient. The clinician should show confidant compassion.

Source: Adapted from Lyman (2021).

Empowerment

Helplessness and feelings of being unseen and powerlessness have negative impacts on the pain experience (Woo et al. 2008; Rosenburg et al. 2022). Rosenburg et al. (2022) write that 'a patient who is cared for, is one who is noticed'; the patient becomes seen. Learned helplessness, where people have learnt to expect that they will not succeed, leads to powerlessness in decision-making. Such feelings may result in emotional states such as depression and these negative emotions combined with feeling threatened can give rise to expectations of pain and suffering. Conversely, empowerment and having a sense of control should have a positive impact. Reframing beliefs and encouraging choices contributing to leading a healthy lifestyle, with an emphasis on sleep, socialising and healthy diets, will have beneficial effects. Dezutter et al. (2015) when looking at meaning in patient profiles found that 'the ability to find meaning and purpose despite physical challenges can change the lens through which the individual views the destabilising events of his/her life', so that the threat of chronic pain is replaced with a perspective of challenge.

Staying active is vital for patients with lower limb ulceration and oedema. Avoiding activity often begins with reacting to and anticipating pain rather than seeking choices to help manage it. Activity will not only be a technique for distraction, influencing expectations and feelings of empowerment, but will also be an essential element in improving the physiological elements of underlying pathologies. Increasing ankle range of motion will have a positive impact on reducing pain, for instance (Chapter 4).

In determining psychosocial support for patients, it is helpful to be reflective and consider what information would be helpful (see Box 6.6). Being reflective on clinician interaction will also assist in developing a therapeutic relationship that aims to offer a safe place for further discussion and partnership working.

Box 6.6 Questions to Ponder

- Is my patient housebound or restricted in lifestyle?
- How much social interaction do they have?
- What activities are they involved in?
- Is my patient inclined towards low moods?
- In what ways do I hinder my patient when they are made to feel non-compliant?
- How do I engage with my patient during visits, especially during dressing changes?
- What words do I use with my patient? Are they positive and affirming?
- How do I introduce therapies and treatments?
- Are there opportunities to introduce distraction?
- Are there any activities that can be introduced or promoted?
- Do I have a therapeutic relationship with my patient built on trust? This will include being a competent practitioner with the necessary knowledge and skills.

Key Management Messages That Will Make a Difference to Patients

This is not an exhaustive list, but Table 6.5 outlines the key areas of managing the patient with lower limb conditions and where decisions can be made to prevent and manage painful episodes in patients.

CONCLUSION

Pain experience is complex and multifactorial. A great deal of the pain experienced by patients could be avoided if leg ulcers, erosions and oedema were managed early and swiftly. It is clear that poor or inconsiderate management can set up pain as a defining characteristic for patients. Yet pain should not be a tolerated and accepted feature in the lives of leg ulcer patients. Severe life-changing and debilitating pain can be avoided, or at least reduced, in patients with lower limb conditions. Systems need to be able to support effective management, but practitioners must also partner with patients to help engage in creative solutions.

The pain experience is individual and so pain management strategies must be individualised. The practitioner can play a large part in mitigating pain by listening, validating experience and intervening with appropriate evidence-based regimens. Competent and knowledgeable practitioners help to promote therapeutic relationships built on trust.

REFERENCES

Acton, C. (2007). The holistic management of chronic wound pain. *Wounds UK* 3 (1): 61–69.

Anekar, A.A., Hendrix, J.M., and Cascella, M. (2023). WHO analgesic ladder. In: *StatPearls*. Treasure Island, FL: StatPearls Publishing https://www.ncbi.nlm.nih.gov/books/NBK554435.

Bair, M.J., Robinson, R.L., Katon, W., and Kroenke, K. (2003). Depression and pain comorbidity: a literature review. *Archives of Internal Medicine* 163: 2433–2445.

Ballantyne, J.C. and Sullivan, M.D. (2015). Intensity of chronic pain–the wrong metric? *New England Journal of Medicine* 373 (22): 2098–2099. https://doi.org/10.1056/NEJMp1507136.

Berszakiewicz, A., Kasperczyk, J., Sieroń, A. et al. (2021). The effect of compression therapy on quality of life in patients with chronic venous disease: a comparative 6-month study. *Advances in Dermatology and Allergology.* 38 (3): 389–395. https://doi.org/10.5114/ada.2020.92277.

Boxall, S.L., Carville, K., Leslie, G.D., and Jansen, S.J. (2019). Compression bandaging: identification of factors contributing to non-concordance. *Wound Practice and Research* 27 (1): 6–20.

Briggs, M., Bennett, M.I., Closs, S.J., and Cocks, K. (2007). Painful leg ulceration: a prospective, longitudinal cohort study. *Wound Repair and Regeneration* 15 (2): 186–191. https://doi.org/10.1111/j.1524-475X.2007.00203.x.

Briggs, M., Nelson, E.A., and Martyn-St James, M. (2012). Topical agents or dressings for pain in venous leg ulcers. *Cochrane Database of Systematic Reviews* 11 (11): CD001177. https://doi.org/10.1002/14651858.CD001177.pub3.

Carter, B. and Simons, J. (2014). *Stories of Children's Pain: Linking Evidence to Practice.* London: Sage.

Colloca, L. and Beneddetti, F. (2007). Nocebo hyperalgesia: how anxiety is turned into pain. *Current Opinion in Anaesthesiology* 20 (5): 435–439.

Davies, J.A., Bull, R.H., Farrelly, I.J., and Wakelin, M.J. (2007). A home-based exercise programme improves ankle range of motion in long-term venous ulcer patients. *Phlebology* 22 (2): 86–89. https://doi.org/10.1258/026835507780346178.

Dezutter, J., Luyckx, K., and Wachholtz, A. (2015). Meaning in life in chronic pain patients over time: associations with pain experience and psychological well-being. *Journal of Behavioral Medicine* 38 (2): 384–396. https://doi.org/10.1007/s10865-014-9614-1.

Dueñas, M., Ojeda, B., Salazar, A. et al. (2016). A review of chronic pain impact on patients, their social environment and the health care system. *Journal of Pain Research* 9: 457–467. https://doi.org/10.2147/JPR.S105892.

Ehrlich, B. (2022). Mysterious butterflies of the soul. *Scientific American* 326 (4): 50–57.

European Wound Management Association (EWMA) (2002). *Pain at Wound Dressing Changes.* https://ewma.org/fileadmin/user_upload/EWMA.org/Position_documents_2002-2008/position_doc2002_ENGLISH.pdf

Feldt, K. (2000). The checklist of non-verbal pain indicators (CNPL). *Pain Management Nursing* 1 (1): 13–21.

Flanagan M, Vogensen H, Haase L. (2006). Case series investigating the experience of pain in patients with chronic venous leg ulcers treated with a foam dressing releasing ibuprofen. World Wide Wounds. http://www.worldwidewounds.com/2006/april/Flanagan/Ibuprofen-Foam-Dressing.html

Frescos, N. (2018). Assessment of pain in chronic wounds: a survey of Australian health care practitioners. *International Wound Journal* 15: 943–949.

Green, J., Jester, R., McKinley, R., and Pooler, A. (2017). Chronic venous leg ulcer care – are we missing a vital piece of the jigsaw? *Wounds UK* 13 (1): 32–40.

Hall, K.R.L. and Stride, E. (1954). The varying response to pain in psychiatric disorders: a study in abnormal psychology. *British Journal of Medical Psychology* 27: 48–60. https://doi.org/10.1111/j.2044-8341.1954.tb00848.x.

Hellström, A., Nilsson, C., Nilsson, A., and Fagerström, C. (2016). Leg ulcers in older people: a national study addressing variation in diagnosis, pain and sleep disturbance. *BMC Geriatrics* 16 (1): 25. https://doi.org/10.1186/s12877-016-0198-1.

Hockenberry, M., Wilson, D., and Winklestein, M. (2005). *Wong's Essentials of Paediatric Nursing*, 7e. St Louis, MO: Mosby.

Hoffman, H.G., Chambers, G.T., Meyer, W.J. 3rd et al. (2011). Virtual reality as an adjunctive non-pharmacologic analgesic for acute burn pain during medical procedures. *Annals of Behavioral Medicine* 41 (2): 183–191. https://doi.org/10.1007/s12160-010-9248-7.

Hollinworth, H. (2005). The management of patients' pain in wound care. *Nursing Standard* 20 (7): 65–66. https://doi.org/10.7748/ns2005.10.20.7.65.c3988.

Hopkins, A. and Worboys, F. (2005). Understanding compression therapy to achieve tolerance. *Wounds UK* 1 (3): 26–34.

Indovina, P., Barone, D., Gallo, L. et al. (2018). Virtual reality as a distraction intervention to relieve pain and distress during medical procedures: a comprehensive literature review. *Clinical Journal of Pain* 34 (9): 858–877. https://doi.org/10.1097/AJP.0000000000000599.

International Association for the Study of Pain (2019). Pain assessment in dementia. https://www.iasp-pain.org/resources/fact-sheets/pain-assessment-in-dementia

Jenkins, S. (2020a). The assessment of pain in acute wounds (part 1). *Wounds UK* 16 (1): 26–35.

Jenkins, S. (2020b). The assessment of pain in chronic wounds (part 2). *Wounds UK* 16 (4): 36–44.

Katz, J. and Rosenbloom, B.N. (2015). The golden anniversary of Melzack and Wall's gate control theory of pain: celebrating 50 years of pain research and management. *Pain Research and Management* 20: 285–286.

Krasner, D. (1998). Painful venous ulcers: themes and stories about living with the pain and suffering. *Journal of Wound, Ostomy, and Continence Nursing* 25 (3): 158–168.

Leren, L., Johansen, E., Eide, H. et al. (2020). Pain in persons with chronic leg ulcers: a systematic review and meta-analysis. *International Wound Journal* 17: 466–484.

Lyman, M. (2021). *The Painful Truth*. London: Transworld Publishers.

McCaffery, M. (1968). *Nursing Practice Theories Related to Cognition, Bodily Pain, and Man-Environment Interactions*. Los Angeles: University of California at Los Angeles Students' Store.

Melzack, R. (1996). Gate control theory: on the evolution of pain concepts. *Journal of Pain* 5: 128–138.

Melzack, R. and Wall, P.D. (1965). Pain mechanisms: a new theory. *Science* 150 (3699): 971–979. https://doi.org/10.1126/science.150.3699.971.

Molnár, Z. and Brown, R.E. (2010). Insights into the life and work of Sir Charles Sherrington. *Nature Reviews Neuroscience* 11: 429–436.

Morales, M.E. and Yong, J. (2021). Racial and ethnic disparities in the treatment of chronic pain. *Pain Medicine* 22 (1): 75–90.

Mudge, E. and Orsted, H. (2010). Wound infection and pain management made easy. *Wounds International Journal* 1 (3): 1–5.

National Institute for Health and Care Excellence (NICE) (2022). Neuropathic pain – drug treatment. https://cks.nice.org.uk/topics/neuropathic-pain-drug-treatment

Nicholas, M., Vlaeyen, J.W.S., Rief, W. et al. (2019). IASP taskforce for the classification of chronic pain. The IASP classification of chronic pain for ICD-11: chronic primary pain. *Pain* 160 (1): 28–37. https://doi.org/10.1097/j.pain.0000000000001390.

Phillips, P., Lumley, E., Duncan, R. et al. (2018). A systematic review of qualitative research into people's experiences of living with venous leg ulcers. *Journal of Advanced Nursing* 74 (3): 550–563. https://doi.org/10.1111/jan.13465.

Price, P., Fogh, K., Glynn, C. et al. (2007). Managing painful chronic wounds: the wound pain management model. *International Wound Journal* 4 (Suppl. 1): 4–15. https://doi.org/10.1111/j.1742-481x.2007.00311.x.

Price, P.E., Fagervik-Morton, H., Mudge, E.J. et al. (2008). Dressing-related pain in patients with chronic wounds: an international patient perspective. *International Wound Journal* 5 (2): 159–171. https://doi.org/10.1111/j.1742-481X.2008.00471.x.

Raja, S.N., Carr, D.B., Cohen, M. et al. (2020). The revised International Association for the Study of Pain definition of pain: concepts, challenges, and compromises. *Pain* 161 (9): 1976–1982. https://doi.org/10.1097/j.pain.0000000000001939.

Rosenburg, M., Lindqvist, G., Tuvesson, H., and Fagerström, C. (2022). Experiences of undergoing venous leg ulcer management: a reflective lifeworld research study. *International Wound Journal* 20 (6): 1857–1865. https://doi.org/10.1111/iwj.14044.

Sandkühler, J. (2009). Models and mechanisms of hyperalgesia and allodynia. *Physiological Reviews* 89 (2): 707–758.

Skuse, A. (2021). *Surgery and Selfhood in Early Modern England: Altered Bodies of Identity*. Cambridge: Cambridge University Press https://doi.org/10.1017/9781108919395.

Taverner, T., Closs, S.J., and Briggs, M. (2011). Painful leg ulcers: community nurses' knowledge and beliefs, a feasibility study. *Primary Health Care Research & Development* 12 (4): 379–392. https://doi.org/10.1017/S1463423611000302.

Taverner, T., Closs, S.J., and Briggs, M. (2014). The journey to chronic pain: a grounded theory of older adults' experiences of pain associated with leg ulceration. *Pain Management Nursing* 15 (1): 186–198. https://doi.org/10.1016/j.pmn.2012.08.002.

Treede, R.D., Rief, W., Barke, A. et al. (2015). A classification of chronic pain for ICD-11. *Pain* 156 (6): 1003–1007. https://doi.org/10.1097/j.pain.0000000000000160.

Upton, D. (2014). Psychological aspects of wound care: implications for clinical practice. *Journal of Community Nursing* 28 (2): 52–57.

Upton, D. and Andrews, A. (2013). Sleep disruption in patients with chronic leg ulcers. *Journal of Wound Care* 22 (8): 389–394. https://doi.org/10.12968/jowc.2013.22.8.389.

Upton, D. and Solowiej, K. (2010). Pain and stress as contributors to delayed wound healing. *Wound Practice and Research* 18 (3): 114–122.

Upton, D. and Upton, P. (2015). *Psychology of Wounds and Wound Care in Clinical Practice*. Cham, Springer International.

Wager, T.D., Scott, D.J., and Zubieta, J.K. (2007). Placebo effects on human mu-opioid activity during pain. *Proceedings of the National Academy of Sciences of the United States of America* 104 (26): 11056–11061. https://doi.org/10.1073/pnas.0702413104.

Walshe, C. (1995). Living with a venous leg ulcer: a descriptive study of patients' experiences. *Journal of Advanced Nursing* 22 (6): 1092–1100. https://doi.org/10.1111/j.1365-2648.1995.tb03110.x.

Woo, K.Y. (2010). Wound related pain: anxiety, stress and wound healing. *Wound UK* 6 (4): 92–98.

Woo, K.Y. (2015). Unravelling nocebo effect: the mediating effect of anxiety between anticipation and pain at wound dressing change. *Journal of Clinical Nursing* 24 (13–14): 1975–1984.

Woo, K.Y., Harding, K., Price, P., and Sibbald, G. (2008). Minimising wound-related pain at dressing change: evidence-informed practice. *International Wound Journal* 5 (2): 144–157. https://doi.org/10.1111/j.1742-481X.2008.00486.x.

World Union of Wound Healing Societies (WUWHS) (2004). *Principles of Best Practice: Minimising Pain at Wound Dressing Related Procedures. A Consensus Document*. London: MEP.

Wulf, H. and Baron, R. (2002). The theory of pain. In: *Pain at Wound Dressing Changes*. European Wound Management Association https://ewma.org/fileadmin/user_upload/EWMA.org/Position_documents_2002-2008/position_doc2002_ENGLISH.pdf.

Wynn, M. and Holloway, S. (2019). The impact of psychological stress on wound healing: a theoretical and clinical perspective. *Wounds UK* 15 (3): 20–27.

Zhang, J.M. and An, J. (2007). Cytokines, inflammation, and pain. *International Anesthesiology Clinics* 45 (Spring, 2): 27–37. https://doi.org/10.1097/AIA.0b013e318034194e.

CHAPTER 7

Personalised Care in Leg Ulceration

ALISON HOPKINS AND CHARLOTTE SMITH

Within clinical practice an understanding of effective evidence-based clinical management is essential. It can be rightly expected by people who have leg ulceration and is mandated within clinical governance structures (NICE 2021; www.nationalwoundcare strategy.net). However, effective leg ulcer management goes far beyond the cornerstones of clinical practice discussed in this book: clinical assessment, care planning, treatment implementation and evaluation. To create an effective healing environment, it is imperative that practitioners understand the social, environmental and cultural context of health and health inequalities and of care provision – that is to say, practitioners need to develop an understanding of the wider determinants of health if they are to offer truly personalised care. Understanding of the wider determinants of health is critical to understanding health inequalities and the resulting health outcomes and behaviours, and is therefore crucial to creating the conditions for health improvement for people with leg ulceration. See Table 7.1 for an overview of the social, environmental and cultural context of health that shapes this chapter.

Lower Limb and Leg Ulcer Assessment and Management, First Edition.
Edited by Aby Mitchell, Georgina Ritchie, and Alison Hopkins.
© 2024 John Wiley & Sons Ltd. Published 2024 by John Wiley & Sons Ltd.

TABLE 7.1 The social, environmental and cultural context of health.

The wider determinants of health and health inequalities.
The culture of leg ulcer management and the perceptions of practitioners.
The importance of a personalised approach to care delivery.
Tools for health practitioners to support self-management and undertake
   effective, outcome-improving conversations with the person with
   leg ulcers.

THE WIDER OR SOCIAL DETERMINANTS OF HEALTH

The World Health Organization (n.d.) defines the social determinants of health as:

> the non-medical factors that influence health outcomes. They are the conditions in which people are born, grow, work, live, and age, and the wider set of forces and systems shaping the conditions of daily life.

These powerful influences are known as the wider, or social, determinants of health and are depicted in Figure 7.1.

Accounting for the wider determinants of health is important for practitioners, as healing happens in the places where people live, work and grow. Furthermore, the experience of the patient extends far beyond contact with practitioners. Where health services play an important part in contributing to health and well-being, they are only one of the determinants of health in Dahlgren and Whitehead's model – there are many more influences that contribute to health and well-being. Health is complex in nature; clinical management must take into account this complexity and consider the psychological, social, emotional, practical and political influences on the patient's health and well-being and the management of their condition.

Applying Dahlgren and Whitehead's model to a person with a leg ulcer can help practitioners to understand people's personal experience more holistically. Table 7.2 identifies some of the wider determinants of leg ulcers.

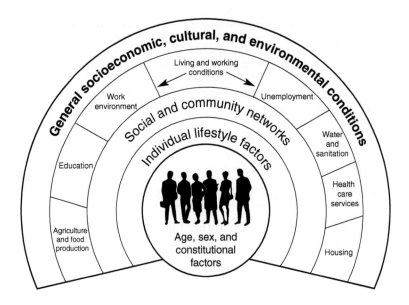

FIGURE 7.1 The wider or social determinants of health.
Source: Dahlgren and Whitehead (1991) / John Wiley & Sons / CC BY 4.0

TABLE 7.2 Examples of the wider determinants of health that affect leg ulcer occurrence and healing.

Increasing age
Obesity
Immobility
Personal or family history of varicose veins
Personal history of deep vein thrombosis
Female sex
Multiple pregnancies
Sedentary lifestyle
Prolonged standing, often linked to occupation

Source: Adapted from NICE (2021).

Furthermore, people from certain demographics may be less likely to receive equitable healthcare in general. People from the global majority have been negatively impacted by poor-quality or discriminatory treatment from health services and by a lack of accessible services (Kapadia et al. 2022). Within education on wound and skin care white bias has been identified, with information and illustrative images overwhelmingly focusing on white skin, which has further contributed to a lack of knowledge of assessment and treatment of skin, wounds and ulceration for people with brown or black skin, further compounding the issues of inequality they face (Wounds UK 2021).

Another group found to be at higher risk of venous disease and less likely to receive evidence-based care is people living in poverty or in areas of high deprivation. What this means for practitioners is that for people who are living in poverty there is a 'socio-economic gradient in venous leg ulcer disease', with those who have less consistently being disadvantaged (Petherick et al. 2013) and at risk of delayed wound healing (Wounds UK 2022).

These examples illustrate that the wider determinants of health and the influence of health practitioners can result in poor health outcomes for the people we care for. To further understand health behaviours that have negative impacts on the healing process, it is necessary to consider the underpinning causes of these behaviours and the interlink between the factors shown in Table 7.3.

Table 7.3 offers just a flavour of the complex relationship between these factors – many more are observed within practice. The social determinants of health are thus interconnected and each can affect a person's ability to participate in treatment or heal.

Some aspects of health are determined prior to or at birth. For example, women who are vulnerable, minoritised or disadvantaged have an increased risk of maternal death (Jones et al. 2022), and babies who are born at low birthweight are at increased risk of poor health outcomes from birth onwards (Office for National Statistics 2023b). Other health outcomes might be determined or influenced by environment. For example, living in a cold home increases the risk of heart attack and stroke, respiratory illness, falls and accidents (Office for National Statistics 2023b) and fuel poverty affects 13.4% of UK households (Department for Business, Energy and Industrial Strategy 2019). As such, how much choice a person has to mitigate the increased risk of heart attack, stroke and other associated illnesses is dependent on the availability of resources and money to heat their home. In the same way, the ability to avoid a leg ulcer is dependent on a range of determinants; women are more likely than

TABLE 7.3 Examples of the inextricable links between the social determinants of health, leg ulceration risk and delayed healing.

Obesity	People with obesity are more likely to develop leg ulceration through reduction in calf muscle function and mobility, as well as increased intra-abdominal pressure (Meulendijks et al. 2020).	People with lower income (also referred to as lower socioeconomic status) are at risk of delayed healing (Gethin et al. 2022).	Lower income is adversely associated with obesity (Kim and Knesebeck 2018).	Obesity-related hospital admissions for women from the most deprived areas are nearly twice as high as for women from the least deprived areas (Holmes 2021).
Smoking	People who smoke are more likely to develop leg ulceration (Wounds UK 2022).	People living in the most deprived areas of England are four times more likely to smoke than those living in the least deprived areas (Office for National Statistics 2023a).	Smoking is related to several other co-morbidities such as circulatory disorders, for example peripheral arterial disease, chronic respiratory disease, kidney or liver disease and anaemia, all of which may be a factor in delayed healing (Wounds UK 2022).	In 2019–2020 there were an estimated 506k smoking-related hospital admissions in the UK (Office for Health Improvement and Disparities 2022).

| Mental health and well-being | Stress is known to have an impact on wound healing and can contribute to delayed healing (Wynn and Holloway 2019; Gethin et al. 2022). Factors such as unemployment, low income, food and fuel poverty are very stressful. | People with lower incomes are more likely to report their health as 'bad' or 'very bad' (Health Foundation 2022). | The body is dependent on the right nutrition and hydration to heal wounds (Wounds UK 2022). People who have less money may not have food security. Food security is when we know we have enough nutritious food to feed ourselves and our family. Not having food security is stressful. | If a person's mental health and well-being are low this may affect their ability to participate in leg ulcer treatment. |

men to experience a leg ulcer, and choices such as smoking and dietary intake, which are influenced by wider determinants such as poverty, also contribute to incidence.

WIDER DETERMINANTS OF ENGAGEMENT WITH TREATMENT

Just as they have impacts on health outcomes, the wider determinants of health can also create or limit a person's capacity for engagement with leg ulcer treatment. For example, telling people who are obese that they need to lose weight in order to expedite wound healing is likely to have limited success if that person has limited mobility, restricted access to affordable healthy food (for example, they do not live near a supermarket and rely on takeaway or convenience foods), works in a sedentary job and has a low income or is not near any green spaces. Similarly, wound healing may not appear to be as high a priority for the person with leg ulcers as the practitioner. For the practitioner, wound management may be the focus of their interaction with the person. For the person with leg ulcers, the wound may be one among many issues occurring in their life that requires their attention, and it may not be the most urgent or important by comparison. An example of this may be that if a person has fuel poverty and is at home cold, this may be the part of their life that is upsetting them the most, with the ulcer taking less of a priority. To navigate this and reach a concordant decision for a management plan, understanding wound management in the context of the wider determinants of a patient's health and life is essential. A lack of understanding can lead to what tend to be called 'issues with compliance' or 'non-compliance'; this is a harmful term that is explored later in this chapter.

It is evident, then, that there are many factors that influence health behaviours and outcomes for people with leg ulcers. Considering these helps us to understand the conditions people experience and the choices they make in response. Furthermore, acknowledging the complexity of health and its determinants demonstrates the limited impact that health practitioners alone might have on preventing and managing wounds. A response more reflective of this complexity of need is required, one that views lower limb health as a public health issue. Public health can be defined as 'the science and art of promoting health, preventing disease, and prolonging life through the organized efforts of society' (Acheson 1988).

When leg ulcers are considered within the context of public health, the 'organised efforts of society' from a public health perspective are required to prevent and manage the problem. What this means is that from a public health viewpoint the response extends beyond one practitioner and one patient to the contribution of wider stakeholders. Table 7.4 illustrates some examples of how a public

TABLE 7.4 Examples of how public help interventions could prevent lower limb ulceration or increase healing rates.

Employers discouraging sedentary working practices.	We know that sitting or standing in one position, all day, every day causes venous hypertension and in the long term, chronic venous insufficiency, which may lead to venous disease and subsequent leg ulceration.
	Examples of employment groups here may be a person employed on a production line in a factory, who is required to stand upright and in a limited floor space area for long periods of time, or a person seated and sedentary in a call centre all day.
Healthy food at affordable prices.	We have explored earlier in this chapter the links between obesity and poor lower limb health.
	A public health approach here would be healthy food at affordable prices, and robust, accessible education on how to shop and prepare healthy meals.
The government addressing fuel poverty.	Fuel poverty is linked to generally poorer mental and physical health.
	Particularly within the context of lower limb ulceration, fuel poverty is linked to increased risk of respiratory infections, which can affect oxygenated blood supply, which in turn is linked to delayed healing.
Local authorities ensuring residents have access to green spaces for activity.	Being active reduces the risk of functional venous hypertension.
Family, friends and colleagues supporting patients and reducing isolation.	This can support shared care and self-care in lower limb management.

TABLE 7.5   Five key areas of public health practice for the lower limb.

Presence of a leg ulcer(s)
Presence of lymphoedema of the lower limb (excluding cancer related)
Cellulitis of the lower limb
Chronic oedema of the lower limb
Diabetic foot ulceration and foot ulceration

Source: Adapted from Sandoz and Walton (2021).

health approach may be achieved in leg ulcer management. Once again, it is important to acknowledge that this is just a snapshot of the public health interventional possibilities and that many more exist.

Leg ulcers do not feature highly on the public health agenda, and within clinical practice there is often a lack of recognition by senior leadership of leg ulceration as a serious and commonly occurring public health issue. In contrast, it is a highly visible issue to those whose daily role is caring for people with leg ulcers (Sandoz and Walton 2021). Local authorities have multiple complex health issues to commission for and cuts to funding, coupled with the Covid-19 pandemic aftermath, mean that services are likely to be even further stretched in the coming years. As such, leg ulcers may not be recognised in their complexity and their full effect on a person's health, especially when competing with other equally important public health issues such as mental health, cardiovascular disease, antimicrobial resistance and diabetes – even though lower leg ill-health may be directly related to these issues (Sandoz and Walton 2021). Practitioners are well placed to raise awareness of leg ulcers as a complex public health issue, and part of their role in clinical management might also include feeding back information about the prevalence and wider impact of leg ulcers to senior managers or service commissioners.

Sandoz and Walton (2021) have successfully implemented and described a public health needs assessment that supports service redesign and new pathways of management focused on six key areas of public health practice for the lower limb. This is explained in Table 7.5.

MAKING EFFECTIVE CHANGE

As has been discussed, a purely clinical response to a person who is experiencing a leg ulcer is likely to have limited success. A health professional's typical response might be to offer solutions and try to 'fix' problems. However, it is often the case that people know what they *need to do* in order to improve their health outcomes; it is *actually doing it* that might require support or guidance. See Box 7.1 for some reflection on this.

Box 7.1   Reflection Point

Think of an issue in your own life that you need to address (this could be anything, for example losing weight, doing 10 000 steps a day, taking more time to relax, managing your finances better) in relation to the following questions:

1. Do you know what you need to do to make the improvements you require? (If not, do you know where to get the information you need?)
2. Do you follow the advice and information you have been given exactly? If not, why not?
3. What do your responses to 1 and 2 tell you about what facilitates/prevents people from following advice and guidance?

As explored in Box 7.1, there is a significant difference between knowing that change is needed and taking action to make change happen. Understanding the process of change can be helpful to both practitioners and the person with leg ulcers, as this can better prepare them to plan, implement and maintain change in a manner that takes into account the wider determinants of health for people with leg ulcers. Prochaska and DiClemente (1983) propose a model of change that might help both patients and practitioners to assess their situation and plan interventions accordingly.

Prochaska and DiClemente's (1983) model suggests that change is a cyclical process. Table 7.6 maps out how we can apply each stage of the cycle to support people with leg ulceration.

Considering this model in alignment with healing might suggest to practitioners that there are optimum times in the cycle for intervention, and that intervention is likely to be different at different stages of the cycle. For example, there would be little point in

TABLE 7.6   Applying the cycle of change to support people with leg ulceration.

The cycle may start with the person not even contemplating the need for change, but the practitioner will recognise this.	
Pre-contemplation and contemplation stages – both might go on for prolonged periods of time	Practitioners might intervene to increase understanding around leg ulcers, compression therapy and lifestyle to begin with.
Preparation stage	Practitioners might support patients to access the correct equipment, resources and information in order to make an informed decision about taking action.
	Examples: addressing some of the wider determinants of health – smoking, income, access to transport and others.
Action stage	The patient takes action to address their wound healing.
	Action might be undertaken in partnership with the practitioner in the form of a mutually agreed management plan, or a patient may choose to follow their own course of action (including taking no action).
Maintenance stage	Here the practitioner has the opportunity to support the patient to maintain the action – to continue with the management plan.
	This might involve revisiting some of the wider determinants of health identified in the preparation stage, assessing their impact on maintaining the plan and making any necessary amendments to support maintenance.
Possible relapse	Relapse is included as a possible stage of the process.
	Here, the patient may find it difficult to maintain the plan and temporarily or permanently cease to engage with it.
	The practitioner and patient can use this as a learning opportunity, exploring the reasons for relapse and planning how to mitigate them when the plan is re-established.

Source: Authors' elaboration based on a model from Prochaska and DiClemente (1983).

teaching a person how to apply compression effectively if they were currently in the pre-contemplation stage. Instead, a useful intervention might be to spend some time listening to the person in an attempt to build a relationship with them, in order to move on to more proactive discussions later on. There are effective tools to support practitioners in assessing people to identify what stage of engagement they are at, which will be discussed later in this chapter.

WHAT INFLUENCES PRACTITIONERS' DECISION-MAKING IN LEG ULCER MANAGEMENT?

Just as patients' health-related decisions and behaviours are influenced by wider determinants, so too are those of practitioners. Unwarranted variation in wound management is well documented and there are multiple influencers for this; the National Wound Care Strategy was initiated to address the issue of sub-optimal wound care (www.nationalwoundcarestrategy.net). Internal factors such as practitioner knowledge, skills and social influences, and external factors such as workload, resource and availability of services all have impacts on decision-making in wound management (Gray et al. 2018). Concerningly, Gray et al.'s (2018) study also identified that colleagues, patients and the pharmaceutical industry were more likely to influence decision-making than research and evidence.

However, there are also individual, personal and professional influences on practice. Many practitioners will be familiar with the expressions 'We've always done it that way' or 'We've tried that before and it didn't work', both of which at times suggest a reluctance to change or even open oneself to new evidence or a different way of working. In other words, practitioners may avoid change because it involves a lot of work (Arsenault Knudsen et al. 2021) or perhaps because they have become weary of change. Although this is by no means acceptable, it is perhaps understandable in the context of today's practice, where workload, staffing and lack of resources and time all present barriers to opportunities for learning and development. Practitioners are human beings, subject to wider determinants of health and health beliefs just as patients are, and doing what we have always done in order to meet the ever-increasing demands of modern-day healthcare in stressful and challenging circumstances seems to make sense, in the short term at least. However, this is a false economy – longer healing times, wound deterioration, disengagement with services and dissatisfied patients and clinicians may all use more time and resource in the long term. Time taken to expose oneself to evidence, engage in clinical peer support and challenge practice where appropriate might well turn out to be the less labour-intensive option.

It can be difficult to challenge cultural practice, particularly when it is well established. However, practitioners are bound by their code of conduct (Nursing and Midwifery Council 2018) to practise safely and effectively, to prioritise people and to promote professionalism and trust. As such, we have a duty to lead and influence decision-making and challenge ineffective practice. Evidence suggests that implementation of impactful, evidence-based practice occurs in situations when there are a number of facilitative factors, including:

- Practitioners having a clear understanding and confidence in the effective impact of a proposed change for patients (Mathieson et al. 2019).
- Managerial support (Teodorowski et al. 2019).
- Ongoing education (Teodorowski et al. 2019).
- Access to resources (Teodorowski et al. 2019).

It can be agreed, then, that there are a range of intrinsic and external factors that influence practitioners' decision-making and practice. Identifying these influential factors in our own practice is integral to taking care of ourselves as well as the people we care for.

THE INFLUENCE OF CONFIDENCE, COURAGE AND COMPETENCE

Having the right levels of confidence, courage and competence can be a challenge within lower limb practices, due to the influence of local culture or arguably due to the myths that have developed particularly around compression therapy (Wounds UK 2022). These myths are discussed later in the chapter. Effective practice and

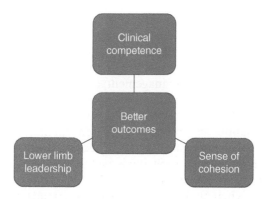

FIGURE 7.2   A framework on which to base confident and competent leg ulcer practice.

therefore better outcomes for people with leg ulceration are under-pinned by three key themes, as illustrated in Figure 7.2.

Clinical competence means the development of a combination of effective technical skills and a personalised approach to care in lower limb management. An example may be effectively applying a bandage and understanding both the scientific theory of the therapy as well as the art of the application in sculpting the person's limb. Clinical competence in technical skills is discussed in more details in Chapter 8. It is suggested that the basis for clinical competence comes from a combination of theoretical knowledge development and organic clinical experience. Being a reflective practitioner is essential for clinical competence. The Nursing and Midwifery Council (NMC) advocates that complexities should be weighed and reviewed in the light of actions taken; beliefs about evidence of efficacy can emerge from this and shape clinical practice. Courage to use compression therapy comes from this knowledge and growing competence.

The second theme is a *sense of cohesion* in lower limb management. Healing rates are linked to social capital and a sense of cohesion, which brings in a participatory public health approach and personalisation. A practitioner's knowledge must be balanced with the lived experience of the person with leg ulcers. This sense of cohesion and appreciation of the complexity provide the courage practitioners need in order to empower citizens, not tell them what to do.

Lower limb leadership, like any type of clinical leadership, means encouraging each other in terms of leadership at all levels. This moves the practitioner from managing one person well to the health of the population. Examples may include developing leadership skills in lower limb management, challenging the narrative or the myths around compression therapy discussed later in this chapter, bringing data together to identify variation in outcomes or health inequalities and introducing the concept that 'change begins with me'. Leadership requires courage because the practitioner will challenge the power of individuals or the system; it requires the practitioner to articulate their knowledge and explore the local evidence even when they feel they lack the competence or confidence to do so.

A PROBLEMATIC CULTURE WITHIN LEG ULCER MANAGEMENT

A number of myths exist in the culture of leg ulcer management that are not helpful and distort a focus on personalised and holistic care (Wounds UK 2022). These have also been the focus in other chapters, for example the myths that foot compression should be avoided or that compression during and after deep vein thrombosis is dangerous are explored and challenged in Chapter 8.

Practitioners should be aware of the prevailing culture in which they work, especially where myths are seen to effect clinical activity. Mannion and Davies (2018) describe organisational culture as shared ways of thinking, feeling and behaving, which are driving forces that can act for change or undermine improvement initiatives (Mannion and Davies 2018). Unhelpful perceptions in the culture of leg ulcer management can generate a culture of blame for the person with leg ulcers and can prevent the practitioner from challenging their peers or indeed challenging themselves in their need to change practice. Table 7.7 describes some of the common prevailing views in leg ulcer management; these are explored in more detail in Chapter 8.

In addition to unhelpful perceptions or myths, system delays in obtaining the right care at the right time can have significant impacts on the trajectory of the person's wound and their lived

TABLE 7.7 Common views of leg ulcer management.

Myth	Reality
Some people see a benefit to keeping their wound unhealed.	With the exception of factitious injuries, there is no evidence of this within lower limb research.
Compression to the foot must be avoided.	The foot needs to be compressed so that the foot pump is enhanced and oedema is not forced down to the foot from compression in the gaiter area. Compression also supports the foot better and aids in walking.
A little compression is better than none.	Most people with non-ischaemic leg ulcers and lymphorrhoea need effective strong compression to heal swiftly. When compression is mild and non-therapeutic, this allows deterioration and poor management of exudate. Pain can thus be severe where there is mild compression.
Strong compression above a moderate 40 mmHg is a risk.	Like all therapy, risks need to be assessed and proactively managed. If moderate compression is not healing the ulcer or managing exudate, the actual risk of non-healing and having poor quality of life is high. Non-standard limbs (long/wide) need a non-standard approach and strong compression to heal.
When compression therapy is painful, it is not suitable for the person with leg ulcers or compression dosage must be reduced.	Compression needs to be applied well and comfortably, then it will be tolerated and all the benefits of therapeutic compression will be received. Why it is painful requires exploration and to be acted on. The common reason for lack of tolerance is poor application technique or the use of a product not suitable to the person's lifestyle. The importance and rationale for compression need to be explained to allay the person's fears, increase their knowledge of this vital therapy and encourage acceptance. Dosage of compression should only be reduced to gain trust and then swiftly increased; be aware of the risk of deterioration with non-therapeutic levels of compression.

TABLE 7.8 System delays that will have impacts on patient outcomes.

Local systems may not respond swiftly to the effective management of a skin tear on the lower leg (LeBlanc and Baranoski 2014), which presents the risk of deterioration to an open leg ulcer.

The primary care nurse may not have been trained in the use of compression despite the national guidance on provision for effective management, leading to an inexperienced workforce (Broadhead et al. 2018).

Delays in initiating compression therapy such as reduced access to diagnostics or the ankle brachial pressure index (ABPI) can allow deterioration and pain to take hold (Hopkins and Samuwiro 2022).

experience (Table 7.8). Practitioners should recognise the challenges this generates: inadvertently compounding existing health issues, allowing wound deterioration and unmanaged oedema or preventing opportunities for management and timely healing. Delays and inadequate system responses will certainly make a standard plan more difficult to tolerate and thus have significant impacts on the person's health outcomes.

It is useful to review the antiquated idea of the 'social ulcer': the prevailing view that some people with leg ulcers want to 'keep' their ulcers for the social gain this brings. This view can be perpetuated by giving it an official title, the 'social ulcer' making the concept feel legitimate. This term started with an article by Wise with that title (Wise 1986). The author described their perspective on the relationship of social isolation to non-healing or recurrence, accepting anecdotal stories of 'the knitting needle syndrome' where patients create wounds to keep the nursing visits. Despite the unsubstantiated claims, the term resonated for many and is still used within the community and by industry, giving credence to this belief, despite lack of evidence. Phrases like this can take on a life of their own and it is incumbent on practitioners to bring critique to the underlying beliefs, as such a catchphrase halts conversations and prevents deeper discussion with the patient to understand their viewpoint or how it is for them to experience leg ulceration. Morgan and Moffatt (2008) conclude that such 'perceptions have resulted in the labelling of patients, which has negatively influenced the care and management of this patient group'. Yet people's lives are disrupted and they have to develop a variety of coping mechanisms to manage this change (Hopkins 2004).

CHALLENGING NON-COMPLIANCE

A key topic in the healthcare culture of leg ulcer management that we need to expose and address is the prevailing view on non-compliance. Similar terms are 'non-adherence' or 'non-concordance'. Hobden's examination of the term concordance (Hobden 2006) was that it 'has evolved from terms such as non-compliance and non-adherence and reflects a shift in the culture of health care interventions, aiming to empower patients'. That may be so from a more academic viewpoint, but the prevailing language used within leg ulcer management is that of poor compliance and difficult patients. Whichever term is used, practitioners need to understand the power differential in the practitioner–patient relationship. Practitioners do expect the patient to take on the 'sick role' and to take and adhere to the practitioner's advice. The conflict comes when this does not happen and at this point the patient can be labelled as 'bad, difficult, disobedient' (Morgan and Moffatt 2008).

When practitioners are asked about what prevents good outcomes, 'non-compliance with treatment' is often raised (Hopkins and Samuriwo 2022). Examples are typically provided of all the tactics and products used in order to achieve compliance, alongside a comment that 'we have tried everything'. These patients could be described as 'unpopular, difficult or "heartsink", without actually being aware of such marginalisation themselves or the impact that such a "label" may have on their subsequent care' (Green and Jester 2019). See Box 7.2 for one person's experience.

Practitioners may sometimes be quick to accept the hesitancy of a person with leg ulcers about compression, rather than exploring the reasons behind it more thoroughly. The assumption is that it is the person's fault for their lack of tolerance, whereas it is the practitioner's duty to assess, plan and implement care in a personalised way, which maximises tolerance and utilises their knowledge and understanding of what can work for the patient. Hughes and Green (2019) examined the root cause of poor 'compliance' with compression hosiery. The themes they identified were discomfort and pain, issues

Box 7.2   A Patient's View on the Term 'Non-compliant' – Tracy, Legs Matter Patient Partner

I had never heard the term before and did not know what non-compliance meant! So the thought that I could have been labelled as non-compliant or non-concordant is actually quite upsetting as I believe I am a good patient. I have put up with so much over the years in terms of pain and discomfort and I have always tried any treatment I have been offered. However, there have been times when it has been too much for me and I have pulled my compression hosiery off (or cut the bandaging off in the early days). I would challenge anyone to be 100% compliant all of the time. Life gets in the way and coping with chronic pain is really hard at times. When I had a painful dressing, I would absolutely dread it because I knew I would be in extreme pain for the whole day and all night. I would cry all night because the pain was so bad, because I was so tired and knew I would struggle the next day looking after my children. I am ashamed to say that I would take extra pain relief because I was so desperate for a good night's sleep. There would only be so much I could deal with and after a few weeks, I would ask the nurse to try a different dressing. Patients don't choose to be ill or to need medical treatment and it is very hard to remain 100% perfect when your quality of life is gradually disappearing down the drain. If this meant that I was non-compliant, then this is hard to accept when I am only human.

What I would ask clinicians to reflect on:

- To discuss this with the patient so they are not given a label they are unaware of; it is not fair treatment.
- To ask why they are not able to adhere to the treatment; there may be multiple answers than can be managed.
- To avoid this type of labelling, to understand that a patient's life can be hugely complex and they have a lot to adjust to.
- Has the reader ever not adhered to the advised treatment plan or instructions that they know would improve their personal health? If yes, reflect on why that was and bring that learning into leg ulcer management.

with application, education and understanding, and aesthetic issues with the hosiery. The topics that led to the primary themes were very personal and included embarrassment, reliance on others, pain and limited belief in the efficacy of the hosiery. Thus, people with leg ulcers can express both intentional and nonintentional non-compliance (Moffatt et al. 2017). This demonstrates the inadequacy of the term non-compliance within the clinical situation: it does not help to address the multifaceted underlying issues or the fact that, within their view of the world, the lack of adherence may be a sensible option for them in their context of their social environment, comfort and balancing the management of their life. The clinician needs to see beyond the term non-compliance in order to have an open and creative personalised discussion so that a co-created management plan can be developed. Box 7.2 provides the lived experience of someone with leg ulcers.

It is well-established that the achievement of comfortable compression is key to leg ulcer management, and that applying compression effectively is a skilled procedure that needs consistent provision. When these are lacking, the person should not be blamed – rather, practitioners should seek to address the issues that are creating barriers to effective compression. In the same way that we need to believe that there will be a successful outcome to going to the gym, changing our diet or walking more, the person with leg ulcers needs to see and believe in the power of compression therapy to create the healing they desire. Practitioners and the person with leg ulcers need to understand that application is more than a task, and that the focus of intervention and desired outcome should be making treatment tolerable and effective. Such demonstration and understanding will have a beneficial impact on the culture of leg ulcer management.

It is evident then that personalised care and an understanding of the impact of social determinants contribute to the holistic approach required to create an effective healing environment. A shared approach to care planning is needed if care is to be truly holistic. Starting from, or at least taking into consideration, the person's experience provides the foundation for the delivery of effective care and education that supports empowerment and self-management. It is essential that practitioners develop awareness of and start to challenge the barriers to care within the culture of nursing and healthcare delivery in order to achieve this.

UNDERSTANDING THE LIVED EXPERIENCE

Practitioners must make themselves aware of what it is like to live daily with a leg ulcer. Arguably, it may be possible to become de-sensitised when working with people with leg ulceration daily. Numerous qualitative studies explore people's experience and the impact of having a venous leg ulcer (Green et al. 2014; Cunha et al. 2017; Hopkins 2004; Phillips et al. 2018; Leren et al. 2020). These studies identify that people with leg ulcers experience significant pain, sleep disturbance, difficulties with footwear, problems with odour and exudate, and mobility issues. This can result in significant negative social and psychological impacts, and in severe cases can lead to social isolation, a negative body image and even loss of work. Green et al.'s (2017) study participants described the impact of exudate and odour on their daily lives, creating 'embarrassment, shame and stress'; in order to bring some control into their life they 'may make a conscious decision to limit social contact, creating an almost self-imposed isolation'. This is because they feared others' reactions and this therefore altered their daily lives (Green et al. 2017). Some patients are more marginalised than others and this is explored further by Geraghty (2021) when listening to the lived experience of patients who inject drugs.

There is a growing narrative in leg ulcer management that people with leg ulcers primarily want to have better symptom management rather than healing. It is difficult to argue against this need for improved symptom management, but in reality very few people want to live without hope of healing. The majority of people with venous leg ulcers should indeed heal if the healthcare system worked swiftly, allowing fast use of compression therapy; healing is the outcome that services should be aiming for. Thus, practitioners should listen carefully to the underlying assumptions being made within publications and case studies where this secondary focus of improved life is elevated above healing, leading again to the belief that healing is not achievable.

Unfortunately unless the health system allows early intervention and excellent use and review of high compression, then many more people are destined to descend into painful leg ulceration. People often agree to tell their story, to reflect on their issues, in order to provide learning from their experiences to prevent others from having the same. There is now sufficient evidence and knowledge to enable the vast majority of leg ulcers to be managed effectively. We need to ensure that the healthcare system is joined up and that determinants of health are considered holistically if we are to safeguard future lives. To move away from the medical model of care, other resources, tools and approaches can be drawn on to create greater agency for the person with a lower limb condition.

SUPPORT PERSONAL HEALTH MANAGEMENT THROUGH PATIENT ACTIVATION

Patient activation is an umbrella term for helping the person with leg ulceration to manage their own health and care, but it is important to break this down so that we can see the steps, the influence and also what it is not. Table 7.9 explains this.

A review on patient-centred intelligence (Strategy Unit and Ipsos MORI 2021) provides a useful tool from which to evaluate a patient activation and engagement strategy. The review describes three steps: the easy to implement such as communication, patient letters and care planning; the organisational change such as patient access to records and shared decision aids; and the final and more complex

TABLE 7.9 The rationale for patient activation.

Patient activation identifies patients' willingness and ability to take their own actions to manage their health and care. The Patient Activation Measure (PAM) tool helps identify where they are in this process and will help in practitioners' understanding.

Activation is not a focus on getting the person to comply with the advice given. The focus is on the development of skills, knowledge and confidence in order to support this.

Activation is part of an engagement strategy. Practitioners have different ways of engaging patients in this journey and they range from the simple to the more time-consuming.

Source: Adapted from Hibbard and Greene (2013).

offer that will be suitable for a specific cohort such as peer support and motivational interviewing. Thus, one size does not fit all, but has to be tailored to the needs of the patient.

PATIENT ACTIVATION MEASURE

PAM is a validated questionnaire designed to measure the knowledge, skills and confidence a person has to manage their health and well-being (NHS England 2019b). Importantly, this tool captures their belief about their ability and the *likelihood* of them acting on this belief. This is very much linked to understanding where a patient believes their level or locus of control is, whether it is internal belief (and within their control) or resides externally through others such as health practitioners (Ingleby 2020). Addressing this locus of control therefore is by activating the patient through building their knowledge and confidence in creating change. The PAM tool provides an individual activation score of 1–100 with four levels of activation and is described in Table 7.10. The higher the score, the more engaged or activated the person is to bring in actions to improve their health.

SHARED DECISION-MAKING

A plan of treatment needs more than clinical knowledge. With the exception of some clinical tasks or diagnostics, the person you are working with has to live all the time with the treatment plan you devise. For this to work for them they need to believe that it will be effective, that the difficulties they encounter will be worth it in the end, that they will see the good effects of the treatment plan and that underpinning all of this is that their humanity is recognised. The plan of treatment needs to resonate or meet with their understanding and a clinician needs to create a space for that to work.

Shared decision-making is both a philosophy and a process (Health Foundation 2010). By allowing time to explore the person's world view and their understanding, there is a subtle shift in the power dynamics: you are emphasising that their views on what will or will not work will be listened to and taken account of. Delivery of

TABLE 7.10 Patient activation scoring in the patient activation measure.

Level 1: Disengaged and overwhelmed.
Consider that they may have too many health or social concerns to focus on the leg ulcer at the moment.
Level 2: Becoming aware but still struggling.
You may hear them express their desire to change an action but the behaviour does not meet this.
Level 3: Taking action.
You may see that a suggestion is acted on or their own simple goal is met.
Level 4: Maintaining behaviours and pushing further.
These citizens are simply easy to work with as they are taking control of their health because they have the knowledge, skills and confidence to do this.

Source: Adapted from NHS England (2019b).

tasks such as compression are adjusted to what the patient believes works for them or needs to be tackled.

Exploring and listening are the basis from which to progress from improving the person's knowledge, thereby building self-confidence and enabling steps to be taken in their self-management and empowerment; these are the steps needed to create change or greater control. Within the prevailing healthcare culture, people with leg ulcers and their families need to have information to be advocates for themselves and to be influential in their own health outcomes. This requires a move away from a medicalised model of care delivery where 'dialogue may be paternalistic and imposed rather than negotiated', encouraging people with leg ulcers to disengage from their care-givers as they do not perceive themselves as equal partners (Green and Jester 2019).

To enable shared care, knowledge flow between the practitioner and patient needs to increase. Both need to be active participants in this change. Practitioners need to move from passively attending study days and knowing how to apply a compression regime, to actions that include bringing critique to the culture they work within, actively listening and sharing in the setting of treatment goals and plans with their patients. People with leg ulcers need to move from being passive recipients of care to feeling encouraged to listen to their body, identify what helps or hinders their tolerance and be bold in describing this and asserting their needs.

SOCIAL PRESCRIBING

Social prescribing is now a well-developed strategy within primary care, with social prescribing link workers assisting in signposting to meet personalised needs. Social prescribing is a key component of the NHSE universal personalised strategy (NHS England 2019b): 'it is an approach that connects people to activities, groups and services in their community to meet the practical, social and emotional needs that affect their wellbeing'. Thus this strategy formally sits within population health, and involves understanding the social determinants of health and identifying the person's needs with them. If they have identified housing as an issue and barrier, for instance, the link worker will direct them to sources of help. If they identify the need to walk more with company, then they will be prescribed a local walking or cycling group, and so on.

The clinician needs to know more about local services and who to link into. Social prescribing can profoundly change people's lives and support activation and self-management.

MOTIVATIONAL INTERVIEWING

Motivational interviewing (MI) is 'an approach that aims to engage people's intrinsic motivation to change their behaviour' (Health Foundation 2011). It is a style of discussion that helps people set their own goals and identify any discrepancies between what they say they wish to see and what they are doing to create the change. This style is aligned to coaching, but within healthcare there are often training programmes available, especially within primary care, focusing on the behaviour changes needed to enable effective self-management of long-term conditions. The evidence of efficacy of MI against more traditional patient education styles is limited (Health Foundation 2011) and may be influenced by the style and personality of the practitioner. However, being trained in MI techniques will help improve conversations and shared decision-making. MI can be transformational (see Box 7.3) and training is often on offer. Of course it requires more resources in training and time, but where simple information is not enough, using these tools will benefit both patient and practitioner.

Box 7.3   Motivational Interviewing – Anna Swinburn, Lymphoedema Specialist

The power of being fully heard by a clinician cannot be underestimated. Patients are experts of their experience and clinicians can gain a wealth of understanding through subtle changes to their conversations, the tone of the interaction, evocative questions, and encouragement for the steps someone is taking without advisory lectures for the steps they have yet to take. These skills and techniques are brought together in the art of motivational interviewing (MI). MI has helped me to explore patient fears and perceptions of change, and to utilise their own strengths to work through challenges. By listening with thoughtful attention to their narrative, harnessing the spirit of MI of collaboration and compassion, I have been able to have truly transformative conversations and support patients in their journey towards wellness and recovery.

SUPPORTING SELF-MANAGEMENT

Supported self-care is a growing trend in leg ulcer management and very much fits with the promotion of personalised care and the development of a person's confidence in their own health management; this is an ambition of the NHS Long Term Plan (NHS England 2019a). Supported self-management is a person-centred approach that 'supports people to develop the knowledge, skills and confidence they need to effectively manage and make informed decisions about their own health-care' (Dowsett 2021); this focus provides quality-of-life improvements as well as clinical and economic benefits. The suitability for this approach needs to be assessed and it is not for everyone. Dowsett (2021) suggests it is for those with simple wounds only and McDonald et al. (2020) found that only 50% of new patients with leg wounds were eligible for self-care. Hallas-Hoyes et al. (2021) report healing rates for venous leg ulcers of 88% using the self-care model with hosiery kits and a six-weekly review; other outcomes included no increase in infection rates, reduced spend on dressings, reduced

TABLE 7.11   The benefits of supported self-management.

The earlier introduction of compression hosiery increases the probability of healing fast and reduces the risk of complexity and deterioration.

Hosiery provides consistent levels of compression therapy; however, its efficacy must be evaluated.

Hosiery requires less bulky dressings and gives fewer footwear issues.

Greater access for bathing, skin care and emollients reduces itching and increases comfort.

Simple self-management increases awareness of what works for the individual and there is less fear associated with the ulcer itself, bringing empowerment and confidence.

Self-management increases confidence, as long as there is responsive and encouraging support from the nursing team.

Self-management increases the knowledge and skills of the patient when used alongside education, skills training and provision of suitable explanatory information leaflets and guides.

travel and reduced nursing activity by 90%. Identifying the cohort (see Table 7.11) who will truly benefit from self-management and not deteriorate in their progress to healing is likely a productive use of time and resources for both patient and practitioner.

Ongoing evaluation is critical to the success of this approach and a person with leg ulcers should not be left to fend for themselves (Hopkins 2020). Organisational support and regular check-ins are essential, and knowing what the red flags are and having a responsive service if these are raised are critical.

The National Wound Care Strategy has a growing portfolio of resources to use alongside outcome data as the programme develops. The Legs Matter coalition has resources and stories to raise awareness and enable greater understanding (see the next section). The medical device industries also have a growing portfolio of tools that are not product specific and thus can be used to support people with lower limb conditions.

As a rule, self-management is effective for early intervention and smaller accessible ulcers on the gaiter region because a standard hosiery regime is often used (see Table 7.12). In contrast, self-management may not be the right plan for those in significant pain, those with a retro malleolal ulcer or those who need an extra-strong compression regime.

TABLE 7.12 Characteristics of people with leg ulcers who are deemed suitable for self-care.

They understand why they have the wound and the diagnosis.
They could identify if their wound became infected, they know who to contact and the importance of doing so.
They know what their treatment plan is and why, and can carry it out.
They can carry out their treatment in a safe and supportive environment.

Source: Adapted from Hallas-Hoyes et al. (2021).

LEGS MATTER COALITION: RAISING AWARENESS OF LOWER LIMB CONDITIONS

The role of Legs Matter (https://legsmatter.org) is an important one in providing a resource for people to have their questions answered and to enable them to know more so that they can be advocates for themselves. This will also mean that they are less reliant on the system working perfectly and help them navigate the health system more effectively.

Legs Matter has been bold in describing the unacceptable situation that people with leg conditions are in, and that the lack of accountability for delays is a patient safety issue and creates daily harm. This delayed care also has significant impacts on the workload of nursing staff and is an avoidable cost to the health system (Atkin et al. 2021). There are many resources available on the Legs Matter website to increase health practitioners' understanding and encourage better conversations, all aimed at delivering a more personalised approach to care that improves outcomes.

PEER SUPPORT GROUPS

Peer support is a range of approaches through which people with similar long-term conditions 'give or gain support from each other to achieve a range of health and wellbeing outcomes' (NHS England 2017). Unlike diabetes or cancer-related illnesses, peer advocacy is rarely used for lower limb conditions. This is likely because there is not one disease for people managing their lives with leg ulcers or lymphoedema. Networks are often informal and linked to attendance at leg ulcer clinics. It is hoped that this form of advocacy will increase with the provision of regional strategies for these conditions with Integrated Commissioning Boards or similar.

The Lindsay Leg Club Foundation, a registered charity, provides a network of Leg Clubs across the country aiming to provide care for people suffering or at risk of chronic leg disease within a psychosocial model of care (Lindsay 2022). The model aims to provide peer and social support, reducing the stigma and isolation associated with leg ulcers.

USING POSITIVE LANGUAGE TO PROMOTE A POSITIVE CULTURE

There is a need for practitioners to look beyond the medical model of care and appreciate the complexities of people's lives and the context in which care is managed. The health culture of leg ulcer management has developed against the background of poorly funded community health services, where leg ulcers are not seen as a medical priority or have been considered the domain of older people, who are often impacted by a stigmatised approach to their age (see the earlier section on myths).

The words we use influence both clinical practice and the patient's experience. The context is important and thus there is a growing realisation that words and the way the person with leg ulcers is described are significant and may need to be challenged. Table 7.13 explores this further through the Wounds UK Best Practice Document (Wounds UK 2022), which identifies the assumptions underlying certain negative descriptors.

TABLE 7.13 Negative terminology

Chronic – suggests that the wound will remain unhealed for a long time.
Complex – suggests that the wound will be too difficult to heal.
Hard-to-heal – suggests that healing is not possible or difficult.
Long-standing – suggests that the wound will be present for a long time.
Static – suggests that the wound will not progress.

Source: Adapted from Wounds UK (2022).

TABLE 7.14 Using positive descriptors to generate action and confidence.

Acute leg ulceration – this introduces an urgency of approach and an expectation of healing.

When referencing a patient's leg ulcer, the term must always be described with its aetiology or cause such as venous leg ulcer or vasculitic leg ulcer – this identifies the vital need for aetiology and for this diagnosis to drive treatment.

Use 'difficult to tolerate' instead of non-compliance – this suggests that clinicians need to actively aid tolerance in the treatment plan and through collaboration.

Not just compression but make it therapeutic compression – this suggests that compression is more than a bandage but provides a therapeutic intervention.

Identify the desired compression dosage – this suggests the need to identify a personal level of therapeutic compression and enables the clinician to question whether this is being achieved.

Bring 'courage to compress' into the team conversation and culture – this recognises the need for clinicians to bring critique to the healthcare environment and culture of care for the benefit of people with leg ulcers.

Greater awareness of our use of language in this field is important and allows us to challenge the descriptors and also contribute a more positive influence to this speciality, bringing more optimism and confidence to the experience of people with leg ulcers and practitioners. Table 7.14 offers some more positive alternatives.

CONCLUSION

This chapter has examined the complexity of leg ulcer management in the context of the lived experience of people with leg ulceration, the wider determinants of health and the culture of healthcare practice. It has also identified leg ulcers as a public health issue that requires the organised efforts of society to address and places the person at the centre of their healing. The chapter has sought to review the growing focus on the provision of personalised care and empowerment that will support patient engagement and activation within leg ulcer management. These are critical for many people with leg ulcers, who are struggling to heal and need greater understanding; together solutions can be found that also support greater ownership of their health and self-management to improve their well-being. All of these will help system delivery, resource management and the workforce, creating a positive culture of effective leg ulcer management.

REFERENCES

Acheson, E.D. (1988). On the state of the public health [the fourth Duncan lecture]. *Public Health* 102 (5): 431–437.

Arsenault Knudsen, É.N., King, B.J., and Steege, L.M. (2021). The realities of practice change: nurses' perceptions. *Journal of Clinical Nursing* 30: 1417–1428. https://doi.org/10.1111/jocn.15693.

Atkin, L., Bullock, L., Chadwick, P. et al. (2021). Making legs matter: a case for system change and transformation in lower-limb management. *Journal of Wound Care*. 30 (Sup11): S1–S25. https://doi.org/10.12968/jowc.2021.30.Sup11.S1.

Broadhead, R., Livesey, J., and Ritchie, G. (2018). The courage to compress. *Wound Care Today* September. https://www.woundcare-today.com/journals/issue/wound-care-today/article/courage-compress

Cunha, N., Campos, S., and Cabete, J. (2017). Chronic leg ulcers disrupt patients' lives: a study of leg ulcer-related life changes and quality of life. *British Journal of Community Nursing* 22 (Sup9): S30–S37. https://doi.org/10.12968/bjcn.2017.22.Sup9.S30.

Dahlgren, G. and Whitehead, M. (1991). Policies and strategies to promote social equity in health. In: *Background Document to WHO Strategy Paper for Europe*. Copenhagen: Institute for Futures Studies.

Department for Business, Energy & Industrial Strategy (2019). Fuel poverty factsheet 2019. https://www.gov.uk/government/statistics/fuel-poverty-factsheet-2019

Dowsett, C. (2021). Transforming venous leg ulcer management: opportunities for self-care solutions. *Wounds UK* 17 (1): 49–55.

Geraghty, J. (2021). Marginalised voices in wound care: experiences of people who inject drugs living with leg ulceration *"The Gutter, the Nick or a Box!!"*. *Journal of Tissue Viability* 30 (4): 499–504.

Gethin, G., Touriany, E., van Netten, J., and Sobotka, L. (2022). The impact of patient health and lifestyle factors on wound healing, part 1: stress, sleep, smoking, alcohol, common medications and illicit drug use. *Journal of Wound Management* S1–S41. https://doi.org/10.35279/jowm 2022.23.01.sup01.01.

Gray, T.A., Rhodes, S., Atkinson, R.A. et al. (2018). Opportunities for better value wound care: a multiservice, cross-sectional survey of complex wounds and their care in a UK community population. *BMJ Open* 8 (3): e019440. https://doi.org/10.1136/bmjopen-2017-019440.

Green, J. and Jester, R. (2019). Challenges to concordance: theories that explain variations in patient responses. *British Journal of Community Nursing* 24 (10): 466–473. https://doi.org/10.12968/bjcn.2019.24.10.466.

Green, J., Jester, R., McKinley, R., and Pooler, A. (2014). The impact of chronic venous leg ulcers: a systematic review. *Journal of Wound Care.* 23 (12): 601–612. https://doi.org/10.12968/jowc.2014.23.12.601.

Green, J., Jester, R., McKinley, R., and Pooler, A. (2017). Chronic venous leg ulcer care – are we missing a vital piece of the jigsaw? *Wounds UK* 13 (1): 32–40.

Hallas-Hoyes, L., Williamson, S., Kerr, A. et al. (2021). An advanced self-care delivery model for leg ulcer management: a service evaluation. *Journal of Wound Care* 30 (9): 751–762. https://doi.org/10.12968/jowc.2021.30.9.751.

Health Foundation (2010). Implementing shared decision making in the UK. https://www.health.org.uk/publications/implementing-shared-decision-making-in-the-uk

Health Foundation (2011). Evidence scan: training professionals in motivational interviewing. https://www.health.org.uk/publications/training-professionals-in-motivational-interviewing

Health Foundation (2022). Relationship between income and health. https://www.health.org.uk/evidence-hub/money-and-resources/income/relationship-between-income-and-health

Hibbard, J.H. and Greene, J. (2013). What the evidence shows about patient activation: better health outcomes and care experiences; fewer data on costs. *Health Affairs* 32 (2): 207–214. https://doi.org/10.1377/hlthaff.2012.1061.

Hobden, A. (2006). Concordance: a widely used term, but what does it mean? *British Journal of Community Nursing* 11 (6): 257–260. https://doi.org/10.12968/bjcn.2006.11.6.21221.

Holmes, J. (2021). *Tackling Obesity: The Role of The NHS in A Whole-system Approach.* London: King's Fund https://www.kingsfund.org.uk/sites/default/files/2021-07/Tackling%20obesity.pdf.

Hopkins, A. (2004). Disrupted lives: investigating coping strategies for non-healing leg ulcers. *British Journal of Nursing* 13 (9): S6–S8.

Hopkins, A. (2020). Supported self-care not fending for themselves. *British Journal of Nursing* 29 (15): 556–563.

Hopkins, A. and Samuriwo, R. (2022). Comparison of compression therapy use, lower limb wound prevalence and nursing activity in England: a multisite audit. *Journal of Wound Care.* 31 (12): 1016–1028.

Hughes, G. and Green, J. (2019). Factors that impact compression hosiery concordance post healing. *Wounds UK* 15 (5): 36–43.

Ingleby, A. (2020). Knowledge, pain and depression: impact on adherence in individuals with venous leg ulceration. *Wounds UK* 16 (3): 30–36.

Jones, G.L., Mitchell, C.A., Hirst, J.E. et al. (2022). Understanding the relationship between social determinants of health and maternal mortality. *BJOG* 129: 1211–1228. https://doi.org/10.1111/1471-0528.17044.

Kapadia, D., Zhang, J., Salway, S. et al. (2022). Ethnic inequalities in healthcare: a rapid evidence review. NHS Race and Health Observatory. https://www.nhsrho.org/wp-content/uploads/2022/02/RHO-Rapid-Review-Final-Report_Summary_v.4.pdf

Kim, T.J. and von dem Knesebeck, O. (2018). Income and obesity: what is the direction of the relationship? A systematic review and meta-analysis. *BMJ Open* 8 (1): e019862. https://doi.org/10.1136/bmjopen-2017-019862.

LeBlanc, K. and Baranoski, S. (2014). Skin tears. *Nursing* 44 (5): 36–46. https://doi.org/10.1097/01.NURSE.0000445744.86119.58.

Leren, L., Johansen, E., Eide, H. et al. (2020). Pain in persons with chronic venous leg ulcers: a systematic review and meta-analysis. *International Wound Journal* 17 (2): 466–484. https://doi.org/10.1111/iwj.13296.

Lindsay, E. (2022). The continuous evolution of a person-centred charity. *Wounds UK* 18 (3): 61–62.

Mannion, R. and Davies, H. (2018). Understanding organisational culture for healthcare quality improvement. *BMJ* 363: k4907. https://doi.org/10.1136/bmj.k4907.

Mathieson, A., Grande, G., and Luker, K. (2019). Strategies, facilitators and barriers to implementation of evidence-based practice in community nursing: a systematic mixed-studies review and qualitative synthesis. *Primary Health Care Research & Development* 20: e6. https://doi.org/10.1017/S1463423618000488.

McDonald, M., Bailey, R., and Birch, E. (2020). Improving wound services through a shared care pathway. *Journal of Community Nursing* 34 (5): 36–40.

Meulendijks, A.M., Franssen, W.M.A., Schoonhoven, L., and Neumann, H.A.M. (2020). A scoping review on chronic venous disease and the development of a venous leg ulcer: the role of obesity and mobility. *Journal of Tissue Viability* 29 (3): 190–196. https://doi.org/10.1016/j.jtv.2019.10.002.

Moffatt, C., Murray, S., Keeley, V., and Aubeeluck, A. (2017). Non-adherence to treatment of chronic wounds: patient versus professional perspectives. *International Wound Journal* 14 (6): 1305–1312. https://doi.org/10.1111/iwj.12804.

Morgan, P.A. and Moffatt, C.J. (2008). Non healing leg ulcers and the nurse-patient relationship. Part 2: the nurse's perspective. *International Wound Journal* 5 (2): 332–339. https://doi.org/10.1111/j.1742-481X.2007.00372.x.

National Institute for Health and Care Excellence (NICE) (2021). Leg ulcer – venous. https://cks.nice.org.uk/topics/leg-ulcer-venous

NHS England (2017). Community capacity and peer support. https://www.england.nhs.uk/publication/community-capacity-and-peer-support

NHS England (2019a). The NHS Long Term Plan. https://www.longterm plan.nhs.uk/wp-content/uploads/2019/08/nhs-long-term-plan-version-1.2.pdf

NHS England (2019b). Universal personalised care: implementing the comprehensive model. https://www.england.nhs.uk/publication/univer sal-personalised-care-implementing-the-comprehensive-model

Nursing and Midwifery Council (2018). The code: professional standards of practice and behaviour for nurses, midwives and nursing associates. https://www.nmc.org.uk/globalassets/sitedocuments/nmc-publicat ions/nmc-code.pdf

Office for Health Improvement and Disparities (2022). Smoking and tobacco: applying All Our Health. https://www.gov.uk/government/publica tions/smoking-and-tobacco-applying-all-our-health

Office for National Statistics (2023a). Adult smoking habits in the UK: 2022. https://www.ons.gov.uk/peoplepopulationandcommunity/health andsocialcare/healthandlifeexpectancies/bulletins/adultsmoking habitsingreatbritain/2022

Office for National Statistics (2023b). Child and infant mortality in England and Wales: 2021. https://www.ons.gov.uk/peoplepopulationandcom munity/birthsdeathsandmarriages/deaths/bulletins/childhoodinfant andperinatalmortalityinenglandandwales/2021

Petherick, E.S., Cullum, N.A., and Pickett, K.E. (2013). Investigation of the effect of deprivation on the burden and management of venous leg ulcers: a cohort study using the THIN database. *PLoS One* 8 (3): e58948. https://doi.org/10.1371/journal.pone.0058948.

Phillips, P., Lumley, E., Duncan, R. et al. (2018). A systematic review of qualitative research into people's experiences of living with venous leg ulcers. *Journal of Advanced Nursing* 74 (3): 550–563. https://doi.org/10.1111/jan.13465.

Prochaska, J.O. and DiClemente, C.C. (1983). Stages and processes of self-change of smoking: toward an integrative model of change. *Journal of Consulting and Clinical Psychology* 51 (3): 390–395. https://doi.org/10.1037/0022-006X.51.3.390.

Sandoz, H. and Walton, S. (2021). A healthier future for tissue viability – an initiative to improve outcomes for patients with lower limb issues. *Journal of Tissue Viability* 30 (4): 505–508. https://doi.org/10.1016/j.jtv.2021.07.010.

Strategy Unit and Ipsos MORI (2021). Patient-centred intelligence: a guide to patient activation. https://www.strategyunitwm.nhs.uk/sites/default/files/2021-03/Subproduct-8-Patient-activation-final.pdf

Teodorowski, P., Cable, C., Kilburn, S., and Kennedy, C. (2019). Enacting evidence-based practice: pathways for community nurses. *British Journal of Community Nursing* 24 (8): 370–376. https://doi.org/10.12968/bjcn.2019.24.8.370.

Tsakos, G., Watt, R., and Guarnizo-Herreno, C. (2023). Reflections on oral health inequalities: theories, pathways and next steps for research priorities. *Community Dentistry and Oral Epidemiology* 51 (1): 17–27. https://doi.org/10.1111/cdoe.12830.

Wise, G. (1986). The social ulcer. *Nursing Times* 82 (21): 47–49.

World Health Organization (n.d.). Social determinants of health. https://www.who.int/health-topics/social-determinants-of-health

Wounds UK (2021). Addressing skin tone bias in wound care: assessing signs and symptoms in people with dark skin tones. https://wounds-uk.com/best-practice-statements/addressing-skin-tone-bias-wound-care-assessing-signs-and-symptoms-people-dark-skin-tones

Wounds UK (2022). Best practice statement: Active treatment for non-healing wounds in the community. https://www.wounds-uk.com/resources/details/active-treatment-non-healing-wounds-community.

Wynn, M. and Holloway, S. (2019). The impact of psychological stress on wound healing: a theoretical and clinical perspective. *Wounds UK* 15 (3): 20–27. https://salford-repository.worktribe.com/output/1350826/the-impact-of-psychological-stress-on-wound-healing-a-theoretical-and-clinical-perspective.

CHAPTER

Clinical Management of the Lower Limb

GEORGINA RITCHIE

Effective treatment of lower limb ulceration is underpinned by both the art and the science of clinical practice. The National Institute of Health and Care Excellence (NICE 2023) advocates that all people presenting with a venous leg ulceration should have access to a healthcare professional with expertise in wound management, and arguably this advice goes beyond the most common type of ulceration observed in practice (venous) and should be the case for all lower limb ulceration. Professional expertise requires a good understanding of how to apply both art and science within the context of lower limb management and is fundamental to ensure effective clinical practice.

The research tells us that outcomes for patients in terms of faster healing rates, less frequent infection and less bilateral ulceration are usually better when lower limbs are managed in specialist settings such as leg ulcer clinics (Patton 2009; Hughesden 2021). Also, the presence of a multidisciplinary approach including medical practitioners, allied health professionals (for example from podiatry) and nursing professionals improves outcomes for patients (Nuttall and Rutt-Howard 2020). Arguably in practice this is frequently not the case, with nurses often being left alone to manage complex

Lower Limb and Leg Ulcer Assessment and Management, First Edition.
Edited by Aby Mitchell, Georgina Ritchie, and Alison Hopkins.
© 2024 John Wiley & Sons Ltd. Published 2024 by John Wiley & Sons Ltd.

healthcare needs such as ulceration outside of specialist settings, frequently within patients' own homes, where care can be delayed if ulceration assessment and management are not prioritised (Queen's Nursing Institute 2019).

To apply the science, it is necessary to understand principles such as Laplace's law and Pascal's law; these explain the differing factors that will affect the dose of compression therapy applied and are explained later in this chapter. Furthermore, it is necessary to understand the components of each of the various compression treatment systems, to ensure that the person who has lower limb complications receives the correct type and dose of the therapy. The different systems are constructed in different ways and so work differently on the body. Examples of the various therapies include bandages, hosiery and wraps and again these are discussed later in the chapter. The art of practice within the context of lower limb management is to understand techniques for application of compression to the limb and to ensure the correct dosage of compression and support is applied. Thus, the art and the science are inextricably linked and once an understanding of the two is developed, effective clinical treatment can be achieved in partnership with the patient, leading to faster Medi healing rates, fewer infections and a better overall experience for the patient.

All people who present with ulceration should be considered for surgical intervention. In the case of venous leg ulceration this may be for superficial venous surgery such as endovenous ablation (NICE 2023) (discussed in more detail in Chapter 9) and in limbs that have arterial compromise it may include surgery to restore oxygenated blood flow. However, it is important to acknowledge that surgery may not be an option for all people. This may be for a variety of reasons such as frailty, which may mean that the person is too unwell or too vulnerable to undergo surgery, or it may be because the condition they present with is not one that may be rectified through surgical intervention, for example in those who present with post-thrombotic syndrome, where significant damage has occurred to the deep veins. In cases such as this, the damage to the venous system from previous deep vein thrombosis (DVT) is within the deep veins and not the superficial veins and so surgery would not rectify the cause of the ulceration, thus lifelong strong compression is required.

Therefore, in people for whom surgery is not an option, the underlying cause of the ulceration should be treated as a long-term condition that requires long-term management by the multidisciplinary team (MDT). While the ulcer can be treated and, in most people, healed, the underlying cause frequently remains. See Figure 8.1, which depicts lower limb ulceration as a long-term condition in which the individual can heal and may relapse. Chapter 9 discusses in more detail how to prevent reoccurrence of ulceration.

To manage the long-term condition the toolbox approach to compression therapies (discussed later in this chapter) is advocated; see Table 8.1. What the toolbox approach means is that depending on where in the disease trajectory (from prevention, in the acute phase, or in the healed stage) the patient is, the patient and practitioner can select and use the best tool for lower limb management. If we view the cause of leg ulceration as a long-term condition, the patient and practitioner together can use and interchange the tools in the toolbox to manage the lower limb in the long term.

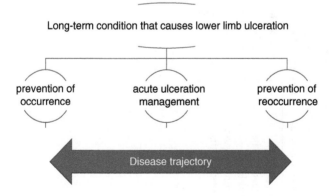

FIGURE 8.1 Recognition of leg ulceration as a symptom of a long-term condition.

TABLE 8.1 Tools in the toolbox.

Name of tool	Also known as	What is this tool used for?	When is this tool not appropriate?	Top tips	Illustration
Compression hosiery kits	Leg ulcer hosiery kits Two-layer compression hosiery kits	Small ulceration that can be dressed with a small non-adherent dressing. Normal-shaped limbs. Low levels of exudate. Self-management.	Presence of complexities such as a distorted limb shape or deep skin folds. Medium to higher levels of exudate. Wounds requiring super-absorbent pads.	Compression hosiery kits should not be confused with compression hosiery stockings.	FIGURE 8.2 Compression hosiery kit. *Source:* Courtesy of Medi.

| Adjustable wraps | Compression wraps | Normal-shaped limbs. Low to moderate levels of exudate. Self-management. Can be used if there is some distortion due to oedema. | Deep skin folds. High levels of exudate. | Wraps can be used in combination with other tools, for example a knee wrap may be helpful to manage swelling around the knee above the top of the bandage line. |

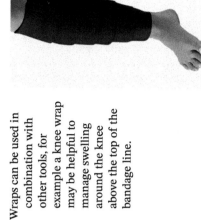

FIGURE 8.3 Compression hosiery wrap. *Source:* Courtesy of L&R.

(*Continued*)

TABLE 8.1 (Continued)

Name of tool	Also known as	What is this tool used for?	When is this tool not appropriate?	Top tips	Illustration
Compression bandages	Multilayer bandage systems Inelastic bandage Elastic bandage The differences are discussed later in the chapter	Can be used on all lower limbs subject to a holistic assessment.	Self-care is unusual.	Compression bandages are effective at managing the acute phase of ulceration and swelling and an intensive course of bandaging can be effective at reshaping the limb before transition to other tools in the toolbox.	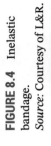 **FIGURE 8.4** Inelastic bandage. *Source:* Courtesy of L&R. 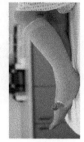 **FIGURE 8.5** Elastic bandage. *Source:* Courtesy of Urgo.

| Compression hosiery stockings | Compression hosiery Compression socks Compression tights | Can be used in early intervention, to prevent ulceration or reoccurrence of ulceration after healing. See Chapter 9 for a more in-depth explanation of hosiery. | Not to be used as a single-layer stocking or sock for acute ulceration. | Compression hosiery stockings or socks can be layered to increase dose and stiffness, but this should only be done by experienced practitioners. |

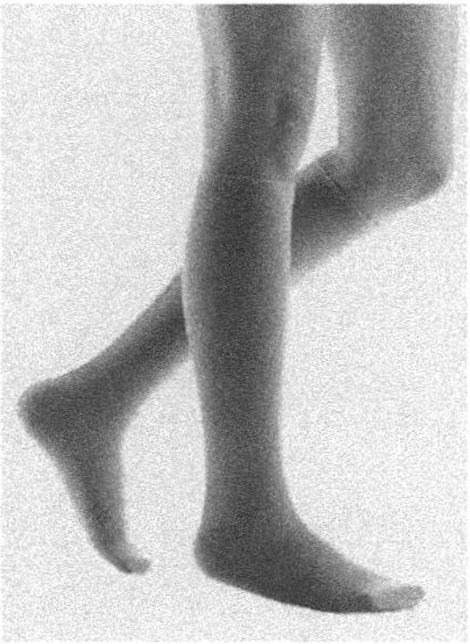

Source: Adapted from Wounds UK (2016).

FIGURE 8.6 Compression hosiery stockings. *Source:* Courtesy of Medi.

THE CASE FOR EARLY INTERVENTION

'Prevention is better than cure' is a widely accepted statement within healthcare practice, and leg ulceration is no exception. Thus, before we examine the clinical management of leg ulceration, we should first explore the need for early intervention to prevent ulceration. The National Wound Care Strategy Programme (www.nationalwound carestrategy.net) advocates that mild compression therapy of up to 20 mmHg can be applied to the lower limb in the absence of red flags. These red flags are acute infection of the leg or foot (e.g. increasing unilateral redness, swelling, pain, pus, heat), symptoms of sepsis, acute or chronic limb-threatening ischaemia, suspected acute DVT and suspected skin cancer. These red flags will exclude the person from early intervention and an immediate referral is needed for treatment.

Application of mild compression is usually achieved through the application of British Standard Class 1 hosiery stockings. In more advanced practice it may be achieved through the application of certain bandages, but this is not discussed in this book. The application of the British Standard Class 1 stocking will usually prevent deterioration of the leg ulcer, but it is unlikely to create healing, and as such should be used until a full assessment is possible. In cases where the leg is an usual shape, has deep skin folds or a loss of sensation, or if there is a large amount of exudate, then again the application of a British Standard Class 1 hosiery stocking or sock is not advocated. Chapter 9 discusses hosiery in more detail.

CLINICAL MANAGEMENT

Following the holistic assessment discussed in Chapter 5, the lower limb management plan should follow three key steps, as detailed in Table 8.2. The overarching key to management of each of these areas is to employ effective compression therapy in partnership with the person.

Step 1: The Person

A holistic approach to the person's health and well-being is important. Factors that affect the whole person and therefore indirectly the leg ulceration and potential healing, such as obesity, pain and

TABLE 8.2 Lower limb management plan.

The person	The limb	Wound bed preparation
The person may require support with their overall health and well-being. This may include management in collaboration with other professionals such as physicians, for example if medication management is required (discussed later in this chapter) or specialist dermatology services for unusual aetiologies of ulceration (discussed in Chapter 3). The wider determinants of health, such as social and economic status, have a significant impact on the person and a direct effect on healing of leg ulceration. See Chapter 7 for a deeper exploration of this area.	The limb overall requires management. This is because with lower limb ulceration the ulcer itself may be the most visible symptom, but ulceration is a symptom of a leg with an underlying pathophysiology, such as chronic venous insufficiency. This may include management in collaboration with other healthcare professionals such as podiatrists for support with gait, mobility and biomechanics (discussed in Chapter 4). Limb management will include managing the skin, any exudate for example, and identifying or eliminating any other significant pathophysiology, such as deep vein thrombosis as part of the differential diagnosis and safety netting. This chapter will examine management of the limb overall.	The wound itself will require management, through wound bed preparation and the selection of an appropriate primary dressing to manage local symptoms. This chapter will examine wound management.

mobility to name just a few, require a shared approach to management and are discussed elsewhere in this book, as are the wider determinants of health. Medication management is part of the wider approach to assessment of the person and is discussed here.

Medication Management

Gathering information about the patient's previous medical and surgical history is an important part of the holistic assessment described in Chapters 4 and 5. It includes asking the patient what medications they are currently prescribed, even for conditions that may not, it would appear, be related to the lower limb problems they are experiencing, and so understanding the medications that are important in lower limb management is an essential component of effective practice. The medications that it is important to know about have been categorised into three areas: medications that may cause foot and leg ulceration, medications to treat ulceration and medications that can cause or exacerbate swelling in the ankle and lower limb (also known as ankle oedema).

Medications That May Cause Leg and Foot Ulceration

Several medications are related to the development of lower limb ulceration. Often this is linked to delayed healing caused by medicines such as corticosteroids, non-steroidal anti-inflammatories and immunosuppressants (NICE 2023). Broadly speaking these medications are linked to delayed wound healing and increased susceptibility to infection, which contribute to the overall pathophysiology of a hard-to-heal ulcer. However, two medications are identified as directly causing leg and foot ulceration, and therefore it is important that clinicians working within leg ulcer practice have an awareness of them.

Nicorandil

Nicorandil, a vasodilatory oral medication (tablet form) that is widely used in the treatment of stable angina (BNF 2023a), has been identified as a cause of ulceration (NICE 2023). Nicorandil works by relaxing and widening circulatory blood vessels; this in turn increases the supply of blood and oxygen to the heart, which serves to reduce the chest pain that angina causes. Frequently nicorandil is linked to mucosal ulceration, and typically these ulcerations are observed in mucosal areas, such as the peri-anal region, nose, eyes and the oral cavity, with skin ulceration being seen less often (BNF 2023a). However, when skin ulcerations are present, 60% of occurrences are observed on the leg (Babic et al. 2018).

The ulcers are often described by patients as painful. On assessment they are frequently localised in nature and may extend into the deeper tissues. There is also usually little evidence of granulation activity in the dermal bed (Patel and Harding 2010). A direct link between dose and occurrence of skin ulceration is apparent and so clinicians should be mindful not just of those patients who have recently commenced taking nicorandil, but also those who have had a recent dose increase (Patel and Harding 2010). The treatment of a nicorandil-induced ulcer is to cease taking nicorandil; however, this course of action is a multidisciplinary decision that should be made in partnership with the patient. An alternative medication to manage the angina should be prescribed. A full medication review should be led by an appropriately qualified and experienced prescriber.

Hydroxycarbamide

Hydroxycarbamide is a cytotoxic oral medication (tablet form) that is used mainly in the treatment of cancers; it is also used in the treatment of psoriasis and sickle cell disease (BNF 2023b). Hydroxycarbamide (formerly known as hydroxyurea) has been identified as a cause of lower limb ulceration (NICE 2023). It is recognised as having other dermatological side effects beyond leg ulceration, such as dry skin, scaling of skin, erythema and hyperpigmentation. Hydroxycarbamide interferes with cell growth, which is a welcome effect within cancer management, but this process also damages basal keratinocytes and can interrupt the growth of collagen too, which causes dermatological side effects and can occasionally result in complications such as hydroxycarbamide-induced ulceration. This is because hydroxycarbamide can cause red blood cells to become deformed and enlarged in size, which can impair the flow of oxygenated blood into the microcirculation, which leads to ulceration, particularly where there is co-existing trauma to the limb (Swain 2014).

Ulcers caused by hydroxycarbamide are frequently described as painful, and clinical assessment will often identify fibrotic ulceration, with trophic, peri-ulcerative skin. In up to 25% of hydroxycarbamide ulcerations it is reported that necrosis may be present (Swain 2014). The most common sites for this type of ulceration are at the tibial crest or retro malleolar area. However, ulcers are not limited just to this area and can also appear on the plantar or dorsum aspects of the foot.

Similarly to nicorandil, the treatment for this form of ulceration is to cease administration of the medication, but it is imperative that this is done under the direction of the MDT. It is also worthy of note that even after the ulcer has healed, recommencing hydroxycarbamide will lead to reoccurrence of the ulceration in most cases.

It is important in leg ulcer management to note that if an ulcer is not healing as you would expect it to, despite the optimum treatment being employed, question why. Have you achieved a correct diagnosis for the cause of the ulceration? Do you need to revisit the principles of holistic assessment, including previous medical history, unusual presentation and currently prescribed medications?

Medications Used to Treat Venous Ulceration

Pentoxifylline is an oral medication (tablet form) that may be prescribed to aid in the healing of venous leg ulceration in some patients (BNF 2023c). It has multiple effects on the circulatory system, such as causing a decrease in blood viscosity and decreased platelet aggregation and adhesion, which assists in improving blood flow and peripheral tissue oxygenation (Hassan et al. 2014). It also has anti-inflammatory effects, since pentoxifylline can inhibit the production of inflammatory cytokines. These actions make it a useful treatment in venous leg ulceration (Annamaraju and Baradhi 2022).

However, pentoxifylline has several contraindications and cautions that make it unsuitable for many of the patients seen within daily lower limb practice. These contraindications and cautions include people with cardiac arrhythmias, hypotension, coronary artery disease, diabetes and severe hepatic and/or renal impairment (NICE 2023; BNF 2023c). Pentoxifylline also interacts with many of the commonly prescribed medications in patients who present with leg ulceration, for example antihypertensives, antidiabetics and warfarin (Annamaraju and Baradhi 2022). Older patients are at particularly high risk of the side effects from pentoxifylline, as they frequently have co-morbidities and polypharmacy, which can put them at higher risk of hypotension, falls and hypoglycaemia (Annamaraju and Baradhi 2022). What this means for clinical practice is that while NICE (2023) recommends that pentoxifylline can be a useful adjunct therapy in the management of venous leg ulceration, in practice it is seen less widely used outside of specialist MDTs.

Non-venous Ulceration – Managing Medications

Ulcers that present due to other aetiologies, for example pyoderma gangrenosum, sickle cell ulceration and ulceration secondary to other conditions, such as rheumatoid arthritis, require medication management as the primary intervention to manage symptoms and promote healing. These less common causes of ulceration are discussed in Chapter 3.

Medications That Can Cause or Exacerbate Swelling in the Ankle and Lower Limb

Swelling and treatment of swelling are vital components in the overall comprehensive management of the lower limb. Further information on chronic oedema and lymphoedema can be found in Chapters 1 and 2. However, within the context of medication management, it is important to examine medications that can cause or exacerbate swelling in the ankle and lower limb. See Table 8.3 for a list of medication categories that should be considered when swelling is present. This is most commonly observed in calcium channel blockers, for example amlodipine and nifedipine. Calcium channel blockers are usually prescribed to treat conditions of the heart and blood vessels, for example angina, hypertension, certain heart arrhythmias and less frequently Raynaud's phenomenon (a long-term condition that causes painful and cold fingers and toes due to narrowing of the arteries that provide blood supply in the hands and feet). Calcium channel blocker–induced ankle and lower limb oedema appears to be due to redistribution of fluid from capillaries to interstitial spaces.

TABLE 8.3 Medications that can cause or exacerbate swelling in the ankle and lower limb (ankle oedema).

Medication	Examples
Calcium channel blockers (calcium channel antagonists)	Amlodipine
Sex hormones	Hormone replacement therapy
Corticosteroids	Prednisolone
Antipsychotics	Risperidone
Antidiabetics	Pioglitazone
Proton pump inhibitors	Esomeprazole

Source: Adapted from Keeley (2018) and Specialist Pharmacy Service (2020).

This occurs despite the diuretic nature of some calcium channel blockers (Keeley 2018).

It is also worthy of note that certain diuretic medications that are used to treat oedema in heart failure are not indicated in chronic oedema and lymphoedema, as they are clinically ineffective in this type of swelling. In cases of chronic oedema and lymphoedema, prescribing loop diuretics may exacerbate the swelling through causing an increase in the oncotic pressure of the oedema fluid. This is due to an increase in interstitial protein concentration because of reduced water entry through capillary filtration. This, in turn, can exacerbate the formation of fibrosis (hardening) of the oedema in the long term. Inappropriate use of diuretics can also put patients at risk of dehydration in the short term (Keeley 2018).

Step 2: The Limb

A thorough assessment of the limb is necessary and gait, mobility, biomechanics and the potentially adversarial relationships between them (Farrelly 2018) are explored in Chapter 4, along with more information about how to assess the limb specifically in Chapter 5. This chapter will discuss effective skin care and exudate management, which are essential to overall good limb health, along with effective compression therapy to promote ulcer healing.

The Importance of Good Skincare When Undergoing Compression Therapy

The skin has many important functions. It provides a protective defence against mechanical, thermal or chemical trauma, and functions as an immunological barrier against penetration of the body by micro-organisms. It provides thermostasis, regulating the blood supply to the skin and controlling heat loss due to sweat production. The skin also has a metabolic function in the production of vitamin D (LeBlanc et al. 2018). The skin is a sensory organ: somatic nerve endings provide the body and brain with important information about the external environment and potential hazards such as heat. The skin is a social communicator of colour, temperature, pheromone secretion and texture. Compromises of skin integrity in any part of the body can impair these important functions (LeBlanc et al. 2018) and therefore ulceration could be framed as organ failure, given that the skin is the largest organ of the human body.

Before we consider the application of compression therapy, the first step is to ensure that the person receives good skincare, which is a key component of lower limb management. Robust hygiene and application of a suitable emollient to moisturise the skin will improve the overall condition of the skin, reduce the risk of skin tears and minimise itching and excoriation to the skin, which is frequently a clinical symptom of lower limb ill-health (Ritchie 2018). Omitting basic skincare requirements from lower limb management can affect a person's ability to tolerate compression therapy. Therefore, cleansing and moisturising the limb are fundamental aspects of treatment (Hopkins 2005) that should not be overlooked (Ritchie 2018). Skin washing and moisturising also present an important opportunity to inspect the skin for signs of trauma or damage alongside monitoring for opportunistic infections such as tinea. Table 8.4 explains the three key steps to good skincare.

Once these three key steps have been followed, it is possible to think about the next step in clinical management, the management of exudate if it is present. A more detailed exploration of emollient use in conjunction with compression hosiery stockings and in maintenance/prevention of reoccurrence is offered in Chapter 9.

TABLE 8.4   The three key steps to good skincare.

Step 1 Cleansing	Step 2 Drying	Step 3 Moisturising
The skin requires careful washing to ensure hygiene without compromising skin integrity. A full foot and leg wash should be done three times per week as a minimum, or at each bandage change if the person is receiving compression bandaging for their lower limb treatment. This will remove the build-up of emollients, dirt and micro-organisms from the skin, which can be uncomfortable, pose a risk of infection (Todd 2014) and may affect the person's ability to tolerate compression therapy. The skin should be washed with warm, not hot, water. A non-perfumed soap substitute should be used to minimise the risk of triggering skin sensitivities. Normal soap can cause the skin to become overly dry and disrupt its protective acid mantle (Voegeli 2008). Special care is needed to wash deep folds of skin on the lymphoedematous limb. It is important to ensure that the folds are cleaned of matter that may provoke an infection. The skin can be cleansed effectively using tap water, in a bowl lined with plastic, using a clean flannel (Wound Care People 2019). If use of a bowl is not possible, consideration may be given to the use of a disposable wipe and tap water.	The skin should be patted dry carefully after washing, without rubbing, to avoid damaging or tearing fragile skin. After washing, it is important to dry in between toes and skin folds thoroughly to ensure no moisture remains that might cause maceration or moisture-associated skin damage (Todd 2014).	Finally, moisturising with the correct emollient therapy is necessary. Emollients will maintain the protective barrier of the skin by 'trapping in' moisture (Penzer 2012). Remember to check for allergies prior to application. Emollients should be applied in the direction of hair growth to avoid folliculitis (Ritchie 2018). Emollient creams are preferred for those using compression hosiery as ointments degrade the stockings. It is important to leave the emollient to dry before putting on the hosiery (Wounds UK 2021).

Exudate Management

Exudate is the fluid that is produced from a wound, lesion, abrasion or area of inflammation as part of the normal healing process (Lloyd Jones 2014). The composition of exudate is complex: it can contain several components such as proteins, nutrients, electrolytes, matrix metalloproteinases, growth factors, inflammatory mediators, neutrophils, platelets, macrophages and cellular waste products, to name just a few (WUWHS 2019). However, wound healing is adversely affected when exudate is overproduced, the composition of the exudate is incorrect or the exudate is leaking beyond the dermal bed onto the peri-wound skin (Moore and Strapp 2015). A thorough assessment of exudate will inform the treatment plan; see Chapter 5 for more information about exudate assessment.

Achieving moisture balance within the wound bed will support healing by providing a moist environment that supports cell migration, nutrition for cell metabolism and cell proliferation. Wounds also require a moist environment to assist with autolysis and removal of non-viable tissue present in the wound bed, but similarly to an overly moist wound bed, an overly dry one can be just as detrimental to wound healing and in particular will inhibit the migration of epithelial cells (Tan and Dosan 2019). Too much exudate can have a destructive effect on the wound bed and the healthy peri-wound skin, causing maceration and skin breakdown, which will increase the size of the wound, cause pain, increase the risk of infection and require more frequent dressing changes. Therefore, achieving moisture balance is key to the management of exudate to promote the optimum healing environment (Nuutila and Erikson 2021).

Exudate presents in a variety of different forms. Examples include a watery liquid, which can be odourless and opaque/clear in colour; it can also be thicker in terms of consistency, which is described as purulent; or with the presence of red blood cells it can be described as haemo-purulent or haemorrhagic (WUWHS 2019). This list is not exhaustive and more detailed information on the types of exudate can be found in Chapter 5.

A change in the appearance and/or the consistency of exudate can provide important information regarding progress or lack of it towards healing, for example an increase in the presence of protein in the wound due to long-term inflammation or the occurrence of infection can cause the exudate to change and become sticky and thickened in consistency. In contrast to this presentation, exudate that is clear and runny has a lower protein content and may be associated with lymphovenous disease or heart failure (Adderley 2008). This information is pertinent in the management of lower limb wounds, where the presence of oedema and swelling must be managed or healing will be significantly compromised. Significant resources are used in the pursuit of exudate management such as super-absorbent pads and nursing time. Optimising compression therapy will manage the oedema and reduce exudate.

Odorous exudate can be attributed to soiled dressings on removal (WUWHS 2019) and some dressing types, for example hydrocolloid dressings, are particularly associated with malodour (WUWHS 2019); however, this type of dressing is used less frequently in the management of lower limb ulceration. Odour is also frequently attributed to the presence of micro-organisms in the wound and poorly managed exudate. Management of micro-organisms through debridement and/or antimicrobial therapy is discussed later in this chapter.

The volume of exudate produced is dependent on several key factors, including wound type, wound location and the presence of micro-organisms within an acute infection, or it can be linked to a wound becoming stuck in the inflammatory phase due to biofilm presence. A lower limb ulceration can produce a greater volume of exudate due to lower limb dependency, which can increase pressure on the circulatory and lymphatic systems causing leakage of fluid into the interstitial spaces (Health Service Executive (Ireland) 2022).

The correctly calculated dose of compression therapy is fundamental for effective exudate management for the lower limb, as reversing the pressure on the venous and lymphatic systems of the lower limb will address the source of the exudate (Wounds International 2015). The importance of the lymphatics in managing swelling and oedema of the peri-wound skin and limb has changed focus in recent years. It was previously thought that reabsorption of the fluid was via the capillary networks back into the circulatory system (Starling 1896). However, more recent research by Mortimer and Rockson (2014) refutes this and indicates that the lymphatic system is the key system in reabsorption of the fluid (see Chapter 2). This reinforces the need to view issues with regard to exudate in particular and the lower limb in general as lymphovenous in nature.

Exudate is not controlled by absorbent dressings, but these provide a way of absorbing and managing the excessive exudate to protect the wound and peri-wound skin, while the compression works to reverse the venous hypertension and presence of fluid in the interstitial spaces of the lower limb. Several dressing options are available to absorb exudate of the lower limb, including gel forming dressings and super-absorbent pads, also known as super-absorbent polymers, all of which are designed to wick away excess moisture from the skin. See Table 8.5 for the threefold approach to dressings for managing exudate.

It is important when applying super-absorbent pads to acknowledge and act on the effect that this will have on the limb circumference, thus reducing the dose of compression therapy. This is rationalised by Laplace's law, discussed later in this chapter.

TABLE 8.5 The threefold approach to exudate management.

Stage	Approach	Reason
Compression therapy	The correct individual dose of compression therapy must be applied following holistic assessment of the patient. Early intervention employing mild compression therapy (of up to 20 mmHg) (NWCSP 2023) can be applied immediately in the absence of red flags or contraindications. This intervention should be maintained until a full vascular assessment is carried out. Early intervention techniques are discussed in Chapter 9.	To address venous hypertension and to ensure fluid is absorbed into the lymphatic system and transported back into the central circulatory system.

(Continued)

TABLE 8.5 (Continued)

Stage	Approach	Reason
Dressing	Initially super-absorbent polymer dressings, which act to absorb and retain exudate under compression therapy, may provide an effective first-line treatment. These dressings work to retain the fluid within the dressing and provide a high moisture vapour transfer rating (MVTR). Once compression has begun to take effect to slow down the exudate, dressings can be stepped down to simple non-adherent dressings, thus reducing the negative effect on the compression dose as the limb circumference is less altered (Ritchie 2018).	To protect the wound and peri-wound skin from maceration.
Skin cleansing, drying and moisturising to remove exudate and protect the acid mantle of the skin are key to protect the skin and prevent infection (Voegeli 2008; Todd 2014).	These three interventions are the cornerstone of good limb management (Ritchie 2018).	Table 8.4 further explores the components of hygiene.

WHAT IS COMPRESSION THERAPY AND HOW DOES IT WORK?

Compression therapy is an essential treatment for people who have a diagnosis of venous disease, venous leg ulceration, lymphovenous disease or mixed aetiology venous/arterial ulceration (for mixed aetiology it is normally at a reduced dose, discussed later in this chapter). Compression therapy is referred to here within the context of these diagnoses. For patients who have significant peripheral arterial disease or limb-threatening ischaemia, it is recommended that referral to a specialist is initiated; if acute limb-threatening ischaemia is identified then an urgent referral for emergency intervention is required. If a person who is diagnosed with diabetes presents with a foot ulceration, they should also be referred urgently for specialist assessment (Wounds UK 2022). See Table 8.6 for contraindications, cautions, and red flags in compression therapy. While compression is a cornerstone of management for lymphoedema, the needs of the more complex patient with lymphoedema are outside the scope of this book.

Compression therapy is also referred to as graduated compression therapy. This term refers to the fact that the dose of compression

TABLE 8.6 Contraindications and cautions in compression therapy.

Contraindications to compression therapy	Cautions in compression therapy
Presence of significant peripheral arterial disease is a contraindication to any compression therapy. This is identified through an absolute pressure value of less than 60 mmHg, an ankle brachial pressure index (ABPI) of less than 0.6 or visual observation of the signs of critical ischaemia (Partsch and Mortimer 2015).	Patients who have a mixed aetiology ulceration, an ABPI of 0.6–0.8 and absolute values of 60 mmHg and above may be considered for a lower dose of compression therapy subject to a holistic assessment (Partsch and Mortimer 2015).
Visual signs of critical ischaemia are a strict contraindication and require an urgent referral. These can be summarised using the 6 Ps approach: Pain at rest, Pallor, Pulselessness, Paraesthesia, Perishingly cold, Paralysis. One or more of these symptoms should trigger an urgent referral.	Deep vein thrombosis (DVT): if the patient is already receiving compression therapy it is necessary to pause the therapy while DVT status is confirmed. Once anticoagulant therapy is commenced, compression therapy may also be recommended (BLS 2021).

(Continued)

TABLE 8.6 (Continued)

Contraindications to compression therapy	Cautions in compression therapy
Patients presenting with a diabetic foot ulceration should be referred to the appropriate local service within 24 hours (NWCSP 2023).	Patients who have diabetes should not be excluded from compression therapy. The practitioner should identify if the patient has a diabetic foot ulceration requiring urgent multidisciplinary team referral (NWCSP 2023) of if they have another type of ulceration, for example venous or mixed aetiology, but with the co-morbidity of diabetes. If this is identified the practitioner should ensure there is no peripheral neuropathy, which can be done by undertaking a 10 g monofilament test or toe touch test (see Chapter 5 for further discussion on this).
Acute deteriorating heart failure: the practitioner should be aware of red flags that may indicate an acute episode of deteriorating heart failure that requires urgent escalation. Symptoms of this may include oedema of the trunk, increasing breathlessness (either at rest or on exertion), a rapid recent increase in weight, increased reports of waking up due to breathlessness or the inability to lay flat due to breathlessness (Atkin and Byrom 2022).	Chronic heart failure: in patients presenting with chronic stable heart failure compression therapy is often necessary to prevent the lower limbs from swelling, lymphorrhoea and infection. A staged approach to compression application may be necessary (Atkin and Byrom 2022) and may require supervision and support from a more experienced colleague.
Suspected skin cancer should be referred immediately for investigation and compression therapy should not be applied (www.nationalwound carestrategy.net).	Known sensitivities or allergies are important to be aware of when using compression therapy, and some manufacturers recommend a patch test prior to the use of their products, for example for bandages containing zinc paste.

reduces from the ankle as it goes up the leg, causing blood and fluid to be pushed back up the leg into the central circulatory system to counteract venous hypertension and swelling in the lower limb. This action of compression therapy and moving fluid is explained later in the chapter using Pascal's and Laplace's laws. Without the correct dose of this essential treatment, wounds on the lower limb will not heal and will almost certainly worsen, putting the patient at risk of further wound breakdown, infection, cellulitis and even sepsis (Hopkins 2020; Wounds UK 2022).

Venous pathophysiology can be further sub-divided into structural pathology, for example venous incompetency and/or venous obstruction or functional venous disease such as calf/foot muscle pump failure or inactivity; many people will present with a combination of both (Wounds UK 2022). Compression therapy will support with both pathologies, but additional referrals for adjunct treatment may also be necessary and helpful for the person (see Table 8.7). Frequently patients will present with a combination of structural and functional challenges that impact and aggravate each other (Wounds UK 2022).

Compression therapy causes actions on the haemodynamic and lymphatic systems to protect homeostasis in the lower limb. Table 8.8 offers an overview of what compression does to the lower limb to

TABLE 8.7 Subdivision of venous pathologies.

Functional venous disease	Structural venous disease
This is normally related to immobility, inactivity, altered gait or biomechanics, which affects the foot and calf muscle pumps (there is more about this in Chapter 4).	This is normally related to valve incompetence or obstruction causing chronic venous hypertension and associate inflammation (there is more about this in Chapters 1 and 5).
Increase in movement and exercise are advocated.	Refer for duplex scan to refute or confirm valve incompetency or obstruction.
Consider referrals to podiatry for orthotics and/or physiotherapy to increase ankle range of motion.	May be suitable for surgery to correct in some cases.

TABLE 8.8 What does compression therapy do?

Increases pressure on the skin and underlying structures to counteract the force of gravity (squeeze) and supports the foot, calf and thigh pumps in moving fluid and blood along the haemodynamic and lymphatic systems.

Improves the overall skin condition, particularly if used in combination with a robust and sustained commitment to skin hygiene, exfoliation and moisturisation.

Prevents backflow of venous blood, which causes venous reflux and pooling of blood in the veins.

Prevents blood components such as proteins from leaking into the surrounding tissues.

Reverses venous hypertension in the superficial veins by reducing vein diameter in elastic systems or occluding the veins in inelastic systems (see Table 8.1).

Manages swelling by supporting the lymphatic system in returning fluid up the limb through reabsorption of interstitial fluid.

Prevents leucocyte adhesion to the endothelial cells, thus addressing inflammation.

promote good leg health and address unwanted pathophysiologies that occur.

Compression therapy should be considered, similarly to any other therapy or medication, in terms of dose. Therefore, it is essential that the correct dose of a therapy is administered by the practitioner to ensure it is effective. For most people where the holistic assessment has ruled out the presence of significant arterial disease, the optimum dose is at least 40 mmHg and anything less than strong compression (see Table 8.9) is a reduced or sub-optimal dose and may be likened to taking half a paracetamol for a headache, thus inadequate and futile. Historically there has been an acceptance within the clinical arena that 'any compression is better than none' or that 40 mmHg is the 'gold standard'. However, this is not the case, with more recent literature highlighting that for many patients the optimum dose, strong compression, is at least 40 mmHg (see Table 8.9) (Wounds UK 2022).

It is also worthy of note that 40 mmHg is not the recommended dose for all patients and that some may require more, for example because they are taller than 180 cm (Wounds UK 2022) or because they have an occupation that requires them to stand for long periods,

TABLE 8.9 The different doses of compression therapy.

Dose	Indications subject to full holistic assessment and ankle brachial pressure index (ABPI) measurement
Mild (<20 mmHg)	Early intervention for mild swelling or wounds to the lower limb. Can be initiated without ABPI if no red flags are observed (www.nationalwound-carestrategy.net). Also see discussion regarding early intervention in Chapter 9.
Moderate (20–40 mmHg)	In mixed aetiology ulceration, can be initiated following a full holistic assessment including ABPI (Vowden et al. 2020). Also see explanation of the pathology of mixed ulceration in Chapter 1 and its assessment in Chapter 4.
Strong (40–60 mmHg)	Suitable for those with venous ulceration subject to full holistic assessment including ABPI (Wounds UK 2022b).
Very strong (>60 mmHg)	Normally used within a specialist setting, or under specialist supervision and in lymphoedema management (Health Service Executive (Ireland) 2022).

Source: Adapted from WUWHS (2008).

for example a chef or hairdresser, who during the day may require an additional dose to counteract the effects of gravity on the limb. In many clinical areas this is considered advanced compression practice, and therefore escalation to a specialist service may be indicated on local treatment pathways and policies. Sub-optimal dosing of compression therapy can be considered as causing harm and if identified without a sound clinical rationale may be considered as harm to the patient (Broadhead et al. 2018). Table 8.9 highlights the different doses of compression therapy as agreed by the World Union of Wound Healing Societies (2008).

When considering the dose of compression therapy there are four areas that it is important to understand. These are listed in Table 8.10 and discussed next.

TABLE 8.10 Four areas to consider when understanding doses of compression therapy.

Area	Explanation	Applicability
Interface pressure (Partsch and Partsch 2005)	Also known as sub-bandage pressure.	Interface pressure is the preferable term as it is applicable beyond bandage use to hosiery and wraps.
Stiffness index (Charles 2012)	Can refer to static stiffness index (SSI) or dynamic stiffness index (DSI).	Stiffness index is applicable to all forms of compression treatment.
Laplace's law (Clark 2003)	Can be applied to compression therapy to explain how the dose can be affected, either deliberately or unknowingly.	This is important when thinking about achieving a therapeutic dose of compression.
Pascal's law (Schuren and Mohr 2010)	Also known as Pascal's principle.	Pascal's law is an important principle because compression therapy is creating a pressurised area to redistribute fluid. This is of particular importance when we think about achieving graduated compression therapy, as we want to ensure we move fluid from the distal part of the lower limb towards the proximal.

Interface Pressure

The interface pressure may also be referred to as sub-bandage pressure. It is the amount of pressure at the interface of the limb and the compression therapy. This is a reliable predictor of the dose of compression the limb receives from the bandage or other compression garment, such as a wrap or compression hosiery stocking (Charles 2012). Effective compression treatment will provide a balance between exerting too little pressure and too much pressure on the lower limb. As discussed earlier in this chapter, for most patients with venous ulceration and subject to a full holistic assessment, a dose of at least 40 mmHg should be applied at the ankle (Wounds UK 2022). Too little pressure (which may also be described as too low a dose) is ineffective in terms of its efficiency as a treatment, as it will not work. This may cause the patient to lose faith in compression as a treatment. Too much pressure (which may be described as too high a dose) may cause pressure damage to the lower limb, in particular to bony prominences, such as the tibial crest or dorsum of the foot, where the interface pressure between the compression and the limb is higher than, for example, softer areas of tissue, such as the calf. Too much or too little compression will affect the efficiency of the therapy and may be uncomfortable for the person, thus achieving the correct dose as with all therapies is of paramount importance.

Compression therapy works on the lower limb to cause a rise and fall in pressure, which is linked to normal movement such as walking, plantarflexion, dorsiflexion or ankle rotation. With the application of an effective compression system during these movements, intermittent pressure of peaks and troughs occurs. These peaks and troughs in pressure serve to massage and support the deep leg veins and more superficial veins to expand and then narrow with the movement of the limb. This movement also causes movement of the lymphatics to promote the movement of lymph fluid. These intermittent pressure peaks provide pressure increases on the veins and lymphatics, which support the damaged or overloaded structures by mimicking the action of a healthy undamaged system (Partsch and Partsch 2005). This interface pressure should be a therapeutic resting pressure and an intermittent high working pressure. What this means is that when the calf muscle is active the compression therapy causes a squeeze on the lower limb and an increase in interface pressure, and when the muscle is resting this pressure decreases.

Stiffness Index

The static stiffness index describes the stiffness of a bandage or other compression system such as compression hosiery. The dynamic stiffness characterises the difference between the working pressures and the resting pressure created by the compression system on the lower limb; that is, the peaks and troughs in pressure when the calf muscle is active and moving or when it is relaxed (resting) and therefore more flaccid (Partsch 2005). This pressure difference occurs in part due to a change in the limb circumference as it expands and hardens during movement and becomes softer and more relaxed during rest. This expansion and relaxation happen during walking or movement of the lower limb.

The stiffness index can be defined as the increase in interface pressure based on the difference of pressure from the resting to the working pressure. Different systems are said to have a higher or lower static stiffness index. Thus, an elastic bandage system is said to have a lower static stiffness as the difference in pressure (measured in mmHg) is said to have less difference between resting and moving. An inelastic bandage is described as having a higher static stiffness index as the stiff nature of the bandage creates high working pressures and low resting pressures (Partsch 2005). Therefore the intermittent raising and lowering of interface pressure is a more pronounced profile. Having a higher static stiffness index indicates a lower resting pressure, which can be more comfortable for the person in compression when they are not active and especially at night (see Figure 8.7).

Laplace's Law

Laplace's law can be applied to compression therapy to explain how the dose can be affected, either deliberately or unknowingly. This is because the pressure exerted by compression therapy is directly proportional to the tension with which the practitioner applies it and the number of layers that are applied, but inversely proportional to the circumference of the limb (Clark 2003). This law is shown in Figure 8.8.

To many this equation can feel quite overwhelming, and this may go some way towards explaining why within the clinical arena many practitioners do not understand how to apply this theory to

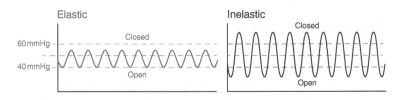

FIGURE 8.7   Static stiffness for elastic and inelastic bandages.

$$P + \frac{T \times N \times 4620 \, (k)}{C \times W}$$

FIGURE 8.8 Laplace's law.

practice. This section aims to break down the application of Laplace's law to encourage evidence-based effective practice.

P is the sub-bandage or interface pressure (as described earlier). However, it is important to appreciate that this pressure or dose can be affected by several factors and as a practitioner it is essential to recognise and understand these if we are to heal ulceration (Clark 2003) (see Table 8.11).

Pascal's Law

Pascal's law (sometimes referred to as Pascal's principle) is the principle of transmission of fluid through the application of pressure. It states that pressure exerted anywhere in a confined container that contains fluid will transmit the fluid equally in all directions throughout the confined container. This is an important principle when using compression therapy because compression therapy is creating a pressurised area to redistribute fluid (Schuren and Mohr 2010). This is of particular importance when we think about achieving graduated compression therapy, as we want to ensure we move fluid from the distal part of the lower limb towards the proximal. Therefore, if we also consider Laplace's law (described earlier), as the leg circumference naturally increases from ankle to thigh graduated compression therapy should be achieved, with the sub-bandage pressure decreasing from the distal aspect of the leg to the proximal, and therefore the fluid is transmitted in the right direction. A further consideration is the need to compress the foot. If adequate compression is not applied to the foot, then fluid will be transmitted from the leg distally towards the foot and toes, which risks causing harm to them.

ANTI-INFLAMMATORY ACTION OF COMPRESSION THERAPY

One of the lesser-known advantages of compression therapy is its action as an anti-inflammatory intervention (see Table 8.12) (Partsch and Mortimer 2015).

TABLE 8.11 Laplace's law explained.

		What does it mean?	Hints and tips	How pressure (dose) is affected
T	Tension	How tightly or loosely the compression therapy is applied can affect the amount of pressure (or dose) applied.	Tension is particularly important when applying a wrap or bandage. When applying a bandage, the practitioner should apply it with consistent pressure and stretch as they apply the bandage from the base of the toe towards the thigh (distal to proximal). This will create graduated compression therapy and move the fluid from the peripheral towards the central circulatory system. Some bandages are applied at 'full stretch', some at less, such as '50% stretch'. Ensure you understand the instructions for the system you are using.	Pressure exerted is directly proportional.
N	Number of layers applied	The number of layers applied will affect the pressure. The more layers the more pressure, therefore the higher the dose.	This is important for bandages as bandages applied in a spiral will create two layers, bandages applied in a figure of eight will create three layers. For other forms of compression such as compression hosiery stockings, this is important as practitioners can add layers of hosiery to achieve the required dose. In some systems such as inelastic bandages, additional layers can also create stiffness, which is useful when effectively encasing the limb.	
C	Circumference of the limb	The higher the circumference of the limb, the lower the pressure or dose of the compression.	A larger limb circumference will receive less pressure. This is particularly important when managing large oedematous limbs where the pressure will be reduced. Similarly, small thin limbs will be subject to higher levels of pressure.	Inversely proportional.
W	Width of the bandage	The narrower the bandage, the higher the pressure applied.		

Source: Adapted from Clark (2003) and Charles (2012).

TABLE 8.12 How compression reduces the inflammatory response in the lower limb.

Reduces inflammatory mediators such as matrix metalloproteinases and cytokines.
Reduces oedema/swelling, part of the unwanted inflammatory response.
Reverses venous hypertension.

Source: Adapted from Partsch and Mortimer (2015).

Wounds that are hard to heal have frequently become 'trapped' in the inflammatory phase of wound healing, leading from the normal sequence of phases in wound healing discussed earlier in the chapter to an extended period of inflammation, causing what is termed 'chronicity'. These wounds will benefit from the anti-inflammatory action of compression therapy. However, the anti-inflammatory effects of compression are important even before the occurrence of a wound. Symptoms such as venous skin changes and swelling can be attributed to the underlying inflammatory responses that are occurring in the lower limb due to venous hypertension raising enzymes such as matrix metalloproteinases and cytokines within the tissues. Thus, the symptoms of irritation that are visible on the skin's surface are due to underlying inflammation that can be reversed with compression therapy. Classic examples of these include venous eczema, oedema, lipodermatosclerosis, itching, aching and heaviness, all of which are signs of venous disease that can occur before the ulceration itself happens. These are listed in Table 8.13 and there is more about how to assess each of these signs in Chapter 5.

It is also important to recognise that wounds and legs that have become hard to heal often have higher than normal levels of colonisation by micro-organisms, which may manifest as biofilms, acute

TABLE 8.13 Signs of inflammation before ulceration may have occurred.

Aching and heaviness
Itching
Venous eczema
Oedema and swelling
Lipodermatosclerosis

---

infection or both. Micro-organisms thrive in environments where the wound has become overly wet, and excessive exudate is triggered in part by inflammation, so again, in combination with cleaning, debridement and the appropriate use of antimicrobial therapies (discussed later in this chapter), using compression to reverse the underlying inflammation and thus oedema is key. Importantly for the person with ulceration, reducing inflammation will also reduce their pain; it is this knowledge that can underpin confidence in commencing compression therapy.

CAUTIONS AND CONTRAINDICATIONS

Compression therapy is contraindicated, or should be used with caution, for some patients. Look back to Table 8.6 for an overview.

Presence of Peripheral Arterial Disease

Compression therapy in the presence of peripheral arterial disease can be further sub-divided into patients who have a mixed aetiology limb and patients who present with critical limb-threatening ischaemia; a significantly different approach to clinical management is required for each. As discussed in Chapter 5, the use of compression therapy is not wholly excluded in those who have arterial disease and it may be used with caution, applying a lower dose in those patients with a mixed aetiology of venous ulceration and presence of some arterial occlusions (Partsch and Mortimer 2015). However, in order to ensure arterial inflow is not reduced, compression pressure should never exceed the local arterial perfusion pressure. This is why we consider absolute values of the ankle pressure, in addition to the ankle brachial pressure index (ABPI). Therefore, a systolic ankle pressure of 50 mmHg or less is a strict contraindication against compression therapy (Partsch and Mortimer 2015) and compression should not be applied in those who have an absolute pressure of less than 60 mmHg due to the presence of significant peripheral arterial disease. For patients presenting with these values or if visual signs of critical ischaemia are observed, then an urgent referral to the local vascular service using local pathways is required without delay.

The decision to recommend a lower dose of compression therapy for patients who have mixed aetiology ulceration, or in the presence of some peripheral arterial disease, should only be undertaken by clinicians who possess knowledge and skills in this area of lower limb management (Ritchie and Taylor 2018). Thus for many clinicians, referral to a senior colleague or specialist is advised if arterial involvement is identified through the holistic clinical assessment.

Presence of Deep Vein Thrombosis

The approach to compression therapy in the presence of DVT can be sub-divided into those who are already wearing compression therapy and those who will require compression therapy due to the damage that occurs to the venous system as a result of the DVT, in order to prevent future lower limb problems. If patients diagnosed with DVT are not wearing compression, it is safe to apply compression once anti-coagulation treatment has been commenced. There is no evidence at present to suggest that risk of pulmonary embolism is increased as a result of appropriately applied compression therapy (British Lymphology Society 2021). If the patient is already wearing compression hosiery when a suspected DVT occurs, a same-day assessment and scan (within 24 hours) are required. Therefore, it is important to follow the local pathway to arrange referral for this. Compression therapy should be paused as soon DVT is suspected, and should be removed until the absence or presence of DVT is confirmed. When the diagnosis is confirmed and anticoagulant therapy has started, compression hosiery can be reapplied, but only if the person can tolerate it; during the acute stage it may be too painful to begin with and so consideration of analgesia is necessary. It is also necessary to ensure a full reassessment, as the DVT may cause volume changes to oedema in the limb, skin changes or possible breakdown of skin integrity (BLS 2021). For practitioners not familiar with compression therapy in the presence or suspected presence of a DVT, escalation to a senior or more experienced colleague for support to maintain patient safety is recommended.

Important Co-morbidities

Other co-morbidities that require a cautious approach to compression include patients who have chronic heart failure, renal impairment, diabetes and patients receiving end-of-life or palliative care. It is important to note that the application of compression therapy should not be ruled out, and a high number of patients with these conditions will certainly need compression therapy, but an awareness of how their other co-morbidities will affect their lower limb management is important to ensure effective clinical therapy.

Compression in Heart Failure

There is a reluctance to apply compression therapy for people who have a diagnosis of heart failure. This is understandable and requires exploration, as frequently the practitioner will be presented with a dichotomy of solutions and challenges in the face of this type of complexity. First, heart failure should be sub-divided into stable or unstable heart failure. Those whose health and condition are unstable require support from the MDT to manage the heart failure in the first instance. For those who have stable heart failure, challenges are also present, but carefully managed compression is advocated. Not to act and treat the person's leg ulceration, oedema or lymphorrhoea constitutes an omission in care. It is not safer or kinder to leave this person with unmanaged lower limb problems, and indeed this places them at risk of further deterioration in their ulceration, infections, sepsis and even death, so not acting is not an option. However, it is acknowledged that fear and lack of knowledge exist in this area at a standard level of practice. Therefore, it is suggested that patients who present with lower limb ill-health and stable heart failure are referred urgently to specialist services such as tissue viability, where measured but progressive compression in heart failure can be instigated and monitored as part of the MDT.

CONSIDERING AND COMMENCING TREATMENT

Once aetiology and an accurate diagnosis are established, and any contraindications or cautions explored, if compression therapy is indicated it is then important to select the correct mode of therapy, for example a particular bandage system or wrap from the selection of tools in the toolbox (see Table 8.1).

Compression Hosiery Kits

Compression hosiery kits, sometimes referred to as leg ulcer hosiery kits, are designed to deliver graduated compression therapy to support venous return. They should not be confused with single-layer hosiery stockings. Compression hosiery kits consist of two stockings, an understocking and an overstocking, which together should offer a dose of at least 40 mmHg at the ankle in people who present with an ankle circumference of 18–25 cm, as well as stiffness that is achieved through the combination of two layers that would not be achieved through a single stocking alone (Ritchie and Freeman 2018).

Different products and brands offer differences in dose for the understocking and overstocking, for example in some kits the understocking delivers approximately 20 mmHg and the overstocking 20 mmHg, totalling an overall dose of 40 mmHg; other brands offer an understocking of approximately 10 mmHg and an overstocking of 25–35 mmHg, again totalling 40 mmHg.

Compression hosiery kits can be considered as first-line treatment for venous leg ulcers that are not complex in nature, for example in people who have a small ulceration, who have a normal-shaped limb and are not experiencing high levels of exudate. People with high volumes of exudate, the presence of deep skin folds or distortion due to established oedema or a very oedematous limb should be excluded from treatment with compression hosiery kits. The advantages and limitations of compression hosiery kits are highlighted in Table 8.14.

Bandages

A variety of bandages are available. It is important to understand how these different bandage systems work and how the dose or pressure is achieved. Regardless of the type of bandage to be used, it is important first to measure the circumference of the ankle just above the malleolus. Within UK clinical practice boundaries regarding ankle circumference are advocated to inform how the practitioner should choose and apply a system, because ankle circumference is normally an indicator of overall leg size and this can affect the dose, as discussed earlier within the framework of Laplace's law. See Table 8.15 for further discussion on this. It is also important to note that very tall people, those >180 cm tall (Wounds UK 2022), frequently need higher levels of compression, and often so do people who have a particularly long limb length between the malleolus and the knee; this is due to the increased effects of gravity on the lower limb. This is not explored here, but be aware that if despite the

TABLE 8.14   Advantages of compression hosiery kits.

Health service outcomes	Person-centred benefits	Other considerations
Possible reduction in costs when used appropriately.	Can be used in self-care, shared care with the health professional and with carer or family support.	Compression hosiery kits are not suitable for all patients, as fragile skin can be damaged when putting them on or taking them off, and some people are unable to do this at all due to compromised flexibility or impaired dexterity. It is important to assess this aspect.
Clinical time can be reduced in terms of frequency of consultations and shorter appointments (Tickle 2015).	Kits may also be more acceptable, as they do not interfere with shoes or clothes, they are more discreet and this may make the treatment easier to tolerate.	More agile patients can remove compression hosiery kits, whereas a bandage is more telling if it has been adjusted or tampered with.
A consistent compression dose is given, which is not affected by practitioner skill or competence (Tickle 2015).	People may become accustomed to compression hosiery kits and may associate this with healing, thus they may be more willing to wear similar therapies in the long term such as hosiery to prevent reoccurrence.	Donning and doffing devices are available and prescribable via the NHS and so practitioners should always consider if these should be supplied in combination with compression hosiery kits.
Training in this type of therapy is less complex than for some other treatments.		

Source: Adapted from Ritchie and Freeman (2018).

TABLE 8.15 Ankle circumference.

Circumference	Size	Bandaging	Cautions	Advice
<18 cm	Regarded as a small ankle.	Bandage carefully and consistently.	Ensure a wadding layer is used to protect the bony prominences, but do not over-pad.	Think Laplace – remember the pressure is higher on a smaller limb circumference.
18–25 cm	Frequently viewed as a normal ankle.	Bandage consistently.	Ensure a wadding layer is used to protect the bony prominences.	
>25 cm	Recognised as a large ankle.	Consider additional layers and using a short stretch inelastic system, as it is most likely that oedema will be present.	Be careful not to over-use a wadding layer.	Think Laplace – remember the pressure will be lower on a larger limb circumference.

correct dose and application of compression a person is not healing and they are very tall or have a long lower leg, you should consider a referral to specialist services for more advanced techniques (Hopkins et al. 2017).

Once the ankle is measured and routine hygiene and skincare are completed (steps in effective skin care are discussed earlier in this chapter), the next step is to add in a simple protective layer under the wadding layer to protect the skin from irritation that can be caused by the wadding layer. This should be a knitted tubular stockinette (Figure 8.9), which should be applied from the base of the toe to just above where the bandage will stop. It is advisable to leave a few centimetres extra at each end so that this may be rolled back over the outside of the compression bandages once applied.

Next is the wadding layer. This is not a bandage and does not apply any compression or pressure. The purpose of the wadding layer is to protect bony prominences, which are subject to a higher interface pressure and are therefore more vulnerable to pressure that may cause discomfort. Beware of over-padding, as this will affect the efficiency of the compression bandages, as explained by Laplace's law. Normally one roll is enough, and in occasional circumstances two. See Figure 8.10 for the wadding layer and how it is applied effectively.

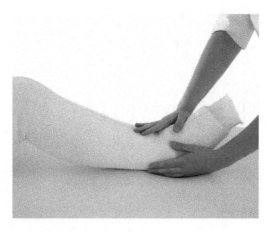

FIGURE 8.9 Tubular stockinette.
Source: Courtesy of L&R.

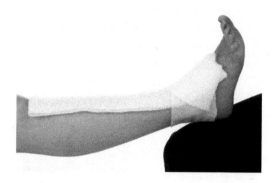

FIGURE 8.10 The wadding layer is applied to protect the bony prominences on the dorsum of the foot.
Source: Courtesy of L&R.

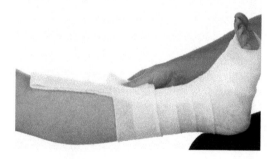

FIGURE 8.11 The wadding layer.
Source: Courtesy of L&R.

Next the wadding layer is applied in a spiral application, overlapping by approximately 50% on each turn around the leg (Figure 8.11).

Following the wadding layer, the compression bandages can be applied. Table 8.16 subdivides the different types of bandages and the variety of terminology used, which can lead to confusion for the novice practitioner. Names such as 'two-layer' and 'four-layer' are not advocated. Compression bandages fall within the type 2

TABLE 8.16 Different types of bandages.

Type	Explanation	Characteristics	Applicability
Type 2 bandages (Hopkins and Worboys 2005). Dose varies according to the variables highlighted in Laplace's law. It is estimated that in a standard limb circumference one layer should achieve 40 mmHg mercury pressure; in a larger ankle circumference a second layer is advised. Other factors may also affect the dose of the compression, for example the person's height, or if they have an occupation where they are standing all day (It is worthy of note that other types of non-compression bandages such as crepe bandages fall within the Type 2 bandage category within the British National Formulary).	Inelastic bandages, also known as short stretch bandages. 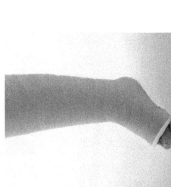 **FIGURE 8.12** Inelastic bandage. *Source:* Courtesy of L&R.	Have limited extensibility and are applied at full stretch. They have no elastomer fibres, but sculpt the limb like a supportive cast. Have low resting pressures and high working pressures. Support the calf muscle pump and lymphatic system in returning blood and lymphatic fluid. Occlude the veins intermittently with movement.	Can be used in the presence or absence of oedema. Can be used in mobile and immobile patients. Can be used for palliative bandaging and sports, but only if additional education in these fields has been undertaken.

The term 'two-layer' should be rejected because in very thin limbs only one layer may be used. Similarly, in advanced practice layering is applied in a specialist manner that does not sit within two-layer frame works. In standard care inelastic bandages are applied at full stretch in a spiral manner with a 50% overlap; in advanced practice this can vary.

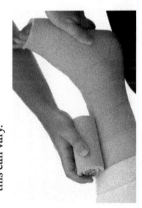

FIGURE 8.13 Applying an inelastic bandage.
Source: Courtesy of L&R.
Brand examples include Actico and Comprilan.

(Continued)

TABLE 8.16 (Continued)

Type	Explanation	Characteristics	Applicability
Type 3 compression bandages Type 3a 14–17 mmHg It is important to note that the dose varies according to Laplace's law. It is predicted that in a standard limb circumference the bandage should achieve 14–17 mmHg mercury pressure; in a larger ankle circumference a different bandage is advised (Hopkins and Worboys 2005).	Elastic bandage. Light compression bandage. Also known as long stretch. Terms such as three- and four-layer should be rejected. In standard care they are applied in a figure of eight at 50% stretch. Brand examples include K-Plus and Profore 3.	Have elastomer fibres making them easily extensible. Have less of a difference in resting and working pressures. Do not fully occlude the vein but cause narrowing. Elastic is always present, therefore pressure is always present.	Not advocated for the management of oedema. Can be used in mobile and immobile patients.
Type 3b 18–24 mmHg Dose varies according to Laplace's law. It is predicted that in a standard limb circumference the bandage should achieve 18–24 mmHg mercury pressure (Hopkins and Worboys 2005).	Elastic bandage. Moderate compression bandage. Also known as long stretch. Terms such as three- and four-layer should be rejected. In standard care they are applied in a spiral manner with a 50% overlap; in advanced practice this can vary. Brand examples include Ko-Flex and Profore 4.		
Type 3c (25–35 mmHg) and Type 3d (extra-high compression) bandages (Hopkins and Worboys 2005).	Elastic bandage. High compression bandage. Not advocated if oedema is present, switch to an inelastic bandage (Wounds UK 2022).		

For the multilayer system a combination of type 3 bandages is selected, dependent on ankle circumference.

and 3 bandage categories, therefore bandages outside of these categories are not discussed.

Adjustable Wrap Systems

Wraps consist of a liner underlayer that serves to protect the skin and an overlayer that is the wrap itself. This is made from a low elastic material section that wraps across and around the limb and is secured with hook and loop or Velcro® fasteners. They are designed for self-application or in partnership with the practitioner and are therefore well suited to self-care and shared care approaches. They are available in different sizes and thus education is necessary for the practitioner to ensure correct measurements. Wraps are available for different areas of the lower limb including foot, calf, knee and thigh pieces (Ritchie and Freeman 2018). There is also a variety of materials available for different uses. The Velcro wrap systems significantly reduce the limb circumference and improve the tissue density, which can be particularly helpful in challenging fibrosed tissues. A combination of wraps can be used to support the lower limb, for example foot and calf. Wraps can also be used in conjunction with other therapies, for example a compression bandage could be used to manage the gaiter ulceration and a knee wrap above may provide treatment for a swollen knee (Ritchie and Freeman 2018).

Whichever tool has been selected, it is important to monitor the effectiveness of the intervention to ensure that the patient heals. Table 8.17 details how to monitor if the therapy is working.

TABLE 8.17 Monitoring whether therapy is working.

Oedema	Wounds
An aim of treatment for swollen lower limbs should be a reduction in swelling leading to a normal limb size and shape.	Aim of treatment should be reduction in wound size leading to healing.
This can be monitored through observing for the presence of guttering (Hopkins and Worboys 2005).	This can be monitored through photography and measuring the wound (Wounds UK 2022).

LOCATION OF THE ULCERATION

The location of a wound frequently brings its own challenges for healing. Within the wider context of the body, wounds for example on the sacrum may be complex due to the risk of cross-contamination with body fluids. The scalp brings its own challenges due to a thin layer of dermis and hypodermis and the presence of hair. Leg ulceration is no different: a wound on the leg will often be harder to heal than a wound on the arm, purely due to the different effects of gravity on the arm compared to the leg. The exact location of the ulceration on the lower limb adds to this complexity. In particular wounds in the retro malleolar area can be difficult to heal. The reason is that for many patients the retro malleolar fossa is deep, and even when effective high compression therapy is applied a 'hammocking' effect can occur, where the ulceration sits deeper within the fossa and so receives little if any compression. In cases such as this more advanced techniques such as fan strapping may be required (Hopkins et al. 2011). These techniques go beyond standard practice and require additional training. If people are identified as not healing and they have ulceration in this area, then referral for bespoke or specialist intervention is needed.

COMPRESSION OF THE FOOT

A myth exists that the foot should not be compressed. This myth requires challenge and comparison if practitioners are fearful. The comparison is that the foot is compressed in leg ulcer hosiery kits, the foot is compressed in compression hosiery stockings, so why would we not compress the foot when using bandages as a therapy? Indeed, not encasing and protecting the foot leaves it vulnerable. Pascal's law assures us that if effective compression therapy is applied on a fluid (such as a muscle group) in a closed container (fascia muscularis and compression bandage), there is an equal increase at every other point in the container (leg) (Schuren and Mohr 2010). However, when the fluid is moved out of the area where compression is applied, there can be a risk to that tissue if not managed as the fluid is shunted there by the compression. This can be the foot, the toes or the knee, so these surrounding areas require protection through skilled compression. Compression to the foot also augments the foot muscle pump and can improve walking (see Chapter 4).

INTERMITTENT PNEUMATIC COMPRESSION

Intermittent pneumatic compression (IPC) is a mechanical device that can be used to aid in the healing of several types of ulcers, including venous leg ulcers (Nelson et al. 2014), and can help reduce oedema in patients with lymphoedema (Desai and Shao 2020). See Table 8.18 for the types of ulceration that an IPC device may be suitable for.

When applied to the lower limb or thigh (depending on which device is used), IPC comes with a sleeve or cuff that is attached to a motorised machine. The sleeve/cuff has cycles of inflation and deflation that vary in time depending on the device used. An IPC device comes in a variety of different cuffs/sleeves ranging from foot, below knee and up to the thigh. In recent years advances in IPC technology mean that the device can be applied to targeted areas of the body. This is an advantage for patients who have lower limb ulceration, as the device can be applied and used without squeezing over the site of pain and ulceration. For example, even if the venous leg ulcer is located on the lower leg below the knee, the application of the IPC device on the thigh is still therapeutic (Partsch et al. 2002).

IPC encourages circulation by decreasing venous stasis and improving arterial flow, improving microcirculation and lymphatic drainage and reducing the production of inflammatory mediators

TABLE 8.18 Types of ulceration for which intermittent pneumatic compression may be suitable.

Venous leg ulceration
Mixed aetiology leg ulceration
Arterial leg ulceration
Lower limb pressure ulceration
Diabetic foot ulceration
Lymphoedema
Pyoderma gangrenosum
Sickle cell disease induced ulceration

Source: Adapted from Young et al. (2021).

TABLE 8.19 Indications and contraindications for intermittent pneumatic compression (IPC) therapy.

Indications	Contraindications
As an adjunct therapy to the application of compression therapy	Signs of acute infection to the limb or sepsis symptoms
Painful wound(s)	Suspected deep vein thrombosis
Unable to tolerate optimal compression dose (note that IPC can be considered, but it is important to explore and address the reasons the therapy is difficult to tolerate and attempt to address this with the person)	Suspected or confirmed skin cancer
Hard-to-heal wounds	Renal failure
	Acute or chronic limb-threatening ischaemia

Source: Adapted from Young et al. (2021).

(Young et al. 2021). Naik et al. (2019) also highlight the biomechanical effects of IPC therapy, when the endothelial cells release antithrombotic, pro-fibrinolytic and vasodilatory properties that aid in the prevention of clot formation. See Table 8.19 for the indications and contraindications of IPC therapy.

IPC is an adjunct therapy to compression therapy. Optimal dose compression therapy should always be considered as the mainstay of treatment in lower limb ulceration. IPC can be used intermittently or for a set period of time as part of the overall treatment plan, not instead of compression therapy (Young et al. 2021).

WOUND BED PREPARATION AND CLINICAL MANAGEMENT

While compression is the key to managing most types of lower limb ulceration, it is also important that appropriate wound bed preparation and dressing selection are undertaken. Chapter 5 explained how to undertake a robust assessment using the TIMES framework. From this assessment three steps to wound bed preparation are advocated, which are explained in Table 8.20.

TABLE 8.20 Three steps to wound bed preparation.

Regular wound hygiene to include wound bed cleansing and debridement (Wounds UK 2022).	Identification of biofilm (IWII 2016) and challenge if present with mechanical debridement and application of a topical antimicrobial (Malone et al. 2017; Wounds UK 2020).	Application of an appropriate dressing.
Wash surrounding limb as discussed earlier in this chapter.	Key indicators of biofilm presence include:	Dressings do not heal wounds; the body heals wounds, given the right nutrition and hydration.
Cleanse the wound to ensure removal of debris, exudate or dressing remnants. This should include the wound bed and wound margins.	■ Recurrence of delayed healing on cessation of antimicrobial administration.	In the case of the lower limb, due to underlying pathophysiology and the effects of gravity, compression therapy is key to healing and should be the key focus, not the type of dressing.
Undertake mechanical debridement to physically remove any devitalised tissue.	■ Increased exudate levels.	Dressings should be selected for their ability to provide a contact layer between the leg and the compression tool being used, to support autolytic debridement, maintain moisture balance and manage exudate (see the earlier section of this chapter for more details on exudate management).
	■ Low-level chronic inflammation.	
	■ Low-level erythema.	
	■ Poor granulation tissue or friable tissue that bleeds easily.	
	■ Hypergranulation.	
	■ Wound breakdown and enlargement.	
	Challenge biofilm by undertaking mechanical debridement at least three times a week to disrupt the protective matrix covering the micro-organisms so that topical antimicrobial can penetrate to the micro-organisms.	
	Apply a topical antimicrobial for a maximum of two weeks, then review.	

CONCLUSION

This chapter has examined clinical management, employing a framework that will assess the person, assess the limb and assess the leg. The overarching aim is to create healing, but it is also important that other goals such as a personalised approach to care are adopted. Ensuring the person is left with as good a limb shape as possible is also a primary consideration, as of course is thinking ahead to the future and the prevention of ulcer reoccurrence caused by this long-term condition. Chapter 9 will examine the prevention of reoccurrence and the use of compression hosiery stockings.

REFERENCES

Adderley, U. (2008). Wound exudate: what is it and how to manage it. *Wound Essentials* 3: 8–13.

Annamaraju, P. and Baradhi, K.M. (2022). Pentoxifylline. In: *StatPearls*. Treasure Island, FL: StatPearls Publishing https://www.ncbi.nlm.nih.gov/books/NBK559096/.

Atkin, A. and Byrom, R. (2022). *The Links between Heart Failure and Leg Oedema: The Importance of Compression Therapy*. London: Wounds UK.

Babic, V., Petitpain, N., Guy, C. et al. (2018). Nicorandil-induced ulcerations: a 10-year observational study of all cases spontaneously reported to the French pharmacovigilance network. *International Wound Journal* 15: 508–518.

British Lymphology Society (BLS) (2021). British Lymphology Society position paper for the management of people with lymphoedema in the presence of deep vein thrombosis (DVT). https://www.thebls.com/documents-library/british-lymphology-society-position-paper-for-the-management-of-people-with-lymphoedema-in-the-presence-of-deep-vein-thrombosis-dvt

British National Formulary (BNF) (2023a). Nicorandil. Indications and dose. https://bnf.nice.org.uk/drugs/nicorandil

British National Formulary (BNF) (2023b). Hydroxycarbamide. Indications and dose https://bnf.nice.org.uk/drugs/hydroxycarbamide

British National Formulary (BNF) (2023c). Pentoxifylline. Indications and dose. https://bnf.nice.org.uk/drugs/pentoxifylline

Broadhead, R., Ritchie, G., and Livesay, J. (2018). The courage to compress. *Journal of Community Nursing* 32 (6): 8.

Charles, H. (2012). The function and composition of next generation bandages. *Wounds UK* 8 (1): s16–s19.

Clark, M. (2003). Compression bandages: principles and definitions. In: *Understanding Compression Therapy* (ed. S. Caine). EWMA position document. https://ewma.org/fileadmin/user_upload/EWMA.org/Position_documents_2002-2008/Compression.pdf.

Desai, S.S. and Shao, M. (2020). Superior clinical, quality of life, functional, and health economic outcomes with pneumatic compression therapy for lymphedema. *Annals of Vascular Surgery* 63: 298–306.

Farrelly, I. (2018). The adversarial relationship between wounds and biomechanics in the lower limb. *Wounds UK* 14 (5): 70–76.

Hassan, I., Dorjay, K., and Anwar, P. (2014). Pentoxifylline and its applications in dermatology. *Indian Dermatology Online Journal* 5 (4): 510–516.

Health Service Executive (Ireland) (2022). All-Ireland lymphoedema guidelines 2022. https://www2.healthservice.hse.ie/organisation/national-pppgs/all-ireland-lymphoedema-guidelines-2022

Hopkins, A. (2005). Leg ulcers: assessment and management plan. *Nursing in Practice* 25: 78–83.

Hopkins A (2020). Why are we still not getting compression 'dosage' right? *Wound Care Today* September. https://www.woundcare-today.com/journals/issue/wound-care-today/article/why-we-still-not-getting-compression-dosage-right

Hopkins, A. and Worboys, F. (2005). Understanding compression therapy to achieve tolerance. Wounds UK. https://wounds-uk.com/journal-articles/understanding-compression-therapy-to-achieve-tolerance-1

Hopkins, A., Worboys, F., Bull, R., and Farrelly, I. (2011). Compression strapping: the development of a novel compression technique to enhance compression therapy and healing for 'hard-to-heal' leg ulcers. *International Wound Journal* 8 (5): 474–483.

Hopkins, A., Bull, R. and Worboys, F. (2017). Needing more: the case for extra high compression for tall men in UK leg ulcer management. *Veins and Lymphatics* 6 (1). https://doi.org/10.4081/vl.2017.6630

Hughesden, C. (2021). The impact of early recognition, prompt referral and high levels of compression to achieve excellent venous ulcer healing rates within a community clinic at Accelerate CIC. Paper presented at the Society of Tissue Viability Conference.

International Wound Infection Institute (IWII) (2016). *Wound Infection in Clinical Practice*. London: Wounds International.

Keeley, V. (2018). Drugs that may exacerbate and those used to treat lymphoedema. *Journal of Lymphoedema* 3 (1): 57–65.

LeBlanc, K., Campbell, K.E., Wood, E., and Beeckman, D. (2018). Best practice recommendations for prevention and management of skin tears in aged skin: an overview. *Journal of Wound, Ostomy and Continence Nursing* 45 (6): 540–542.

Lloyd Jones, M. (2014). Exudate: friend or foe? *British Journal of Community Nursing* 19 (6): S18–S23.

Malone, M., Bjarnsholt, T., McBain, A.J. et al. (2017). The prevalence of biofilms in chronic wounds: a systematic review and meta-analysis of published data. *Journal of Wound Care* 26 (1): 20–25.

Moore, Z. and Strapp, H. (2015). Managing the problem of excess exudate. *British Journal of Nursing* 24 (15): S12–S17.

Mortimer, S. and Rockson, S.G. (2014). New developments in clinical aspects of lymphatic disease. *Journal of Clinical Investigation* 124 (3): 915–921.

Naik, G., Ivins, N.M., and Harding, K.G. (2019). A prospective pilot study of thigh-administered intermittent pneumatic compression in the management of hard-to-heal lower limb venous and mixed aetiology ulcers. *International Wound Journal* 16: 940–945.

National Institute for Health and Care Excellence (NICE) (2023). Clinical knowledge summaries: Leg ulcer venous. https://cks.nice.org.uk/topics/leg-ulcer-venous

Nelson, E.A., Hillman, A., and Thomas, K. (2014). Intermittent pneumatic compression for treating venous leg ulcers (review). *Cochrane Database Systematic Review* 2014 (5): CD001899.

Nuttall, R. and Rutt-Howard, J. (2020). *The Textbook of Non-medical Prescribing*. Chichester: Wiley Blackwell.

Nuutila, K. and Eriksson, E. (2021). Moist wound healing with commonly available dressings. *Advances in Wound Care* 10 (12): 685–698. https://doi.org/10.1089/wound.2020.1232.

National Wound Care Strategy Programme (NWCSP) (2023). Recommendations for Leg Ulcers. NWCSP-Leg-Ulcer-Recommendations-1.8.2023.pdf (nationalwoundcarestrategy.net).

Partsch, H. (2005). The static stiffness index: a simple method to assess the elastic property of compression material in vivo. *Dermatologic Surgery* 31 (6): 625–630.

Partsch, H. and Mortimer, P. (2015). Compression for leg wounds. *British Journal of Dermatology* 173: 359–369.

Partsch, B. and Partsch, H. (2005). Calf compression pressure required to achieve venous closure from supine to standing position. *Journal of Vascular Surgery* 42 (4): 734–738.

Partsch, H., Menzinger, G., Borst-Krafek, B. et al. (2002). Does thigh compression improve venous hemodynamics in chronic venous insufficiency? *Journal of Vascular Surgery* 36: 948–952.

Patel, G.K. and Harding, K.G. (2010). Nicorandil ulcer: moves beyond the mucosa. *Annals of the Royal College of Surgeons of England* 92 (6): 451–452.

Patton, L.R. (2009). Are community leg ulcer clinics more cost-effective than home care visits? *Journal of Wound Care* 18 (2): 49–50.

Penzer, R. (2012). A best practice statement for emollient therapy. *Dermatology Nurse* 11 (4): S1–S19.

Queen's Nursing Institute (QNI) (2019). *The View of District Nurse Team Leaders in the United Kingdom*. London: QNI.

Ritchie, G. (2018). Understanding compression: part 4 – bandaging and skin care. *Journal of Community Nursing* 32 (4): 20–28.

Ritchie, G. and Freeman, N. (2018). Understanding compression: part 3 – compression hosiery stockings and adjustable compression wraps. *Journal of Community Nursing* 32 (4): 20–28.

Ritchie, G. and Taylor, H. (2018). Understanding compression: part 2 – holistic assessment and clinical decision-making in leg ulcer management. *Journal of Community Nursing* 32 (3): 22–29.

Schuren, J. and Mohr, K. (2010). Pascal's law and the dynamics of compression therapy: a study on healthy volunteers. *International Angiology* 29 (5): 431–435.

Specialist Pharmacy Service (2020). Managing peripheral oedema caused by calcium channel blockers. https://www.sps.nhs.uk/articles/managing-peripheral-oedema-caused-by-calcium-channel-blockers

Starling, E.H. (1896). On the absorption of fluids from the connective tissue spaces. *Journal of Physiology* 19: 312–336.

Swain, D. (2014). Treating a rare foot ulcer caused by hydroxyurea. *Podiatry Today* October. https://www.hmpgloballearningnetwork.com/site/podiatry/treating-rare-foot-ulcer-caused-hydroxyurea

Tan, S.T. and Dosan, R. (2019). Lessons from epithelialization: the reason behind moist wound environment. *Open Dermatology Journal* 13: 34–40. https://doi.org/10.2174/1874372201913010034.

Tickle, J. (2015). Managing venous leg ulcers and oedema using compression hosiery. *Nursing Standard* 30 (8): 57–63.

Todd, M. (2014). Self-management of chronic oedema in community. *British Journal of Community Nursing* 19 (4): S30–S36.

Voegeli, D. (2008). The effect of washing and drying practices on skin barrier function. *Journal of Wound, Ostomy and Continence Nursing* 35 (1): 84–89.

Vowden, P., Kerr, A., and Mosti, G. (2020). *Demystifying Mild, Moderate and High Compression Systems – When and How to Introduce 'Lighter' Compression*. London: Wounds International.

World Union of Wound Healing Societies (WUWHS) (2008). *Principles of Best Practice: Compression in Venous Leg Ulcers: A Consensus Document*. London: MEP.

World Union of Wound Healing Societies (WUWHS) (2019). *Wound Exudate: Effective Assessment and Management: A Consensus Document*. London: MEP.

Wound Care People (2019). Chronic oedema: skin care and exercise. *Journal of Community Nursing*. 36 (5): 37–43.

Wounds International (2015). *Simplifying Venous Leg Ulcer Management. Consensus Recommendations*. London: Wounds International.

Wounds UK (2016). *Best Practice Statement, Management of Venous Leg Ulcers*. https://wounds-uk.com/category/best-practice-statements

Wounds UK (2020). Best practice statement: Antimicrobial stewardship strategies for wound management. https://wounds-uk.com/best-practice-statements/best-practice-statement-antimicrobial-steward ship-strategies-wound-management

Wounds UK (2021). Best practice statement: Compression hosiery: a patient-centred approach. https://wounds-uk.com/best-practice-statements/best-practice-statement-compression-hosiery-patient-centric-approach

Wounds UK (2022). Best practice statement: Holistic management of venous leg ulceration (second edition). https://wounds-uk.com/best-practice-statements/holistic-management-venous-leg-ulceration-second-edition

Young, T., Chadwick, P., Fletcher, J. et al. (2021). *The Benefits of Intermittent Pneumatic Compression and how to Use Wound Express™ in Practice*. London: Wounds UK.

CHAPTER 9

Lifelong Management

JANE HARRY

Lower limb wounds represent an important public health problem for people with ulceration, the health system and society in general. This leads to a heavy burden in terms of time and costs for health services, and it does not end once the ulcer is healed. Harding et al. (2015) estimated that 69% of patients with a venous leg ulcer have a recurrence within one year of healing (around 7/10 patients). The wound care burden was highlighted across the United Kingdom by the publication of the Guest data in 2015, which showed the significant burden that wounds pose on the NHS and how clinicians were failing to conduct holistic assessments of wounds. Guest et al. (2015) identified that only 16% of patients were having a full ankle brachial pressure index (ABPI) assessment and that wound care spend was the equivalent to 5% of the total NHS spend. A more recent study identified that only 15% of patients with a lower limb wound had an ABPI measurement documented on their records (Guest et al. 2020). In cases where patients do not have an ABPI obtained and recorded treatment and healing delays are likely to be seen, which in turn leads to increased costs for the NHS, a pull on clinical resources, and a greater burden and chronicity of these wounds (NHS England 2017).

With wound care in the six top spending categories for the NHS and leg ulceration spend being twice as much as any other type of wound, Guest et al. (2020) equated this to the highest spend within wound care and went on to highlight that this problem needs to be

Lower Limb and Leg Ulcer Assessment and Management, First Edition.
Edited by Aby Mitchell, Georgina Ritchie, and Alison Hopkins.
© 2024 John Wiley & Sons Ltd. Published 2024 by John Wiley & Sons Ltd.

addressed. The coronavirus pandemic has brought new issues in caring for patients generally, with long-term conditions and leg ulcer management a particular concern. Guest and Fuller (2023) further stated that healing rates of venous leg ulcers in 2020–2021 decreased by 16% and 42%, respectively, compared with 2019, and time to heal increased by >85%. The number of community-based face-to-face clinician visits decreased by >50% in both years and >35% fewer patients were referred to a specialist. Guest and Fuller (2023) also reported that in 2020 and 2021 up to 20% of patients were prescribed dressings without compression, compared to 5% in 2019. There was a significant trend towards decreasing wound care through the pandemic, which went outside the boundaries of good care. The pandemic also led to unprecedented challenges in delivering wound care and held back the national improvement work of the National Wound Care Strategy Programme (NWCSP) (Adderley 2020). At the same time, some barriers that once limited patients have been lifted through the use of supported self-care and telemedicine (Schofield 2021), but supported self-care is not an option for everyone.

Due to the nature of the underlying disease process, it is common for patients to go through a cyclical process of periods of being healed followed by periods of ulceration and tissue breakdown. The risk of this may increase as the patient ages and their co-morbidities worsen. However, this is an unnecessary cycle if practitioners prevent this reoccurrence through proactive lifelong management. To do this it is important to diagnose the underlying disease and identify the person's needs in terms of prevention of reoccurrence, which is supported by practitioners building sustainable relationships with the patient during diagnosis, treatment and post ulceration (Wounds UK 2022).

The risk of reoccurrence and the need to manage an increasing population of people requiring lifelong management will continue to increase as the general population ages: the number of people over 85 will increase from 1.7 million people (2.5% of the UK population) to 3.1 million people (4.3% of the UK population) by 2045 (Office for National Statistics 2022), further increasing the public health burden. Overall primary prevention and treating the underlying venous disease prior to any occurrence of leg ulceration will lead in the long term to a lower rate of leg ulceration and therefore a lower impact on people, the health service and the health economy (Wounds UK 2022).

It is a common misconception that people with venous leg ulcers cannot be healed. Myths need to be addressed and awareness raised within the nursing profession and the public. As healthcare professionals we have an opportunity to transform and change perspectives and shape leg ulcer care and well leg management in the future (Atkin et al. 2021). Once the ulcer is healed the maintenance stage should commence; this is just as important as the diagnosis and treatment phase. Education with people who have lower limb problems should start from the very first contact with them about how to manage their condition and equip them with the knowledge and tools of how to prevent further breakdown. Laying the foundations for supported self-care or fully independent self-care and management at the start is key to maintaining well legs in the future. People should be encouraged to see compression and well leg management as a lifelong commitment, and this is how we as practitioners and the wider healthcare community should see it also. Chapter 7 explores personalised care in more detail.

FACTORS INFLUENCING VENOUS ULCER RECURRENCE

There are many factors that can influence if a person's leg ulcer will recur and when. It is not just the person's medical conditions that influence this, but also their commitment and ability to maintain a well leg. In some cases recurrence is due to ceasing compression hosiery or not getting new hosiery when it is damaged, leading to insufficient levels of compression on the limb to reverse venous hypertension and support the veins leading to tissue breakdown. Other causes of recurrence could be new trauma to the limb; uncontrolled venous disease such as varicose eczema, leading to skin irritation; and patients with urinary incontinence, who may develop severe dermatitis leading to ulceration (Moffat et al. 2009). Practitioners may also bear responsibility here: evidence suggests that there are gaps in knowledge about compression hosiery (Heyer et al. 2017: Gong et al. 2020) within clinical practice, with a heavy reliance on off-the-shelf and British Standard hosiery due to a lack of knowledge about bespoke hosiery, which is necessary for many people who have had ulceration and/or chronic oedema and altered leg shape. Education for healthcare professionals is discussed in more detail later in this chapter. Healthcare professionals need to work together with patients to overcome recurrence, heal the ulcer again and educate the person in the self-care methods they can use to prevent further disease progression and recurrence of future ulcerations.

Recurrence in Patients with Peripheral Arterial Disease

Patients with an established arterial component to their ulceration should have a reassessment every three months, or more frequently if there are any changes in the patient's symptoms (such as new pain in the foot, arch or toes, or rapid deterioration of the ulcer), as this could indicate that the peripheral circulation is deteriorating and may require a change in the treatment regimen or onward specialist referral (Wounds UK 2015). Chapter 5 explores assessment of arterial factors in more detail.

Prevention of Recurrence in Patients with Healed Venous Ulceration

It is important to implement an agreed and ongoing self-management plan with the patient, including movement/exercise and a skincare regimen (Wounds UK 2022). People need to be supported in developing their knowledge so that they understand that prevention of breakdown of a healed ulceration is a lifelong commitment. Education with this group of people should start from the first contact when they present with ulceration to a healthcare professional and be revisited regularly during treatment.

When the venous leg ulcer is healed, it is important that the underlying problem that caused the wound to develop in the first instance is addressed – venous hypertension. In order to manage this, ongoing compression therapy is required to reduce the venous pressure and hypertension. Patients should be given an explanation of venous hypertension and understand the role of compression therapy in healing ulcers and then maintaining skin integrity; this helps to prevent recurrence of the venous leg ulceration and reduce the nursing workload (Wounds UK 2022). The National Institute for Health and Care Excellence (NICE 2021) states that patients should be offered the strongest compression that they can tolerate and apply.

To prevent recurrence, compression hosiery should be prescribed (following a holistic assessment including ABPI) British Standard hosiery if no oedema is present, or the European class hosiery if oedema is present. Consider a referral to vascular services to assess the need for venous intervention to reduce the risk of recurrence (NICE 2020; Wounds UK 2022).

The guidelines suggest that compression hosiery is the first option for the maintenance phase (NICE 2020), but there are other options:

- Compression hosiery kits, also known as leg ulcer hosiery kits, which have two layers of hosiery to achieve approximately 40 mmHg. These can also be used while the patient has active ulceration, and this is now suggested as first-line treatment where possible (Wounds UK 2022). The VenUS IV study (Ashby et al. 2014) found that patients who became used to wearing hosiery as an ulcer treatment would be more likely to wear it as a maintenance treatment after healing – appropriate ongoing compression therefore makes recurrence less likely.
- Adjustable compression wraps use Velcro® to make it easier for patients or their carers to apply compression themselves at home, once a trained practitioner has assessed and measured the limb, prescribed the most appropriate wrap, and given the patient/carer instruction in how to apply and wash it. Wraps can be used in either the intensive or maintenance stages of lymphoedema treatment. The advantage of a wrap is that after initial assessment and fitting by a qualified practitioner, the patient and/or their carer can be taught to apply them easily at home when a nurse cannot be present.
- Compression hosiery socks, stocking or tights, discussed later in this chapter.

Both adjustable compression wraps and leg ulcer hosiery kits are discussed in more detail in Chapter 8. Before the correct tool from our toolbox is chosen for treatment, it is first important to undertake a holistic assessment to ensure that effective maintenance hosiery is selected.

HOLISTIC REASSESSMENT INCLUDING ANKLE BRACHIAL PRESSURE INDEX

Reassessments should be carried out:

- For those who continue to have an ulceration.
- For those who have healed and are in maintenance compression therapy – well legs.

TABLE 9.1   Risk stratification for reassessment.

Annual	No cellulitis
	Limited or well-controlled co-morbidities
	Healed ulcer (no recurrence in 12 months)
	Stable oedema
	Able to tolerate treatment with no reported problems with hosiery
	Ankle brachial pressure index (ABPI) >0.9
6-monthly	History of lower leg infection, even if resolved
	Diagnosed with new disease/or new co-morbidities
	History of recurrent lower limb problems
	Multiple morbidities
3-monthly	History of difficulty in tolerating treatment
	Repeated poor fit
	Increasing or unmanaged oedema
	Skin breakdown/ulceration
	Rapidly changing medical condition (for example, the person is having palliative or end-of-life care)

N.B. Expedite a new assessment if there is increased oedema, lower leg pain or new ulceration.
Source: Adapted from Wounds UK (2015).

Assessments should take place as follows:

- Reassessments should take place 3-, 6- or 12-monthly depending on the risk factors for this individual patient (Wounds UK 2015) (see Table 9.1).
- Patients who have active ulceration should be assessed on a four-weekly basis as a minimum to see if their symptoms/wounds are improving with the current care plan and if this remains appropriate (Wounds UK 2022).
- If the leg ulcer has not healed after 12 weeks (Wounds UK 2022), onward referral should be made to rule out another underlying cause. All elements of the holistic assessment for leg ulceration should be revisited at reassessment: history taking, medication review, limb assessment, pain assessment and ABPI. Also, patients should be asked if they have experienced any problems since the last assessment, including with their hosiery.

See Chapter 5 for a more detailed discussion on assessment for acute ulceration.

Reassessment of the person, including ABPI assessment, should occur for the rest of the person's life; leg ulcer prevention is lifelong and the schedule for this is based on the wound history and patient's level of cardiovascular risk (Wounds UK 2022). Both legs should be assessed for lower limb oedema/swelling and haemosiderin skin staining in all at-risk patients (Wounds UK 2022). If a patient has been diagnosed with a venous leg ulcer in one leg that has healed, it is highly likely that the venous disease affects both legs – therefore both legs should be assessed and should receive compression therapy (Wounds UK 2022).

To achieve good adherence to maintenance therapy, people need an informed discussion with the practitioner about the implications of compression hosiery for clothing, footwear, the likely restrictions on travel and exercise, how to manage personal hygiene, skin care and how to take care of the garments. Patients need to understand that although bandages or a wrap may be required in the short term only for intensive therapy, hosiery (or wraps) will be required to maintain the good condition of the limb and prevent recurrence for a long period into the future. A clear plan for maintenance therapy should be agreed between the practitioner and the patient. The plan needs to consider the patient's aims for treatment, their life commitments and their ability to adhere to compression therapy, and the use of suitable footwear and clothing that will enable them to have an appropriate gait for optimal freedom and safety of movement.

Patients should also be supported to develop knowledge so that they are able to be vigilant for any signs that they may need an assessment earlier than scheduled and that they have contact details for the healthcare professional or service who would undertake the assessment (Wounds UK 2022).

ENDOVENOUS ABLATION

All patients with venous insufficiency should be considered for endovenous surgery, as outlined in Box 9.1.

COMPRESSION THERAPY SYSTEMS

Compression is often a lifelong treatment for many individuals who have a venous leg ulcer even after it has healed (Wounds UK 2022). The prescription of compression hosiery is advised to prevent leg

Box 9.1   Endovenous Ablation

Endovenous ablation should be considered for all patients with venous insufficiency with referral to vascular services to assess need for venous intervention and to reduce the risk of recurrence (NICE 2021; Wounds UK 2022).

- Endovenous ablation seals off or 'ablates' the main underlying faulty vein that is feeding the varicosities. This is done either by heat, laser or glue.
- It has the same benefits in terms of vein function compared to traditional surgery, but is less invasive.
- The procedure is done as a day case, under a local anaesthetic, and is viewed as a minimally invasive procedure.
- It should be considered for all patients with venous insufficiency to reduce the risk of ulceration.

Is compression therapy required after surgery?

- Successful endovenous ablation can eliminate the need for long-term compression in patients with purely venous hypertension (i.e. structural venous disease).
- If there is some functional disease (e.g. failure of the calf muscle pump), compression may need to continue with specialist assessment.

Source: Adapted from Wounds UK 2022; NICE 2021.

recurrence after healing and referral to vascular services for venous intervention has been considered (NICE 2021) (see Table 9.2).

Hosiery should be remeasured and replaced according to manufacturer's guidelines, usually every three to six months, three months for British Standard and six months for European Standard (Wounds UK 2021).

The purpose of using compression therapy after ulcer healing is to control lymphoedema/chronic oedema and reduce venous hypertension to prevent further ulceration (Wounds UK 2022). The aim of the compression therapy is also to slow venous disease progression.

TABLE 9.2 Lifelong compression.

Who may require lifelong compression?	Individuals with venous disease where vascular or surgical correction is not possible.
	Individuals with chronic oedema/lymphoedema where the underlying condition has not been corrected (e.g. a valve replacement for heart failure, or someone who has undergone a gastric bypass and now has a healthy body mass index).
Who may not require lifelong compression?	People with a healed traumatic wound with no signs of venous disease. If it is the individual's first episode of a traumatic wound, lifelong compression is not required at this stage.
	Individuals who have had successful endovenous ablation with purely venous hypertension (i.e. structural venous disease).

Source: Adapted from Wounds UK (2022).

Compression therapy has a therapeutic effect by applying external pressure to the lower limb, which supports the superficial veins and counteracts raised capillary pressure. It encourages the lymphatic system to reduce oedema and the venous system to return blood from the limb towards the central circulation (Ritchie and Warwick 2018).

In a healthy leg the valves and the calf muscle pump work in conjunction to ensure that the blood does not slip back down to the foot causing stagnation of the blood in the tissues. Patients who have damaged valves and immobility are at greater risk of the veins coming under pressure and the valves becoming incompetent.

More discussion on how compression therapy works as part of effective clinical management can be found in Chapter 8.

ASSESSING FOR COMPRESSION HOSIERY

Medical hosiery should be selected based on the outcomes of a full holistic assessment, patient preferences and after planning of clear goals and aims of treatment with review dates. People who become familiar with wearing leg ulcer compression hosiery kits to heal their leg ulcers have been found to have a greater willingness to wear compression hosiery to maintain their skin integrity and have a lower recurrence rate in the future (NICE 2020). This may be attributed to them seeing the hosiery help to heal the leg ulceration, building faith in the treatment, and because they may have been able to incorporate compression hosiery wearing into their everyday life successfully (Ashby et al. 2014). Practitioners should consider transition from bandages to leg ulcer hosiery as soon as it is clinically indicated to allow people to take the next steps in recovery and transition to step-down interventions. (These are discussed in more detail in Chapter 8.)

Table 9.3 offers some key steps to consider when assessing for compression hosiery.

TABLE 9.3   Key steps to consider when assessing for compression hosiery.

Step	Approach
Listen and explore	Explore the patient's understanding, concerns and hopes related to medical compression hosiery.
	What do they understand about their current condition and how compression can help?
	Do they require education to help them to understand how the therapy will work?
	Acknowledge the physical and psychological issues that come along with living with a lifelong condition of venous hypertension.
Assess	Assess the limb and the patient to determine the most appropriate medical compression hosiery clinically.
	Involve the patient in choosing the hosiery – they will be more likely to wear it.
	Include a full holistic assessment and ankle brachial pressure index (ABPI).
	You may need to pay particular attention to the limb shape; if there is an unusual limb shape or swelling, bespoke hosiery is required.
	Is there a large amount of swelling, lymphorrhoea or skin fragility? If so, consider other options first to manage the limb and reduce the oedema prior to application of hosiery. Seek specialist help if needed.

TABLE 9.3 (Continued)

Step	Approach
Consider patient's ability	Consider the patient's ability to apply the compression hosiery, for example their manual dexterity and their body size and shape.
	Are they able to put the hosiery on themselves?
	Will they need an aid (see later Table 9.9) to assist or help?
	Might they require a family member or carer to apply the hosiery? Do they have this support available to them?
	What information do the patient and the carer need to receive to enable them to decide?
Check fit	Check how the medical compression hosiery fits on the leg(s), around the ankle(s) and the feet to ensure there is an effective fit that is not too loose or too tight.
	Check that the hosiery is smooth on the leg and not wrinkled or digging in or rolling down.
	Watch the patient apply the hosiery to ensure that it is fitting correctly. This may take several appointments to get them applying the hosiery correctly. Make sure the patient knows to come back if the hosiery gets holes in it or ladders.
	Advise the patient how to care for their hosiery – washing and care instructions.
Patient preference	Ask the patient if they are happy with the appearance and fit of the medical compression hosiery.
	If they are comfortable with the aesthetics of the hosiery, they are more likely to wear the garment. Ask them what would make them more likely to wear the hosiery?

Source: Adapted from Wounds UK (2021).

CHOOSING AND PRESCRIBING HOSIERY

There has been a vast evolution of hosiery over the last few years and there are now more choices than ever before. While this means increasing choice for people who need to wear compression hosiery garments, this may also lead to confusion for practitioners with multiple brands, measurements required and measurement forms to choose from. Garments should be prescribed by an appropriate practitioner (Health Service Executive (Ireland) 2022). The practitioner who measures and prescribes compression hosiery must have sound knowledge of how to measure and select the correct compression hosiery garments to ensure effective treatment.

Inconsistencies have been observed in the prescribing and provision of compression garments (Health Service Executive (Ireland) 2022). In part this may be owing to the large variety of products available. Practitioners need to undertake careful assessment and choose the most appropriate treatment option.

All decisions and prescriptions need to be fully documented, including in the patient's notes, along with limb measurements and the type of garment selected, its size and class. During prescribing and dispensing, it is important to refer to the manufacturer's recommendations and measurements to ensure that the most appropriate garment is chosen. The manufacturer's ordering instructions should be consulted to ensure the person receives the correct product. The brand name, garment style and compression class, as well as the manufacturer's codes for the garment and its style, should be recorded on the prescription (Wound Care People 2019). As there is a large variety of products available, practitioners may prefer to prescribe from a smaller range of hosiery from the local formulary initially, in order to gain experience of appropriate use, therapeutic performance and acceptability to people.

British and European Standards

Differences exist between British, French and German hosiery, as explained in Table 9.4.

Each of these standards has its own testing methods and all use laboratory testing. This enables them to repeat the test with validity and give measured results when testing new products for design, build and then classification.

Differences Between Flat-Knit and Circular-Knit Hosiery

Circular-Knit Garments

The fabric for this type of garment is knitted on a cylinder with circular needles. The way they are made means there is no seam to the

TABLE 9.4 Difference between British, French and German Standard hosiery classes.

Compression class	British Standard 40 (BS-661210), 3-month guarantee (Partsch 2003)	French Standard (AFNOR NF 30.102A) (Levick 2003)	German Standard (RAL GZ 387/1), 6-month guarantee (Földi and Földi 1983)
Class 1 – Mild compression	14–17 mmHg	10–15 mmHg	18–21 mmHg
Class 2 – Moderate compression	18–24 mmHg	15–20 mmHg	23–32 mmHg
Class 3 – Strong compression	25–35 mmHg	20–36 mmHg	34–46 mmHg
Class 4 – Extra-strong compression	Not available	>36 mmHg	>49 mmHg

Source: Adapted from Wounds UK (2021).

garment. Many patients prefer them as they are more cosmetically acceptable and there is a great choice in colour, finish and styles.

These types of garments are used for ready-to-wear hosiery, which is best suited to patients where there is no oedema present and minimal limb distortion (Anderson and Smith 2014), it predominantly acts on the veins to promote venous return rather than on tissue pressure that will address oedema. Circular-knit hosiery is elastic and so inappropriate for managing moderate or severe lymphoedema/chronic oedema, in the presence of limb distortion or if there is a risk of rebound oedema. The circular knit makes the stocking liable to expand in response to increasing swelling of the limb. It may also cause damage to the limb by the hosiery rolling or digging into the flesh, forming a tourniquet that can result in skin breakdown and trauma (Wound Care People 2019).

Flat-Knit Garments

The fabric for these garments is knitted flat on a machine and then the edges are sewn together and inlaid with a thicker yarn, creating a seam. Flat-knit hosiery primarily works to increase tissue pressure, which manages swelling and oedema within the limb, but has a secondary function on the veins to support venous return. With these types of garments the fabric is relatively thick and stiff, meaning that it lies across skin folds without cutting into the skin. This construction creates a semi-rigid fabric that resists the swelling of the limb and is particularly suitable for those with chronic oedema. Its reduced elasticity and stretch support the limb, applying pressure to the lymphatics. This provides a micro-massage effect and is less likely to move on the limb or into deep skin folds.

This type of garment is usually used for made-to-measure garments because it can be easily adapted to an altered limb shape (International Lymphoedema Framework 2006; Wounds UK 2021).

Choosing the Most Effective Treatment

Overall, an understanding of the materials used in a given compression garment and the accessories available to improve the therapeutic effect of garments helps inform clinical decisions about the optimal garment to choose for the most effective treatment for the patient's presentation of lymphoedema/chronic oedema.

One consideration is stiffness, which is defined as the pressure increase produced by the compression hosiery per 1 cm of increase in leg circumference. It is the ability of the bandage/hosiery garment to oppose the muscle expansion during contraction (Mosti 2012). This therefore affects the levels of compression exerted by different types and classes of hosiery. Circular-knit garments are said to have a lower static stiffness index, with flat knits having a higher static stiffness index (Wounds UK 2021). There is more information about stiffness and the static stiffness index in Chapter 8.

Table 9.5 offers suggestions for medical compression hosiery and additional treatments for venous insufficiency and oedema, based on the CEAP classification (see Chapter 5).

Limb Size and Shape

Every effort should be made to reduce the oedema of the limb prior to measurement and application of compression hosiery.

If the limb shape is altered or unusual, then off-the-shelf hosiery is not an option, but there is the option of made-to-measure hosiery and wraps these can be complicated to measure for the practitioner must understand and have the skills for this. It is important for the practitioner to have knowledge of the hosiery garments that are

TABLE 9.5 Treatments for venous insufficiency and oedema.

	Clinical indications	Medical compression hosiery suggestion	Additional treatment suggestions
Venous insufficiency CEAP classification (Lurie et al. 2020)	C0 No visible signs or palpable signs of venous disease C1 Telangiectasis or reticular veins	No treatment required	No treatment required
	C2 Varicose veins C2r Recurrent varicose veins C3 Oedema	Circular-knit, off-the-shelf, RAL standard compression CC1 (18–21 mmHg) or CC2 (23–25 mmHg) may be appropriate For patients who do not fit in standard sizes, made-to-measure, circular-knit, RAL standard options should be considered. If there is significant shape distortion, flat-knit, made-to-measure hosiery in CC1–3 should be considered.	Daily skincare and emollient regimen to maintain skin integrity. Simple ankle/calf exercises to enhance calf muscle pump function. Increase activities/mobility, such as short walks or water exercises (e.g. walking in shoulder-high water, aqua-aerobics or aqua cycling, but not swimming). A GP referral scheme may be available in some areas. Limb elevation on resting. Weight loss/maintenance (referral to dietician or bariatric services). If oedema is venous related and is persistent or worsening, patients should be seen by a vascular specialist to explore venous interventions to aid symptoms (NICE 2021).
	C4 Changes in skin and subcutaneous tissue secondary to CVD C4a Pigmentation or eczema C4b Lipodermatosclorosis or atrophie blanche C4c Corona phlebectatica C5 Healed ulcer	Circular-knit, off-the-shelf, RAL standard compression CC2 (23–25 mmHg) may be the most appropriate. For patient not fitting into standard sizes, circular-knit, made-to-measure, RAL standard hosiery should be considered.	
	C6 Active venous ulcer C6r Recurrent active venous ulcer	Two-layer compression hosiery kit or compression bandaging providing a combined 40 mmHg should be used.	

(Continued)

TABLE 9.5 (Continued)

	Clinical indications	Medical compression hosiery suggestion	Additional treatment suggestions
Oedema classification (International) Society of Lymphology) 2016)	Chronic oedema/lymphoedema stage 0–2 (latency mild or moderate)	Circular-knit, off-the-shelf, RAL standard compression may be suitable in the early stages. Flat-knit, made-to-measure, RAL standard hosiery should be considered in most cases. CC1–4 may be most appropriate according to the holistic assessment of the individual and their circumstances.	Daily skincare and emollient regimen to maintain skin integrity. Simple ankle/calf exercises. Avoid sitting with legs dependent or sleeping in a chair at night-time; this may undermine all compression treatment/management. Increase activities/mobility, such as short walks or water exercises (e.g. walking in shoulder-high water, aqua-aerobics or aqua cycling, but not swimming). A GP referral scheme may be available in some areas. Limb elevation on resting. Consider simple/manual lymphatic drainage.
	Chronic oedema/lymphoedema Stage 3	Flat-knit, made-to-measure, RAL standard compression hosiery with high SSI is often most suitable. CC3 (35–45 mmHg) or CC4 (>49 mmHg) may be most appropriate, however CC2 (25–35 mmHg) may be considered according to the holistic assessment of the individual and their circumstances.	As for chronic oedema/lymphoedema stage 0–2. Weight loss/maintenance (referral to dietician/bariatric services).

CC, compression class; CVD, cardiovascular disease; SSI, static stiffness index.
Source: Adapted from Wounds UK (2021).

available on their trust's formulary, and those that are best suited to the individual, as not all garments will be available to them. The practitioner also needs to know where to refer patients on when specialist advice is needed in choosing and measuring a patient for compression hosiery.

Compression therapy is only effective if the patient's limbs are measured properly and the garment is applied correctly. Inappropriately measured and applied compression can cause trauma and pressure and damage the skin, particularly if the garment rolls during wear or is too tight and digs into the skin (Robertson et al. 2014). Experiences like these can lead to patients not wanting to continue with treatment.

Made-to-Measure Hosiery

This should be considered when:

- The limb does not fit within the measurement guide.
- The limb is an unusual shape.
- The measurement around the malleolus is particularly wide.
- Flat knit is required for the management of lymphoedema and chronic oedema.

The clinician may also need to consider other types of materials for garments to be made from, for instance in the case of allergy to latex the patient may need cotton-rich garments (Wounds UK 2021).

These garments require a greater number of measurements to be taken to ensure they fit the patient correctly. It is possible for some styles of these garments to have zips up the back that can aid in application, but care must be taken not to cause trauma to the skin and the patient's dexterity needs to be considered. Each manufacturer will have a different type of measurement form and measurements that are required.

Measuring people's legs for bespoke hosiery can be difficult to begin with and so seeking support to develop your practice or accessing extra training to be able to measure and fit for made-to-measure garments may be recommended, but once you have achieved competence they are a vital tool in the tool kit when transitioning people who have established oedema from bandages to hosiery.

Off-the-Shelf Hosiery

This type of hosiery is simpler in terms of the amount of measurements required, but it remains vital that correct measurements are taken to ensure the person receives effective and tolerable maintenance therapy. Again the practitioner must ensure fit of the hosiery and that the patient can don and doff the hosiery correctly.

Measurement

Whether using off-the-shelf or made-to-measure garments, once the type of product has been selected, accurate measurement of the limb needs to take place and be documented correctly to ensure that the garment will fit properly and provide therapeutic levels of compression. The practitioner needs to ensure that they have the correct measurement chart for the garments and manufacturer and as the points of measurement vary by manufacturer, the practitioner needs to be confident in the measurement of limbs to prescribe the correct garment. The measurement should be entered into the patient record for reference and another copy be kept with the order/prescription for the garment. Measurement should ideally be taken in the morning, immediately after removal of compression bandaging, or after a period of limb elevation to ensure optimum fit (Wounds UK 2021).

Tips for hosiery measurement include the following (Wounds UK 2021):

- Take measurements as early in the morning as possible when oedema is at a minimum.
- Take measurements directly against the skin to ensure accuracy (use a skin marker to ensure reproducibility and accuracy).
- Take measurements for both legs, as they may differ.
- Take measurements when the patient is sitting down, with their feet flat on the floor.
- Use the correct and current measuring guide for the brand of hosiery to be prescribed, as each manufacturer will differ.
- If the patient has skin folds due to oedema, or the limb is particularly misshapen, a specialist flat-knit garment and therefore referral for specialist assessment may be required for limb reduction prior to the application of a compression garment.

TABLE 9.6   Location for leg measurement for leg compression hosiery.

Measuring site	Hosiery type	
	Below knee	Thigh length
Top of thigh		Y
Thickest part of the calf	Y	Y
Narrowest part of the leg above the ankle	Y	Y
Length from heel base to top of calf	Y	Y
Foot length from toe to heel (if closed toe)	Y	Y

- If the patient feels uncomfortable or embarrassed when having their legs measured, try to make them feel at ease by:
  - Taking the measurements in a private area.
  - Explaining how you are going to measure their legs before you start, including how far up the leg you will need to measure for thigh-length hosiery and answer any questions the patient may have.
  - Explain why it is important to get the right size of hosiery so that it works properly.
  - Explain to the patient what you are doing at each stage.

Across different brands of made-to-measure and off-the-shelf garments different measurements are needed and thus it may be necessary for practitioners to access products available on their local wound care formularies. Table 9.6 offers a broad overview of some of the measurements required and Figure 9.1 illustrates the sites for measurement.

OTHER CONSIDERATIONS WHEN CHOOSING A COMPRESSION THERAPY SYSTEM

When assessing the patient during the limb assessment, the whole leg should be examined, not just the lower limb, for oedema in knee and thigh. Examination of the whole limb is recommended as varicose veins in the thigh will give an indication of the length of hosiery that will be required.

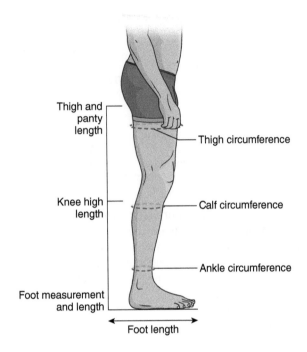

FIGURE 9.1   Sites to measure limb circumference for compression hosiery.

Thigh Length or Knee Length?

Compression therapy is likely to be lifelong so the patient's tolerance of the garment is important. The choice of length of hosiery should be based on patient choice, but also on the clinical presentation of the limb.

Below-knee compression hosiery is recommended:

- To prevent reoccurrence of venous leg ulceration in patients where leg ulceration healing has been achieved.
- When the swelling is limited to the lower leg, or if use of thigh length is not possible or desirable.

Consider thigh-length hosiery in people with severe varicose veins above the knee or who have swelling that extends above the knee (NICE 2022).

Open or Closed Toe?

There are a few other considerations to consider when deciding whether a patient should have open- or closed-toe garments. The healthcare practitioner should be able to guide the patient in making this decision. Assessment of the patient's gait should also be considered to ensure patients are picking up their feet correctly, as if this is not being done it can push the hosiery up the foot, which can lead to tissue damage or oedema in the toes or dorsum of the foot.

People may require open-toed garments for several reasons:

- The patient has arthritic or clawed toes.
- The patient has a fungal infection or is prone to fungal infections of the toes and interdigital spaces such as athlete's foot/tinea pedis.
- The patient prefers to wear a sock over the hosiery.
- The patient has a long foot compared to the size of the calf (some garments do have a longer foot option).
- The patient requires regular podiatry/chiropodist appointments.
- There is no oedema present in the toes and the patient prefers open-toed hosiery (NICE 2021).

Contraindications for Stockings, Garments and Hosiery

Compression stockings/garments and hosiery should *not* be offered to patients who have any of the following red-flag symptoms (NICE 2022; Wounds UK 2021; National Wound Care Strategy 2020):

- Symptoms of sepsis.
- Acute or chronic limb-threatening ischaemia.
- Suspected or proven peripheral arterial disease.
- Peripheral arterial bypass grafting.
- Peripheral neuropathy or other causes of sensory impairment.
- Any local conditions in which compression stockings may cause damage (for example fragile skin, dermatitis, gangrene or recent skin graft).
- Known allergy to the material of the stockings/hosiery.
- Severe leg oedema.
- Major limb deformity or unusual leg size or shape preventing correct fit.
- Acute infection of the leg or foot (increasing unilateral redness, swelling, pain, pus, heat).

■ Suspected acute deep vein thrombosis.
■ Suspected skin cancer.

Onward referral to the vascular team, dermatology or a tissue viability nurse should be considered for these patients.

Fitting and Care of Hosiery

Once the measurements have been taken and the hosiery garment ordered, the healthcare professional should ensure that the garment is well fitting on the first application. The patient should have a further appointment for an application and fitting check. This may take time and the patient should be given the opportunity to practise this new skill until they are confident in donning and doffing the hosiery. Patients should not be given a prescription under the assumption that they can check and ensure correct fitting of the garment unless they have had the same hosiery previously and the healthcare professional is confident in the patient's application technique.

Table 9.7 is a guide to good fit, which could be given to patients as an aide mémoire.

Patients need to understand how to care for their hosiery to ensure that it has the maximum life expectancy for the garment and should be given hints and tips and shown how to apply the hosiery correctly. The healthcare professional should support the patient

TABLE 9.7   Quick guide for good medical compression hosiery fit.

Hosiery should fit well and not feel too loose.
Hosiery should not be twisted, rolled, creased or folded down.
Hosiery should sit two fingers' width below the knee crease, or four fingers' width below the gluteal fold in thigh-length garments.
The fabric should be evenly distributed over the length of the garment.
Hosiery should not pinch the skin or cause pain.
If numbness or pain occurs while wearing medical compression, the hosiery should be removed and reported to the clinician who prescribed it for review.
The patient should be given the information to remove the hosiery and seek advice from there healthcare professional.
Hosiery should not cause shortness of breath. If this occurs, remove the compression and seek medical review of the patient.

Source: Adapted from Wounds UK (2021).

until they are confident in the application and removal of their hosiery garment independently. Information should also be provided in written form so that the patient can refer to it if needed (see Table 9.8 for a suggested check list).

The healthcare practitioner should prescribe at least two pairs of hosiery (one for wearing and one for washing) and ideally provision

TABLE 9.8 Dos and don'ts of compression hosiery.

Do ✓	Don't ✗
Take care when donning and removing hosiery over areas of hard skin that can damage the garment or while wearing jewellery. Ensure that the hosiery is smooth and free of creases. Wearing gloves can help. Hosiery should be fitted well and not loose. Hosiery should sit two fingers below the back of the knee or four fingers below the thigh (gluteal fold). Hosiery should be evenly distributed along the limb with no gathered areas.	Do not roll, twist or fold down compression stockings during wear, it hampers circulation and increases the risk of a blood clot and cause damage to the skin.
Ensure legs are dry before putting on hosiery, to protect the skin and garment integrity. If the skin is fully intact and in good condition, consider patting the legs dry to absorb excess moisture prior to application of the hosiery.	Avoid applying emollients (e.g. lotions or creams) just before application of hosiery, as it could make the garment harder to put on, allow the emollient to be absorbed prior to application.
Speak to the GP, nurse or a pharmacist or other relevant specialist if compression hosiery is not fitting well, has laddered or has holes in it.	Do not cut holes into the elastic or hold-up bands of the compression hosiery, these can cause them not to work as efficiently.
Follow the manufacturer's instructions for washing and care of hosiery. Note: some garments can go in a normal machine wash cycle at lower temperatures, although the label may say hand wash.	Do not cut the feet off the hosiery – discuss options with the GP, nurse or pharmacist or other relevant specialist.

(Continued)

TABLE 9.8 (Continued)

Do ✓	Don't ✗
Air-dry hosiery to maintain elasticity unless stated otherwise. Check manufactures guidelines.	Do not wear compression stockings while sleeping unless specifically advised otherwise by a healthcare professional. Hosiery should be re-applied when walking or straight after a shower.
If applying or removing compression hosiery is too difficult, speak to the GP, nurse, pharmacist or healthcare professional about being prescribed a new application aid. See table 9.10. Patient many also benefit from a further fitting appointment to gain tips of application with or without an aid.	Do not wear larger-sized compression hosiery without speaking to the GP, nurse, pharmacist or other relevant specialist about alternate options.
If there is new numbness to the toes, remove the hosiery and inform the GP or practitioner who fitted the hosiery as soon as possible. Hosiery should not cause shortness of breath if it does removed immediately and seek immediate help.	Do not buy extra pairs of compression hosiery off prescription unless you have been advised to do so by the relevant practitioner.
Important: See the GP immediately if the leg suddenly swells, there is redness or warmth of the skin, new numbness or tingling in the toes, fatigue in the leg or pain that increases when standing or walking. These are potential signs of life-threatening blood clots or localised cellulitis infection, removal of the hosiery is necessary and seek urgent medical help.	Do not double-layer compression hosiery unless specifically advised to by a healthcare professional. Do not wear compression hosiery that has been prescribed for someone else. Do not keep old hosiery after new pairs have been prescribed, to avoid wearing over-stretched or ill-fitting garments.

Source: Adapted from Wounds UK (2015).

of a third pair is advocated every three to six months with a reassessment prior to the next prescription. This will ensure the effectiveness of the garment (NICE 2022).

Application Aids

The patient's physical ability and dexterity need to be assessed when treatment planning for patients, as the correct application of hosiery is key to the success of the garment. There is also a risk of trauma caused by poor application technique. Healthcare professionals need to ensure that the patient is confident and safe in the application of the garment and that no further trauma is caused to the limb.

There is a vast number of aids that patients can have to help with application of compression therapy (Table 9.9). They are generally either fabric or rigid. A fabric aid is normally made of material that is slippery and therefore aids in the application of the hosiery over the heel and then guides the hosiery up the leg; with this type of application aid the patient still needs to be able to bend to reach their feet. The rigid aids typically provide a frame that the patient applies the hosiery garment to and then steps into. This enables the patient to put the garment on without having to bend (Dilks and Green 2005). However, there is a potential risk of trauma to the limb from a rigid device if care is not taken.

Other options available include roll-on membranes and non-slip mats. Patients can also wear rubber gloves with a soft interior lining, which can help in the application of compression hosiery (Wounds UK 2021).

Patient Education and Promoting Self-care

Patients need to have enough information and education to ensure that they understand the reasons for the treatment prescribed and the benefits to them, as well as support and tools to facilitate self-care on going. Patients can also reduce their risk of recurrent leg ulcers by adhering to the following recommendations (Venables 2015; Wounds UK 2021):

- Understanding why they have been prescribed the hosiery and understanding the underlying condition.

TABLE 9.9 Main examples of hosiery application aids – (BPS-Compression Hosiery: A patient - centric approach, 2021). Health care professionals who prescribe hosiery should be know which aids are available on prescription to help their patients with donning and doffing hosiery.

Fabric applicators	Rigid applicators	Miscellaneous
Fabric applicators work similarly to slide sheets. They are made of slippery material to assist with the application of hosiery therefore helping the hosiery over the heel. They can be used for open-toe and closed-toe hosiery, and are compactable and transportable.	Rigid applicators often consist of a frame with a semi-circular tube to assist with the opening of compression stockings to allow easier application. These types of frames typically have long handle options and may assist those who have difficulty bending forward to reach their foot. Measurement of the ankle is required to ensure the limb fits in the frame correctly.	Anti-slip mats can aid in the application and removal of hosiery. Rubber gloves with soft interior linings help during the application and removal of all types of compression stockings. Roll-on adhesives helps the hosiery 'stick' to the limb and can be washed off with water. Rolling compression aids can be used: the hosiery is folded down over the flexible, doughnut-shaped aid, which is then slid up or down the leg to apply or remove hosiery.

Source: Adapted from Wounds UK (2021).

- Ensuring the hosiery garment is well fitted and they know how to apply and remove it correctly and that the patient understands how to care for the hosiery in line with the manufactures instructions.
- Keeping active.
- Elevating legs when sitting.
- Avoiding trauma.
- Skin care regimen - Using emollients daily.
- Wearing compression hosiery daily.
- Having information on 'red flags' and what to look out for and when to contact a healthcare professional, personalised to their particular history.
- Emergency contact details of the healthcare professional/service.
- Having regular check-ups every 6–12 months with a healthcare professional.
- Knowing when and how to reorder new hosiery.

Patients may also benefit from keeping a self-care journal and being provided with access or signposting as to where to find online materials and support groups/organisations.

Hosiery Care

As part of the information given to patients to promote self-care, they should be given information about care of their hosiery, so that they get the maximum wear time out of the garment and keep the hosiery in good condition. This needs to be in accordance with the manufacturer's instructions for care. Patients also need to know that they should obtain a new garment from their healthcare professional should it get any damage, holes or ladders. This information should be provided in written form for the patient so that they can refer to it later if needed.

Maintaining Skin Integrity: Use of Emollients

A skincare regimen should form part of the patient's daily care plan and the healthcare professional should stress the importance of washing, cleansing and moisturising the skin. This will help with maintaining overall skin integrity (Wounds UK 2022).

The skin is the largest organ in the human body and is very complex. It provides a protection barrier between the body and the surrounding environment and prevents loss of water, reduces chemical exposure and protects against micro-organisms. During the ageing process physiological changes occur, including decreased collagen production, decreased blood circulation, decreased fat content and loss of rete ridges. In intrinsic ageing theory it is suggested that the reparability of the DNA decreases, which in turn leads to the formation of wrinkles, acne, eczema and psoriasis (Putri et al. 2021). There are also factors that affect the role of the skin in intrinsic ageing, such as ethnicity, anatomical variations and hormonal changes. The epidermis thins over time at the dermo-epidermal junction and the melanocytes and Langerhans cells also decrease in number over time. The dermis reduces in thickness as the patient ages, synthesis of collagen and elastin fibres reduces and there is a decrease in the number of blood vessels. The distribution and volume of fat change in the hypodermis of the skin. There is also a decrease in melanin, the number of sweat glands and sebum production falls (Putri et al. 2021). Understanding this is critical within a programme of reassessment in lifelong conditions, as the acceptability or impact of garments and their properties may change.

The use of emollients to promote skin barrier function is critical in the prevention of recurrence of leg ulceration. Emollients help to restore the function of the skin, reduce itching and skin breakdown and increase the level of hydration. Emollients work in one of two ways and this depends on their constituents. The first traps moisture into the skin, which has been shown to slow the evaporation of water; the second actively draws down moisture into the stratum corneum from the dermis through the effects of humectants (Moncrieff et al. 2015). Humectants either mimic or comprise the same molecule as the natural moisturising factors within the skin, such as urea, glycerol or isopropyl myristate (Moncrieff et al. 2015).

In patients with previous leg ulceration, it is essential that a good daily skincare regime - washing, cleansing and emollient application, is embedded in to daily life to reduce the risk of further breakdown. Patients should be taught the correct way to apply emollient in order to prevent folliculitis, and the importance of applying the emollient daily and checking for any changes in their skin. Emollients also pay a key part in the prevention of skin tears (Bale et al. 2004).

At every appointment with the patient, note any skin changes as this may indicate progression of the venous or lymphatic disease process, and educate your patient on what healthy skin is and when to report changes to a healthcare professional. It is important that the practitioner and the patient know how to identify skin changes and early detection can prevent tissue breakdown. The practitioner should be able to identify and treat the following: breaks in the skin, signs of trauma, signs of infection, rashes, pressure damage, varicose eczema, contact dermatitis and fungal infections such as tinea pedis. Particular attention should be paid to any skin folds and between the toes for fungal infection.

Precautions should be taken with regard to skincare under compression therapy garments and bandaging systems. The practitioner needs to identify if the skin is already fragile – skincare needs to form part of the holistic assessment and be included in the treatment planning for the patient.

Patients should be given tools and knowledge of ways to maintain skin integrity, signs and symptoms of skin breakdown and what to look out for, and when to seek help of a practitioner.

Complete emollient therapy should be recommended and encouraged in all patients – this is defined as everything that goes on the skin being emollient based and all soaps replaced with emollient wash products. This includes a combination of wash and leave-on products like creams and ointments. It is also important that patients are given instructions on application methods: emollients should always be applied in a downward direction or the direction of hair growth (Wounds UK 2018).

Patients should use emollients as part of treatment planning to aid in moisture management and should be encouraged to use emollients instead of soap for cleansing as part of their daily self-care regime (daily for humectant-containing emollients, twice daily for all other emollients) (Wounds UK 2018).

A benefit of emollients is that they moisturise the skin while cleansing it, rather than decreasing the moisture within it and prevent the skin from drying. Some emollients are buffered so they maintain normal skin pH. Evidence has also shown that emollients can accelerate regeneration of the skin barrier function and reduce dryness. Most lipid-rich emollients restore the skin barrier rapidly (Held et al. 2001; Moncrieff et al. 2015).

Emollients come in many forms and the one selected must be acceptable to the patient as this will help with concordance with the care regime. These preparations include ointments, creams, lotions, gels and sprays. Most of the greasiest preparations contain paraffin. There is a Medicines Healthcare Regulatory Agency (2020) alert for products containing soft white paraffin at a content above 50% due to safety concerns raised by the creams having contact with dressings, clothing and bedding, as they are highly flammable. This needs to be a consideration when treatment planning for patients who smoke or are on home oxygen.

Ensure that patients have adequate emollient and soap substitute prescribed. Also if patients are prone to skin breakdown, look at the materials used in the hosiery, as it may be that the patient needs a cotton rich bonded garment or skin-friendly undergarments.

Tips for good skincare can be summarised as follows (Wounds UK 2015, 2021):

- Ensure that the legs are dry before putting on medical compression hosiery.
- Avoid applying skincare products (e.g. emollients, topical steroids) just before application of hosiery as this can make application of the garment harder. Applying skincare products 20 minutes prior to the application of hosiery can reduce the difficulty. Or apply skincare products in the evening, after removing hosiery for bed.
- Check skin daily (or as often as possible) for changes, including on the legs, toes/nails and interdigital spaces.
- Check for any breaks in the skin, any signs of athlete's foot (tinea pedis), varicose eczema or red leg syndrome, and signs of cellulitis.
- Hosiery should be applied first thing in the morning, when oedema is at its lowest level, to help prevent skin damage and oedema in the tissues.
- Gently elevate the legs when resting to reduce pooling of oedema that can result in skin damage (high elevation not necessary).
- Keep physical activity to the fullest extent possible, depending on each patient's specific situation. Follow guidance for ankle exercises for chronic venous insufficiency, chronic oedema and lymphoedema as far as possible. Give information sheets of exercises to patients as an aid.

EMPOWERING PATIENTS' SELF-MANAGEMENT FOR LEG ULCER PREVENTION

As healthcare professionals we need to encourage patients to achieve positive outcomes, which includes engagement with the patient, family and carers to be involved in their care to a level suitable for their capacity and capability. This is why it is essential that the healthcare professional considers the patient's views, priorities and expectations around their care (Wounds UK 2022). Promoting self-management for patients is part of the NHS Long Term Plan's Comprehensive Model for Personalised Care to make personalised care standard across the health and care system (NHS England 2020). See Chapter 7 for further exploration.

One of the roles of the healthcare professional is to help patients tolerate compression; most patients can tolerate it more easily when the correct type and size of hosiery have been selected in partnership with them. Labelling a patient as non-compliant, or non-concordant is dismissive to the patient and must be avoided (Wounds UK 2022). A recent study also showed that patients' individual factors were rarely considered when prescribing compression hosiery garments (Schwann-Schreiber et al. 2018). Healthcare practitioners need to understand from patients their concerns over leg management and what their goal for treatment is, and to work with the patient to achieve this many different treatment options and garments may need to be discussed with the patient in order to find an acceptable solution. If patients are to have any faith in and be commitment to a treatment plan, they need to feel that they are part of the planning stage and feel listened to. It is unhelpful to label patients as intentionally non-adherent (Green and Jester 2009); instead, healthcare professionals should work with patients to understand their concerns and their goals for treatment and ongoing management.

Improving patient engagement with personalised prevention methods is beneficial to both the patient, the healthcare professional and the wider health service (Table 9.10). We must understand what the patient knows about the condition of their leg in order to be able to provide the correct information to them so they can make an informed choice about their care going forward. Healthcare professionals need to use language that resonates with the patient and back up the discussion with written information so that the patient may consider everything in their own time and revisit the information for clarification. Table 9.11 offers suggestions for how to educate and involve patients in their care.

It is acceptable to discuss, compromise and plan with patients. This will help to build trust in the healthcare professional–patient relationship over time, which in turn will help the patient to approach the healthcare professional with questions and seek help when needed. During appointments with patients explore other treatment

TABLE 9.10 Supported self-management.

Assess the patient's capacity and capability.
Assess their willingness/desire to participate in supported self-management.
Assess whether there are any safeguarding issues.
Talk to them about previous experiences of supported self-management.
Before encouraging supported self-management, ensure the patient is informed of the following information:

- Treatment plan, practicalities of wound care and using compression garments, and use of emollients in the form of a care contract or leg ulcer/well leg passport.
- Hand washing and limb hygiene.
- Reasons for treatment.
- Signs of deterioration and improvement.
- Signs and symptoms of infection.
- Contact details of who to contact if the patients is concerned.
- When self-supported management may not be appropriate for people with venous leg ulceration.
- Safeguarding issues (e.g. mental health patients in the community living alone.
- Patients who do not or struggle to understand.
- Patients who are not able to tolerate compression therapy (once they are supported to tolerate compression, they could be more involved in self management).
- Patients who have dexterity problems who are unable to apply the hosiery themselves even with an aid and have no support network to help them.
- Where hygiene levels are not appropriate.
- Where they have problems accessing required products.

Review every four weeks if the patient has active ulceration in line with NWCSP (2023) recommendations.
or
Remeasure and replace hosiery according to manufacturer's guidelines, usually every three months for British Standard Hosiery and six months for European Standard Hosiery (Wounds UK 2021).
When self-supported management may not be appropriate for people with venous leg ulceration. Safeaguarding issues (eg mental health patients in the community living alone. Patients who do not or struggle to understand. Patients who ae not able to tolerate compression therapy (once they are supported to tolerate compression, they could be more involved in self management). Patients who have dexterity problems who are unable to apply the hosiery themselves even with an aid and have no support network to help them. Where hygiene levels are not appropriate. where they have problems accessing required products.

Source: Adapted from Wounds UK (2022).

TABLE 9.11 Tips for patient education and involvement.

Involve the patient in the decision-making process from the beginning.

Ask the patient what motivates them and what is important to them to achieve?

Be aware that the patient's view on supported self-care may change over time continue to re-explore this during the patient's journey.

Use positive language and avoid terms like non-concordant, non-adherent and non-compliant, tight (when talking about compression therapy)

Explain treatment and rationale at all stages, establishing patient's and carers' long-term and short-term goals and experiences.

Use information leaflets, online and resources, videos to help patients get the information they need in a wat in which they can understand it to help them make an informed choice.

Use telemedicine (e.g. online video calling, apps, smartphone support).

Suggest patient support groups where appropriate and where available.

Involve friends, family and carers where possible give them the information if they are to be applying the compression hosiery for patients with regards to application of the hosiery, how to care for the hosiery and when to seek healthcare professionals advice.

Encourage continuity of care with consistent messages.

Source: Adapted from Wounds UK (2022).

options that will aid in their tolerance of compression therapy (Wounds UK 2021):

- Different hosiery options – another type of hosiery may be more cosmetically appealing to the patient. They may have a special event coming up, such as a family wedding, and they do not want to wear bandages to the event, for example. Work with them to find a solution – maybe they could have hosiery for that event.
- Skincare regimen: is the patient able to apply the emollient independently? Do they need a family member's help or a foam application aid for its application?
- Elevation: encourage the patient to elevate their legs every time they sit down, whether to rest, to watch television or to read. All elevation will help. Encourage activity, which could be getting up and mobilising with their frame if housebound to encourage calf muscle pump action. Even if they are unable to get up independently, they may be able to do simple leg and foot exercises whilst sat in the chair.

- Encourage patients to have a healthy diet and support them to make the correct choices talk to them about what food is important for wound healing. They may also need dietician review, weight loss or bariatric service referral. Do they have support for shopping if house bound?
- When discussing compression therapy with patients, ask them to consider the future with regard to their lower limb and discuss the possible consequences of not wearing the compression therapy. For example, what might happen if they chose not to wear it? What could life be like in a few years' time? Give the patient time to consider what could happen.
- Are there any support groups locally or nationally that the patient can access Chapter 5 discusses the Lindsay Leg Club model in more detail.

Brown (2013) identified some fundamental steps to support people having compression therapy:

- Ask the patient about their overall well-being.
- The plan or treatment regime designed with the person should be individualised and consider their wishes and concerns.
- Listen to their concerns with regard to their leg care and the issues they have identified as concerns. Try to address these and include them in the patient's prevention and management plan going forward. Find out what the person's expectations are and what they want to achieve; this could be healing, dry sheets in the morning if the exudate levels are high, wearing regular-fitting shoes or trousers again or gaining greater mobility.
- Make the person the centre of the process when assessing, measuring and fitting hosiery involve them in all decisions.
- Ensure you offer the person a choice of hosiery to fit their needs.
- Take the patient's feedback and use this to adapt their treatment plans and the broader service being provided to all patients.
- Involved the wider multidisciplinary team to develop strong patient pathways and referrals on to other services such as tissue viability, dermatology and vascular as required.

There is more about personalised care in Chapter 7.

KNOWLEDGE, STAFF AND TRAINING

Knowledge and training are essential for any clinical skill. If healthcare professionals are to choose the correct compression therapy for patients, they need to have the appropriate awareness and skills in assessment, recognition, knowledge of products and correct application techniques, aids for application and personalised treatment planning in order to provide safe and effective care for their patients. They also need to have an understanding of the different types of compression therapies and their uses in practice and the differences between them. This all needs to be considered in conjunction with the requirements of the patient groups.

Historically, education around compression therapy has been framed within the context of 'training to deliver an intervention e.g. application of a compression bandage. This approach to training has contributed to the current situation within UK practice: sub-optimal doses of compression leading to patients not having adequate levels of compression, variations in practice across the UK, inappropriate selection and measurement of garments, and then blaming the person for not 'complying' with the treatment plan offered. Practitioners deserve good-quality education to help them develop knowledge about the under pinning science and theory of compression therapy, followed by support in clinical practice to grow confidence and competency in the art of measuring, selecting and applying the right treatments together with the person who will be wearing them. Without robust education that focuses on the art and science of the compression therapy, not just a task, practitioners will not be confident and courageous in their practice and sub-optimal provision will continue, unabated.

The NWCSP introduced a core capabilities framework for wound care in 2021 (Figure 9.2) to address inequalities in wound care provision for patients; to enable care that is organised and research informed; to achieve the best possible healing rates, better experience of care for patients and greater cost effectiveness; and to prevent wound incidence and recurrence in health and social care settings. The framework is for a multiprofessional workforce working in wound care and supports practitioners to develop and provide evidence for their knowledge and skills and enables high standards of practice (NWCSP 2021).

The structure of the framework is broken down into 5 domains with 12 core capabilities (Table 9.12). The capabilities are numbered

Tier 1
Capabilities that require a general knowledge and understanding of wound care and the skills which support the provision of care.

Tier 2
Capabilities that enable the provision of wound care independently and with a degree of critical analysis

Tier 3
Capabilities that require a high degree of autonomy and complex decision making, an ability to lead wound care practice, enable innovative solutions to enhance peoples experience and improve outcomes

Notes
- A practitioner may move between the tiers depending on role, setting or circumstance.
- Capabilities are cumulative, therefore a practitioner working at tier 3 will be able to demonstrate the capabilities of tiers 1 and 2, as well as those of tier 3.
- It's important to note that the tiers do not relate to specific roles or pay grades.
- The framework is designed to cover all health and social care settings.
- The framework does not replace local arrangements for service provision, for example in respect of referral pathways and composition of multi-disciplinary teams.

FIGURE 9.2   The core capabilities framework tiers (NWCSP 2021).
Source: Reproduced with kind permission from Skills for Health and the National Wound Care Strategy.

TABLE 9.12   Structure of the core capabilities framework.

Domain	Domain title	Topic/capabilities
A	Underpinning principles	1. Underpinning principles
B	Assessment, investigation and diagnosis	1. Assessment and investigations 2. Diagnosis
C	Wound care	1. Care planning 2. Wound care and interventions 3. Referrals and collaborative working
D	Personalised care and health promotion	1. Communication 2. Personalised care 3. Prevention, health promotion and improvement
E	Leadership and management, education and research	1. Leadership and management 2. Education and research 3. Audit and quality improvement

Source: Adapted from National Wound Care Strategy Programme (2021).

for ease of reference – this does not indicate a pathway for completion, or a prescribed pathway, process or hierarchy. The capabilities are then divided into skills, knowledge and behaviours, which are described for each of the tiers see Table 9.12 (NWCSP 2021).

The core capabilities framework has been designed to identify areas for personal development for healthcare practitioners to help them build there skills for optimum care delivery; areas of service development may also be identified during this process. Leg ulcer prevention and management training combining the core capabilities should be available to all staff caring for patients with this condition. The training should include leg ulcer assessment, diagnosis and management training based on local and national policies and procedures where the clinician is working. Training should also be provided in a variety of delivery methods to make it accessible for all: taught in-person sessions, online lectures, practice skills workshops and assessments of clinical competencies in practice.

PUBLIC HEALTH

Since Lord Darzi published his report 'High Quality Care for All' (Department of Health and Social Care 2008) and the High Impact Actions (NHS Institute for Improvement and Innovation 2010), tissue viability teams across the county have been tasked with measuring the effectiveness of services. This can be difficult to measure as there are so many variances that affect healing rates. The NHS Long Term Plan (2019) is committed to facilitating measurable improvements in public health and reducing health equalities across the country, minimising the impact of the burden of wounds to healthcare in the future and improving care delivered to patients. With this in mind, early prevention, presentation and assessment of patients are key in preventing a further burden in years to come on the health service and for services to meet demands in already struggling workforces. For this to be possible, patient education and self-care are essential moving forward. See Chapter 7 for a greater exploration of the determinants of health.

For some time the NHS has been encouraging patients to manage their own health and long-term conditions, including wounds. This was a concept introduced by the introduction of The Five Year Forward View (NHS England 2014) and further supported as one of the six elements of the personalised care plan in the NHS Long Term

Plan (NHS England 2019). Clinicians should equip patients with a toolbox of information and advice in order for them to manage their conditions independently – in the case of management of well legs, this would be exercise, hosiery application and maintenance, skin care regimen, diet and lifestyle education and advice on when and where to seek a healthcare professional's help between appointments. The wound care agenda was highlighted across the United Kingdom by the publication of the Guest et al. data in 2015 (discussed earlier in the chapter).

Coleman et al. (2017) discovered that there was no national minimum data set for generic wound assessments or leg ulcer assessments which was leading to variations in practice and outcomes for patients. After a literature review and a structured consensus, a set of criteria was set out to improve and standardised wound assessments in clinical practice, which was adapted and adopted by the National Wound Care Strategy to form the lower limb recommendations (2020). The aim was to standardise care for patients.

The NWCSP was commissioned by NHS England and began in 2018 to improve the prevention and management of pressure ulcers, lower limb ulcers and surgical wounds. The goal of the project was to implement a high standard of care for all patients receiving care across England. The lower limb recommendations from the NWCSP (2023) put a greater focus on the importance of patients receiving compression therapy in a timely manor and early endovenous intervention for all suitable, and to achieved by greater public awareness. This would be achieved by reducing variations in practice, improving safety and increasing patient experiences and outcomes.

Commissioning for Quality and Innovation (CQUIN) and NHS England in 2018 set about improving outcomes and quality for patients with leg ulceration managed by community services. CQUIN targets, introduced in 2020–2021, are aimed to reduce unwanted variation in practice across the country for the management of lower limb wounds. The purpose of the CQUIN is to ensure appropriate assessment, diagnosis and treatment for 50% of patients with lower limb wounds, a figure that trusts must achieve in order to benefit from income from CQUIN targets. This will in turn encourage the development and redesign of services and therefore better outcomes for patients and the health economy as a whole.

There also needs to be an increase in patient and public awareness if the general population are to start recognising early signs of venous disease progression and seek early help to slow the progression down. An increase in public campaigns to highlight the importance of leg care would be needed, such as the Legs Matter campaign, Leg Club Model and Lively Legs Model.

The Queen's Nursing institute (QNI) (2019) has described how staffing levels are reducing across community nursing services nationally and this, coupled with the increasing demands on district nursing services, is reducing the capacity for essential training opportunities. The QNI estimated that 46% of the overall highly skilled and experienced workforce is expected to leave or retire in the next five years, which will leave an unskilled workforce in these essential clinical skills, with very few mentors to facilitate learning opportunities in lower limb management and essential skills such as performing Ankle brachical pressure index readings (ABPI) skills. Staff must have training and investment in time must be made in order to be proficient in the skills and support need to deliver the CQUIN targets across community services. The challenge to practitioners is how this is achieved with a reducing workforce, reduction in skill mix and greater demands on services.

A study into the comparison of compression therapy uses by Hopkins and Samuriwo (2022) identified that there was a greater number of patients with lower limb wounds than those that had been recognised, recorded and classified as having leg ulcers within community settings. They also showed substantial variation in access to diagnostics and compression therapy practice between the sites of data collection, and by locations within those local areas. They identified that lack of use of compression increased nursing time by 37% and that where there is a lack of access to therapeutic intervention, the resultant patient harm is not being recognised, reported or documented.

Wound care services had to adapt and change during the Covid-19 pandemic and had to utilise other ways of connecting with patients and healthcare professionals, such as telemedicine or video calls. But with this came a reduction in patient contacts and in the community workforce in the early 2020s, which may well have a longer-term impact on service delivery and patient outcomes.

Evaluation of Service

NHS services are under increasing pressure to prove the value of the service provided to patients to secure ongoing funding and resources – and wound care services are not excluded from this. Evidence is needed to justify and prove the worth of the existence of services and the rationale for the intervention and pathways that support local system change; the provision of system data enhances an anecdotal or case study focus to delivery. The Health Foundation (Jones et al. 2021) defined a quality service as care that is effective, safe and provides as positive an experience as possible for the users by being caring, responsive and person centred. The definition also states that care should be well led, sustainable and equitable, achieved through providers and commissioners working together and in partnership with, and for, local people and communities.

In order to prove the worth of a service a combination of elements need to be used: evidence-based practice, following local policy and this should be updated in line with national guidelines, combined with patient satisfaction surveys alongside wound care audits. These need to be used to provide an improvement plan for service change and development and the cycle then starts again. Auditing should be a continuous cycle.

Over the last 10 years the introduction of CQUINs for wound care, first for pressure ulcers and then leg ulcer services, has driven the audit process through community nursing teams, community leg ulcer services and community tissue viability teams. It concentrates on the evaluations of healing rates although there are many variable with this and waiting times from referral to full holistic assessment. The other important elements of a service audit should not be forgotten, such as quality-of-life audits, patient experience surveys and the link to resource management and consumable (dressing/bandage) usage and cost data. Triangulating this data and information is often insightful into how services are performing.

Plan–Do–Study–Act Cycle

Implementing change in the NHS is not easy (NHS England 2018). For the change to be sustainable and effective, a recognised framework and change model should be used. The Plan–Do–Study–Act (PDSA) cycle (Figure 9.3) is simple to implement for healthcare teams on the ground to use and assists the clinician in testing potential quality improvement on a small scale, which can than allow for any adjustments and changes to be made to a project prior to its wider roll out and implementation. The cycle runs as follows:

- Plan – plan the change to be made.
- Do – carry out the test or change.

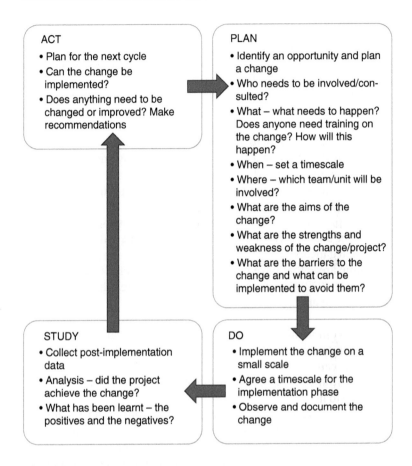

FIGURE 9.3 Plan–Do–Study–Act (PDSA) cycle.
Source: Adapted from NHS England (2018).

- Study – based on measurable outcomes, collect data before and after the change and reflect on the impact of the change and what was learned.
- Act – plan how the change will be fully implemented.

Using a change model that has been validated gives a structured way of organising ideas and identifying potential changes to services and also helps to pinpoint any barriers (NHS England 2018). Using the cycle can also encourage educational opportunities that will help to highlight which ideas will work and which ideas may be less successful going forward. NHS England maintains that using the PDSA cycle can be less disruptive to patients and staff than larger change models, as it allows repeated cycles through the model and changes to smaller pilot studies.

NHS Improvement (2020) suggests answering three sets of questions before testing a change idea:

- What are you trying to accomplish? What is the overall aim?
- How will you know if the change is an improvement? How will you measure success?
- What changes can you make that will result in improvement?

This process and the identified outcomes can support the development of business cases that aims to improve the outcomes of people with leg ulcers.

Some areas that have been suggested for change (Mahoney and Simmonds 2020) within community nursing in relation to leg ulcer management are:

- Poor compliance on the part of the professional with guidance within teams, which can lead to delays in implementing appropriate care.
- Time from referral to first full holistic assessment including ABPI.
- Time to heal.
- Poor holistic assessments, which could result in delay referring patients to the most appropriate healthcare professional for care delays in getting appropriate compression therapy.
- Increased costs of resources through inappropriate and ineffective treatments prolonging the length of stay of a patient on the caseload.
- Costly dressings that were inappropriate.
- Underuse of strong compression bandaging.
- Poor quality of care, patient satisfaction and quality-of-life outcomes.

Audit Process

Audit should be a continually component of all leg ulcer services delivered to patients. It is important for service development and monitoring the of quality of the service, and it gives the healthcare professional outcome measures to see if the service is providing quality, safe, effective care to patients. Prevalence and incidence audits are necessary tools in planning workforce and resource management (Vowden and Vowden 2010; Hopkins and Worboys 2014). Audit can also be used to show what impact changes have had on the service and outcomes for patients, and can be implemented to continually monitor care and measure outcomes. Audit tools need to be standardised across the service/organisation, so that the audit should be able to be repeated at any point within the service or organisation and by any clinician.

If you have not conducted an audit before, starting small this will give you the opportunity to see if your data collection tool works before embarking on a larger audit of patients. Using the PDSA cycle discussed previously in the chapter.

For an audit to be successful you first need to do the following:

- Gather your working group. If you are working within a team, decide on the roles that each of you will undertake.
- Identify your stakeholders. This could be people who have an interest in your service, the district nursing team, GP, intermediate care team, Care Commissioning Group, secondary care.
- Set a timetable for when the different elements of the audit will take place and allocate them to members of the audit team.
- Check to see if your organisation/trust has an audit policy. Who do you need to tell that you are planning an audit? Do you need approval from ethics and governance? There might be certain data that all audits have to collect; there might be an organisational data collection tool or a report format for writing the data up; there might also be a clinical audit team within the organisation that you need to register your audit with. Do you need patient approval for the data you are collecting? Do you need ethics approval for your audit?
- What do you want to find out? The process of audit can be applied to many things, from type of treatment used to healing, patient experiences of pain, patient experiences and opinions of the service, staff knowledge, experience and competencies, or costs spent on treatment for patients. You need to develop your audit questions. For example: How long was the wait from referral to first assessment including Doppler assessment? What was the mean time to healing for a venous leg ulceration with the

service? The answers to both questions can be measured against national data. Wider questions for an organisational audit might include finding out about staff training alongside the audit. There might be a correlation between this and patient assessments if there are not enough staff available with the skills to carry out full holistic assessments for patients.

- Inclusion criteria for the audit. Inclusion and exclusion criteria both need to be specific, or you will find that your audit has too big a scope and the data collected will be hard to analyse and report on. For example, if the inclusion criteria are patients with an ABPI between 0.8 and 1.3 and receiving full compression UK standard compression therapy in line with NICE guidance (40 mmHg), they might have had their assessment within a set period, and you might also want to look at the type of compression they are receiving, such as two-layer bandaging, four-layer bandaging or compression hosiery kits.
- Exclusion criteria for the audit. This is all the patients you do not want to include. For example, if you are looking at patients with a venous leg ulcer you may want to exclude patients who have an ABPI less than 0.8 or greater than 1.3, patients with a diabetic foot wound or patients who have had a pressure ulcer. Be specific, as this will help to narrow down your patient group and give a more reproducible audit tool for the future.
- Limitations of the audit. Document any limitations such as time frames, workforce to conduct the audit or any IT system issues that may affect the data collection process.
- When is the audit going to take place and what is its scope? For instance, is it going to capture a moment in time (this is called a point prevalence audit, e.g. patients seen on a particular day) or will it examine the caseload as a whole?
- Resources needed to carry out the audit. This could be funding for staff to collect data, printing, expertise for data entry and so on.
- How many patients you are going to include and how they will be selected. For example, if the whole caseload is to be included you could number them from 1 to 100, then pick 10 random numbers, which would mean the audit is covering 10% of the caseload. If patients are taken from a sample seen on a certain day, this would be a point prevalence audit looking at a moment in time.

After those aspects have been decided on and documented, move on to the following steps:

- Development of the audit tool. There are some audit tools online or you may find that your organisation has a set pro forma for standard audit collection, to which you can add your service-specific questions. What is the minimum data set that needs to be collected? What questions do you need to include on your audit tool? Are you going to use a spreadsheet or a paper tool to collect the data?
- Data collection. Set aside time to conduct the audit to ensure all data is collected as required. If allocating collection to other members of the team, ensure everyone knows who is collecting what data and when. For example, person A collects data for patients 1–10, person B collects data for patients 11–20, person C collects data for persons 21–30 and so on. This will stop miscollection of data. Also decide prior to data collection how the data will be collected, for example if using a spreadsheet and your question is what type of compression the patient received, you might want to allocate letters to the answers, e.g. A = hosiery kit, B = two-layer compression, C = four-layer compression.
- Data analysis. How will this happen? Will an Excel spreadsheet be used, who will complete it and how long do you plan for this part to take?
- Decide who you will present the data to. Which members of your organisation need to have the data? Do the audit results need to be presented to others such as the local integrated care system group?
- Identify recommendations for change and write an improvement plan based on the audit. Identify good practice and areas for improvement. How can this improvement be achieved? It could be introduction of a care pathway, a new piece of documentation, or training and education for staff in a particular subject. Think about how these could be implemented with the use of the PDSA cycle.
- Set a date for the next audit. For example, re-audit in quarter four.
- Write up the data in a structured format:
  - Outline the scope of the audit.
  - Described the method for data collection – inclusion and exclusion criteria, data collection tool.

- Write up the findings from the audit. Did the data you collected answer your audit questions? Did you experience any limitations on the audit? Identify any pockets of positive or negative practice.
- Recommendations for change.
- Identify anything you would change if you were to conduct the audit again.
- Include who the audit results will be presented to and when.
- Add in the improvement plan.
- Write a conclusion.
- Specify the date for implementing the improvement plan.
- Specify the date for the re-audit.

PATIENT SATISFACTION AND QUALITY OF LIFE

All NHS organisations now regularly conduct friends and family testing to see how patients experience the organisation, services provided and how they feel about living with a condition (NHS 2023). This helps the NHS to make improvements to services.

Patient quality of life is defined by WHO (2012) as an 'individual's perception of their position in life in the context of the culture and value systems in which they live and in relation to their goals, expectations, standards, and concerns'. Quality-of-life surveys should look at four domains: social, psychological, health and function.

Such surveys should be given to patients at certain points of their care: at the beginning of care (first contact) to assess how they feel about their leg ulcer, then monthly throughout the treatment plan, and then once they are healed (Mullings and Merlin-Manton 2018). Conducting surveys regularly through the treatment phase checks if the patient's views or thoughts have changed and if any of the patient's concerns have be addressed.

LEG ULCER PATHWAYS

Leg ulcer pathways came to the forefront of clinicians' minds with NHS England's RightCare scenario featuring Betty's story (2017), which put a national focus on the optimal pathway for patients. NICE implemented the Venous Leg Ulcer scenario (2021), which outlined nationally recognised leg ulcer guidance and focused on best practice.

Pathways have a structured approach, which can provide person-centred benefits to the clinician, patient and the health economy. They enable patients to receive the right evidence-based care at the right time and ensure equitable care for all (correct assessment, primary dressing, compression regimen and reassessment or onward referral). Pathways also need to be auditable and audited to establish if best practice is actually being delivered, with a reduction in recurrence and occurrence demonstrating system-wide improvement or the reverse.

Implementing a clinical pathway for leg ulcer management and care is essential to ensure that there is a standard of care across an organisation and that patients are receiving evidence-based care that considers both physical and psychological impacts of living with a lower limb wound. The pathway should also include the impact on patient quality of life. It needs to be bespoke to support holistic patient care that is specific to local communities while meeting explicit care needs (Mullings and Merlin-Manton 2018). The pathway needs to be broken down into sections for leg ulcer assessment, management and reassessment. Its primary aims should be to reduce time to heal and provide standardised, equitable care to all patients.

Mullings and Merlin-Manton (2018) found that by introducing a standardised approach to leg ulcer care that: time to heal has been reduced, waiting lists have decreased and the patient journey has become more streamlined, therefore providing the best chance to achieve healing quickly.

Atkin et al. (2021) stated that it is essential that health services move towards the elimination of unwanted variations in leg ulcer management. The introduction of leg ulcer pathways (assessment and treatment) reduces the variation in wating times, treatments and outcomes for patients and provides an equitable research-based service to patients across whole organisations.

CONCLUSION

One element is clear: the patient should be at the centre of the process of preventing recurrence of leg ulceration. They need to have the tools and the knowledge to empower them to manage and maintain their well legs independently in the community. Healthcare professionals need have the skills and the knowledge to carry out full holistic regular assessments, including ABPI assessment, for a patient and then plan and implement their ongoing care in collaboration with the patient.

Patients need to be supported throughout their leg ulcer management journey and healthcare professionals need to work with them so that looking after their well legs as this is a lifelong commitment. The choice of hosiery should be that of the patient and the healthcare professional should be there to guide the patient's decision about which garments to choose and which would provide the best clinical outcome for them. If the patient agrees with the prescribed garment and if they have chosen it and accepted its use, there will be an easier road to well legs in the future.

REFERENCES

Adderley, U. (2020). National Wound Care Strategy Programme: looking at the impact of COVID-19. *Wounds UK* 16 (2): 11.

Anderson, I., and Smith, G. (2014). Compression made easy. London: Wounds UK. https://wounds-uk.com/made-easy/compression-made-easy/

Ashby, R.L., Gabe, R., Ali, S., and Adderley, U. (2014). Clinical and cost-effectiveness of compression hosiery versus compression bandages in treatment of venous leg ulcers (venous leg ulcer study IV, VenUS IV): a randomised control trial. *Lancet* 383 (9920): 871–879.

Atkin, L., Hopkin, A., Gardner, S. et al. (2021). Making legs matter: a case for system change and transformation in the lower limb. *Journal of Wound Care* 30 (supp 1): S1–S28.

Bale, S., Tebble, N., Jones, V., and Price, P. (2004). The benefits of implementing a new skin care protocol in nursing homes. *Journal of Tissue Viability* 14 (2): 44–50.

Brown, A. (2013). Self-care support in leg ulcer services should be a priority. *Nursing Times* 109 (4): 11.

Coleman, S., Nelson, E.A., Vowden, P. et al. (2017). Development of a generic wound care assessment minimum data set. *Journal of Tissue Viability* 26 (4): 226–224.

Department of Health and Social Care (2008). High quality care for all: NHS Next Stage Review final report. https://www.gov.uk/government/publications/high-quality-care-for-all-nhs-next-stage-review-final-report

Dilks, A. and Green, J. (2005). The use and benefits of compression stocking aids. *Nursing Times* 101 (21): 32.

Földi, E. and Földi, M. (1983). Die Antomischen Grundlagen der Lymphödembehandlug. *Schweizerische Rundschau fur Medizin Praxis* 72 (46): 1499–1464.

Gong, J.M., Du, J.S., Han, D.M. et al. (2020). Reasons for patient non-compliance with compression stockings as a treatment for varicose veins in the lower limbs: a qualitative study. *PLoS One* 15 (4).

Green, J. and Jester, R. (2009). Health-related quality of life and chronic venous leg ulceration: part 1. *Wound Care* 141: S14–S17.

Guest, J.F. and Fuller, G.W. (2023). Cohort study assessing the impact of COVID-19 on venous leg ulcer management and associated clinical outcomes in clinical practice in the UK. *BMJ Open* 13: e068845. https://doi.org/10.1136/bmjopen-2022-068845.

Guest, J.F., Ayoub, N., McIlwraith, T. et al. (2015). Health economic burden that wounds impose on the National Health Service in the UK. *BMJ Open* 5 (12): e009283.

Guest, J.F., Fuller, G.W., and Vowden, P. (2020). Cohort study evaluating the burden of wounds to the UK's National Health Service in 2017/2018: update from 2012/2013. *BMJ Open* 10: e045253.

Harding, K., Dowsett, C., Fias, L. et al (2015). Simplifying venous leg ulcer management. Consensus recommendations. London: Wounds International. https://woundsinternational.com/consensus-documents/simplifying-venous-leg-ulcer-management-consensus-recommendations

Health Service Executive (Ireland) (2022). All-Ireland lymphoedema guidelines 2022. https://www2.healthservice.hse.ie/organisation/national-pppgs/all-ireland-lymphoedema-guidelines-2022

Held, E., Lund, H., and Agner, T. (2001). Effects of different moisturisers on SLS-irritated human skin. *Contact Dermatitis* 44 (4): 229–234.

Heyer, K., Protz, K., and Augustin, M. (2017). Compression therapy – cross-sectional observational survey about knowledge and practical treatment of specialised and non-specialised nurses and therapists. *International Wound Journal* 14 (6): 1148–1153. https://doi.org/10.1111/iwj.12773.

Hopkins, A. and Samuriwo, R. (2022). Comparison of compression therapy use, lower limb wound prevalence and nursing activity in England: a multisite audit. *Journal of Wound Care* 31 (12): 1016–1028. https://doi.org/10.12968/jowc.2022.31.12.1016.

Hopkins, A. and Worboys, F. (2014). Establishing community wound prevalence within an inner London borough: exploring the complexities. *Journal of Tissue Viability* 23 (4): 121–128.

International Lymphoedema Framework (2006). Best practice for the management of lymphoedema. https://www.lympho.org/uploads/files/files/Best_practice.pdf

International Society of Lymphology (2016). The diagnosis and treatment of peripheral lymphoedema: 2016 Consensus Document of the International Society of Lymphology. *Lymphology* 49: 170–184.

Jones, B., Kwong, E., and Warburton, W. (2021). Quality improvement made simple – what everyone should know about health care quality improvement. London: Health Foundation. https://www.health.org.uk/sites/default/files/QualityImprovementMadeSimple.pdf

Levick, J.R. (2003). *An Introduction to Cardiovascular Physiology.* London: Arnold.

Lurie, F., Passman, M., Meiser, M. et al. (2020). The 2020 update of the CEAP classification system and reporting standards. *Journal of Vascular Surgery: Venous and Lymphatic Disorders* 8 (3): 342–352.

Mahoney, K. and Simmonds, W. (2020). Using health improvement methodology to standardise leg ulcer management. *British Journal of Community Nursing* 25 (Sup 9): S20–S25.

Medicines and Healthcare Products Regulatory Agency (MHRA) (2020). Paraffin-based skin emollients on dressings or clothing: fire risk. https://www.gov.uk/drug-safety-update/paraffin-based-skin-emollients-on-dressings-or-clothing-fire-risk

Moffat, C., Martin, R., and Smithdale, R. (2009). *Leg Ulcer Management.* Oxford: Blackwell Publishing.

Moncrieff, G., Van Onselen, J., and Young, T. (2015). The role of emollients in maintaining skin integrity. *Wounds UK* 11 (1): 68–74.

Mosti, G. (2012). Stiffness of compression devices. *Veins and Lymphatics* 2 (e1): 1–2.

Mullings, J. and Merlin-Manton, E. (2018). Improving patient outcomes through the implementation of a person-centred leg ulcer pathway. *Journal of Wound Care* 26 (6): 378–384.

National Institute for Health and Care Excellence (NICE) (2020). Varicose veins. https://cks.nice.org.uk/topics/varicose-veins

National Institute for Health and Care Excellence (NICE) (2021). Scenario: Venous leg ulcers. https://cks.nice.org.uk/topics/leg-ulcer-venous/management/venous-leg-ulcers

National Institute for Health and Care Excellence (NICE) (2022). Scenario: Compression stockings. https://cks.nice.org.uk/topics/compression-stockings/management/compression-stockings

National Wound Care Strategy Programme (NWCSP) (2021). National Wound Care Core Capabilities Framework for England. https://www.skillsforhealth.org.uk/info-hub/national-wound-care-core-capability-framework-for-england

National Wound Care Strategy Programme (NWCSP) (2023). Recommendations for Leg Ulcers. NWCSP-Leg-Ulcer-Recommendations-1.8.2023.pdf (nationalwoundcarestrategy.net).

NHS (2023). NHS Friends and Family Test (FFT). https://www.nhs.uk/using-the-nhs/about-the-nhs/friends-and-family-test-fft/

NHS England (2014). NHS Five Year Forward View. https://www.england.nhs.uk/publication/nhs-five-year-forward-view

NHS England (2017). NHS RightCare scenario: The variation between suboptimal and optimal pathways. https://www.england.nhs.uk/rightcare/

wp-content/uploads/sites/40/2017/02/nhs-rightcare-bettys-story-app1.pdf

NHS England (2018). Sustainable Improvement Team: The change model guide.https://www.england.nhs.uk/wp-content/uploads/2018/04/change-model-guide-v5.pdf

NHS England (2019). The NHS Long-Term Plan. https://www.longtermplan.nhs.uk/wp-content/uploads/2019/08/nhs-long-term-plan-version-1.2.pdf

NHS England (2020). Universal personalised care. https://www.england.nhs.uk/personalisedcare/comprehensive-model

NHS Improvement (2020). Quality, service improvement and redesign (QSIR) tools. https://aqua.nhs.uk/QSIR

NHS Institute for Innovation and Improvement (2010). High impact actions for nursing and midwifery: the essential collection. https://www.england.nhs.uk/improvement-hub/wp-content/uploads/sites/44/2017/11/High-Impact-Actions-The-Essential-Collection.pdf

Office for National Statistics (2022). National population projections: 2020-based interim. https://www.ons.gov.uk/peoplepopulationand community/populationandmigration/populationprojections/bulletins/nationalpopulationprojections/2020basedinterim

Partsch, H. (2003). Understanding the pathophysiological effects of compression. In: *Position Document: Understanding Compression Therapy* (ed. European Wound Management Association), 2–4. London: MEP.

Putri, K.L., Aryani, I.A., and Nopriyati (2021). Anatomy and histologic intrinsic aging skin. *Bioscientia Medicina: Journal of Biomedicine and Translational Research* 5 (11): 1065–1077.

Queen's Nursing Institute (2019). District nursing today: the view of district nurse team leaders in the UK. https://qni.org.uk/resources/district-nursing-today-the-view-of-district-nurse-team-leaders-in-the-uk

Ritchie, G. and Warwick, G. (2018). Understanding how compression works: part 1. *Journal of Community Nursing* 32 (2): 24–32.

Robertson, B.F., Thomson, C.H., and Siddiqui, H. (2014). Side effects of compression and stockings: a case report. *British Journal of General Practice* 64 (623): 316–317.

Schofield, A. (2021). What have tissue viability services learnt from the coronavirus pandemic? *Nursing Times* 117 (3): 23–25.

Schwann-Schreiber, C., Marshal, M., Murena-Schmidt, R., and Doppel, W. (2018). Long-term observational study on outpatients' treatment of venous diseases with medical compression stockings in Germany. *Veins and Lymphatics* 7: 7560.

Venables, J. (2015). Prescribing compression stockings to prevent recurrent leg ulcers. *Nurse Prescribing* 13 (1): 38–42.

Vowden, K. and Vowden, P. (2010). The role of audit in demonstrating quality in tissue viability services. *Wounds UK* 6 (1): 100–105.

World Health Organization (WHO) (2012). WHOQOL: Measuring quality of life. https://www.who.int/tools/whoqol

Wound Care People (2019). Best practice in the community: Chronic oedema. https://www.woundcare-today.com/uploads/files/files/66774-Best-Practice-Statement.PDF

Wounds UK (2015). Best practice statement: Compression hosiery, second edition. https://wounds-uk.com/best-practice-statements/compression-hosiery-second-edition

Wounds UK (2018). Best practice statement: Maintaining skin integrity. https://wounds-uk.com/best-practice-statements/maintaining-skin-integrity

Wounds UK (2021). Best practice statement: Compression hosiery: a patient-centricapproach.https://wounds-uk.com/best-practice-statements/best-practice-statement-compression-hosiery-patient-centric-approach

Wounds UK (2022). Best practice statement: Holistic management of venous leg ulceration (second edition). https://wounds-uk.com/best-practice-statements/holistic-management-venous-leg-ulceration-second-edition

Index

Lower Limb and Leg Ulcer Assessment and Management, First Edition.
Edited by Aby Mitchell, Georgina Ritchie, and Alison Hopkins.
© 2024 John Wiley & Sons Ltd. Published 2024 by John Wiley & Sons Ltd.